Basic Medical Science for Speech and Language Therapy Students

MARTIN ATKINSON, BSc, PhD
University of Sheffield

STEPHEN MCHANWELL, BSc, PhD, MIBiol, CIBiol
University of Newcastle upon Tyne

GW00649053

W
WHURR PUBLISHERS
LONDON AND PHILADELPHIA

© 2002 Whurr Publishers

First published 2002 by
Whurr Publishers Ltd
19ᴮ Compton Terrace, London N1 2UN, England
325 Chestnut Street, Philadelphia PA19106, USA

Reprinted 2002, 2004, 2005, 2006 and 2010

British Library Cataloguing in Publication Data

A catalogue record for this book is available from the
British Library.

ISBN 13- 978 1 86156 238 8 p/b

Contents

Contents

Dedication

To the memory of Frank White

Preface

Prospective speech and language therapists need a sound working knowledge of the structure and function of the human body to provide a solid foundation for future clinical practice. This has not always proved easy because human communication science students have often had to make do with textbooks written for other groups of students. Through long experience of teaching, we feel our students have been handicapped by the lack of a textbook dedicated to those important areas of anatomy, physiology and neuroscience related to speech and language therapy. This is our attempt to produce a book to fulfil these needs.

It is tempting for students to see the basic sciences as subjects simply to be learned, ticked off and forgotten when the inevitable examination hurdle has been successfully crossed. To divorce basic science from clinical practice is, we believe, both artificial and wrong. The great difficulty for students of anatomy, physiology and neuroscience is knowing how much or little to learn. The great difficulty for writers of a textbook on the same subjects is knowing what to include or omit. This difficulty has increased in recent years with the extraordinary growth of scientific knowledge and the addition of new areas to the repertoire of speech and language therapists. What we have included underpins virtually every aspect of speech and language therapy. We have, however, included sufficient background material so that the principles of structure and function of the human body may be understood; detail fits into place much more easily if the principles underlying the detail are known. Speech and language therapy is not a surgical science so there is little need for anatomical minutiae. Nevertheless, certain important details have to be appreciated to understand how different components work to formulate language and generate speech. Detail has been included only where it has direct relevance. If the application of basic science to clinical practice is made clear, students can see why they need to know the material. To emphasize the interdependence of science and practice, we have used clinical examples liberally throughout the book. We hope the focus on relevant material, the concentration on principle rather than detail and the use of clinical illustrations will make it easier for students to decide what to learn.

The number of hours devoted directly to basic sciences varies considerably in different universities offering human communication science courses, and students at some universities where this component is relatively short may at first be daunted by the amount of material in this book. Do not be fooled. Even if it is not taught under a convenient heading of anatomy, physiology or neurology, much of the content of this book will be encountered sometime during the clinical part of the course or in practice itself; these subjects will be returned to again and again. Unless you are blessed with a superb memory, you are unlikely to remember every detail, but you will know where to look it up when you need this information later in the course or in practice. We have also included some subjects which, even in universities which teach a comprehensive basic science course, are not usually encountered until the clinical part of your course; dysphagia, dysphasia, orthodontics and various examples of pathology fall into this category. We have attempted to make the layout of the book as clear and logical as possible so that the subject matter may be found even if the course taken does not follow the order of this book.

We hope that both undergraduate and postgraduate students and practitioners will find this book useful, that it will give them an understanding of the principles of anatomy, physiology and neuroscience relevant to clinical practice and an appreciation of the underlying importance of basic science for speech and language therapy.

Acknowledgments

And sustain with undiminished poise
That saddest dedication: *lastly my wife, who did the typing.*[1]

This book grew out of one written for dental students by Martin Atkinson and Frank White. Just as they had started to write the new book, sadly, Frank White died. The project went into abeyance until Steve McHanwell offered to add his experience and expertise by joining Martin Atkinson as co-author. Much of the text has its foundation in the contribution Frank made to the original book.

When we started on this project, we believed we knew it all but soon discovered huge gaps in our knowledge. We have learned a great deal while putting this book together, especially from many of our colleagues. We would like to thank Richard Greene and Liz Laude and several of the 2000–1 Master's students in Sheffield and MSc students Victoria Ashburner, Sue Band and Sinead Kennedy in Newcastle who have given us helpful comments on individual chapters. Although we are both experienced teachers of anatomy, physiology and neuroscience, we are not speech and language therapists. This book would not have been possible without the contribution of many of our clinical colleagues who willingly gave us the benefit of their experience in their own specialities within speech and language therapy. Paul Carding in Newcastle and Cheryl Gray, Sara Howard and Rosemary Varley in Sheffield have read drafts of various chapters and have offered valuable comments; Caroline Pickstone, like the proverbial 7th US Cavalry, saved us at the eleventh hour. We would also like to thank Adrian Jowett for his invaluable help and patience in preparing the illustrations.

Martin is fortunate to be married to Diana Syder, a gifted writer and artist as well as a speech and language therapist of considerable

---

[1]From 'The Poet's Companion' by Ursula Fanthorpe; in *Neck Verse*, Cornwall: Peterloo Poets, 1992.

experience and skill. Diana has made an inestimable contribution to the book. She has read virtually all the draft chapters and provided invaluable insights into the work of speech and language therapists to help us make the editorial decisions about what goes in and what goes out. She has also drawn some of the illustrations. Moreover, Diana has encouraged and supported Martin when other things threatened to submerge the whole project. Thanks just doesn't say enough, Diana.

Steve would also like to thank Professor Ruth Lesser, Emeritus Professor and former Head of the Department of Speech in the University of Newcastle upon Tyne, who provided early encouragement for this project. Heartfelt thanks are also due to Wendy Davison who has helped to prepare the Newcastle part of the manuscript. Her unfailing enthusiasm and optimism, especially when other events looked like conspiring to jeopardize the completion of this project, were a constant source of encouragement. Grateful thanks to Steve's partner Jackie, as well as Claire and Tim, who have all provided marvellous support for him in different ways throughout the writing of this book. It has been a long time in gestation and their encouragement has helped to ensure that it became a reality – especially as the manuscript neared completion, when he was characterized more by his absence from home rather than his presence.

Lastly, Steve would like to thank Martin for his patience as Steve made slow progress towards completing his part of the manuscript. Martin's greater experience in completing a task of this nature has been invaluable in ensuring that this book was produced. Collaboration that is effective should result in something that ends up greater than the sum of its parts. We believe that this book has benefited from our joint efforts and reflects something of our different strengths while remedying our different weaknesses and so represents a real effort of collaboration.

Thanks to Whurr Publishers for their encouragement, forbearance and unfailing good humour as the whooshing sounds of deadlines rushed past their ears.

Irrespective of the invaluable help of all these people, the final content is our own: we are culpable for any mistakes and omissions. We welcome comments from our readers which we hope we can incorporate into improved future editions.

Martin Atkinson, Sheffield
Stephen McHanwell, Newcastle upon Tyne
November 2001

Chapter 1

Introduction

The human body is a wonderful piece of design – the design of individual components and their integration to form different organs and systems is fitted exactly to their function. **Anatomy** is the study of bodily structure and **physiology** is the study of bodily function, although the two disciplines are interlinked. **Neuroscience** is the name given to the anatomical and physiological study of the structure and function of the nervous system. Defects in normal structure and function account for many of the abnormalities of speech and language. It follows that several aspects of the structure and function of the body must be understood to comprehend how normal language and speech is generated, how abnormalities may arise, and the rationale underlying possible treatments.

The study of the body

Biochemistry is the study of the chemical level of organization of the body, and although much of it is outside the scope of this book, some fundamental elements are included. **Cell biology** is the study of cells and the cellular level of organization. Cells are grouped together into functional units called tissues. The study of tissues is called **histology** and the principal method used in their examination is microscopy. Relevant topics in cell biology and histology are covered in context. The tissues of the body are combined to form organs and organ systems which have specialized functions. They can be studied in several ways. The commonest method is by dissection of human bodies, carried out either by students or by using prepared specimens. Anatomy is derived from a Greek word meaning 'to cut up'. There are several branches of anatomy: **gross anatomy** is the study of organs and tissues with the naked eye; **microscopical anatomy** is a synonym for histology. Another method used to study the body is **radiography** (X-rays and other imaging techniques). Individual systems often require specialized methods of study. The study

1

of the nervous system is **neuroscience**. **Embryology** is the study of early processes in the development of cells, tissues and organs and the study of their subsequent development is called **developmental anatomy**.

Speech and language

Language is a communication system composed of specific elements. The use of these elements combined in specific orders is governed by sets of rules. For example, the specific meaning of particular words or phrases is governed by **semantic** rules, and **syntactic** rules determine the order of words. Speech sounds, symbols used in writing or sign languages, or symbolic uses of gesture, facial expression and bodily posture are interpreted in the brain using the linguistic rules for the language in question so that we can understand. Likewise our brains use the linguistic rules to construct our reply whether the output is delivered in sound as **speech**, or in writing, or is signed. A simple distinction between language and speech is that thinking of words in your head requires language but does not require speech.

Speech production involves the coordinated movement of a number of structures within the head, neck and thorax. If our language output is as sound, then we need to generate a source of energy to produce these sounds. This is achieved by generating a flow of air through those structures in the head and neck involved in speech production. For the majority of sounds in the languages of the world (and for all sounds in English and Western European languages), sound is produced during exhalation of air from the lungs. Exhalation during speech necessitates significant alteration in the normal pattern of breathing. The volume of air which can be exhaled determines the length of the utterance but, in most cases, the length of utterance desired determines how much air we breathe out. The pressure at which air is exhaled determines in part both the **frequency** and **intensity** of the sound produced; frequency is perceived as **pitch** and **intensity** as loudness.

Breathing out produces a continuous smooth flow of air through the larynx and pharynx in the neck and the mouth and nose (the **vocal tract**). The **larynx** is a constriction in the vocal tract and is narrowest at the vocal folds; these are normally open during exhalation but can be partially or completely closed by muscular action to modulate the continuous airflow. If the vocal folds are closed during exhalation then air pressure will build up below them. As exhalation continues against the closed vocal folds, the pressure will eventually rise sufficiently to overcome the muscular force and air will be released through the vocal folds into the vocal tract above the vocal folds with a consequent fall in pressure below the vocal folds. If the muscular action closing the larynx is maintained, the vocal folds will close. Pressure will once again build up until the folds are forced open. This cycle of opening and closing will be repeated many times a second resulting in a flow of air into the supralaryngeal vocal tract in a series of rarefactions and compressions at a certain frequency depending upon how fast the vocal cords are opening and closing. The frequency determines the pitch. The vibration of the vocal folds is known as **phonation**. Modulation of airflow is not required for all speech sounds; those sounds where vibration of the vocal folds is required are **voiced** and those where there is no vocal fold vibration are **voiceless** (or unvoiced) sounds.

The pulses of air released from the larynx are not in themselves sufficient to produce recognizable sounds without further modification. The cavities above the larynx can be opened or closed or their size and shape can be altered to modify the vibration of air produced by the larynx and produce the individual speech sounds. This involves movement of the tongue, lips, and lower jaw and pharyngeal walls and is termed **articulation**. **Vowels** are produced by varying the size and shape of the mouth and pharynx without unduly obstructing the airflow. The production of **consonants**, however, requires that the airflow is restricted with or without causing turbulence in the airflow or is stopped completely for a brief period. Constrictions that result in turbulence produce consonant sounds known as **fricatives** and consonants produced with closure are **stop consonants**. The changes in the shape and size of the pharynx and oral cavity affect the quality or timbre of the voice by amplifying or damping some of the overtones accompanying the basic frequency generated by the laryngeal vibration. For certain **phonemes**, the individual components of speech, air may be directed through the nasal cavities as well as the oral cavity by movements of the soft palate. The nasal cavities cannot be altered in size or shape but modify the sound by passive resonance.

The **nervous system** is of paramount importance in interpretation and formulation of language and control of speech although many other structures are needed to produce speech. The **ear**, a specialized part of the nervous system, is also necessary to understand the spoken word. The ear is also crucial to monitor what you are saying (**auditory feedback**). Other forms of feedback are also necessary in the control of speech; tactile sensation is required to ensure that articulatory organs such as the tongue are making correct contacts with other articulators and information generated in muscles about their length and force of contraction (proprioception) regulate muscular activity. When normal function of the nervous system is disrupted by trauma or disease, language and speech may be affected with the following effects. Disorders of the areas of the brain concerned with language lead to **aphasia**, the partial or total loss of the ability to use or understand language; often speech sounds are perfectly normal but utterances are semantically and syntactically incorrect so that what the person says is nonsense. Damage to the parts of the nervous system controlling the muscles in the larynx, pharynx and mouth involved in speech produces **dysarthria**, in which inaccurate or defective speech sounds are produced; language is unaffected but it is difficult to understand what the person is saying because of the distorted sounds.

It follows from the brief description of the anatomy and physiology of language and speech that the nervous system is paramount in these activities. However, without an understanding of how nerves function, it is impossible to understand how the nervous system performs these complex activities. To go back one step further, it is difficult to understand how nerves work without some knowledge of the fundamental structure and function of **cells**. By the same token, knowledge of the structure and functions of **muscles, bones** and **cartilages** is required to appreciate how the various muscles of the larynx, tongue, lips, palate and jaws work during phonation and articulation. This knowledge will also help in understanding the respiratory system and its function during speech. Some less obvious aspects of bodily structure and function are needed to understand how the body functions as a whole; in particular, a working knowledge of the **cardiovascular system** is required as nothing works without an adequate blood supply. The **endocrine system**, a series of glands which secrete hormones that have a long range effect on other organs and tissues, controls various aspects of bodily function, some of which are pertinent to speech disorders. Although many abnormalities of speech and language arise as a consequence of disease processes, some are due to disturbances which occur during the development of the body during embryonic and foetal life. An appreciation of the principles underlying development and a more detailed knowledge of the formation of those structures relevant to speech and language is therefore required. Treatment of **dysphagia**, the disturbance of normal swallowing, is now part of the remit of speech and language therapists. An understanding of the anatomy and physiology of the relevant parts of the digestive tract involved in swallowing is needed to appreciate how normal swallowing occurs, how it may be disrupted by various disease processes, and the rationale for various treatments.

This brief outline of speech and language and some of their disorders should illustrate that a practising therapist needs a knowledge of those structures directly relevant to speech and language and an understanding of the underlying principles of how the components of these structures work. Thus, in Chapter 2, an outline is given of the structure and function of cell tissues and organ systems of the body, before presenting a more detailed consideration of the parts of the body directly relevant to speech and language therapy. An overview of each system pertinent to speech and language is presented in Chapters 3 to 7; these chapters are also intended to introduce the subjects to students who have not studied biology in any depth before. Because the nervous system has such overriding importance in the formulation of language and control of speech, this subject is covered in depth in Chapters 8 to 13. We then follow what is often referred to as the **speech chain**: respiration and its modification for speech is covered in Chapters 14 and 15; the structure and function of the larynx and its role in phonation is dealt with in Chapters 16 and 17; the structure and functions of the many components needed for articulation are described in Chapters 18 to 22. This section is the most appropriate place to examine the development of the body – the face and jaws in particular (Chapter 20) – and swallowing and dysphagia as many of the structures used for articulation are also involved in swallowing (Chapter 21). Finally, the structure and functions of the ear are considered in Chapters 22 and 23.

Anatomical terminology

Specific terms are used to describe particular features and the positions of different parts of the body relative to each other. The language of anatomy is not difficult and will become second nature within a short time. So that descriptions may be standardized, they all refer to the body in one specific pose called the **anatomical position** (Figure 1.1), in which the subject is standing erect, feet together, facing the observer with the arms placed at the subject's side and the palms of the hands facing forward.

Planes of the body

The disposition of organs and tissues in the body is related to imaginary planes passing through the body. The midsagittal plane passes vertically through the midline of the body and divides it into equal right and left sides. A plane parallel to the midsagittal plane is called a parasagittal or sagittal plane. The coronal plane is a vertical plane at right angles to the midsagittal plane and thus divides the body into anterior and posterior halves. Horizontal planes run perpendicular to the sagittal and coronal planes and produce a cross-section of the body at a particular level. Sections of the body in any of the three planes are assuming greater importance in the interpretation of images produced by modern imaging techniques (see Chapter 8).

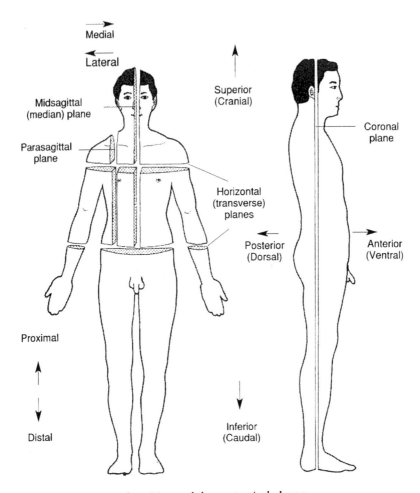

Figure 1.1 The anatomical position and the anatomical planes.

Descriptive terminology

Figure 1.2 should be studied as the terminology is described. Descriptive terms relate to the three planes described, and minimize complex description when used appropriately and accurately. Most of the descriptive terms are paired and it is often implicit in the nomenclature of anatomical structures that if a descriptive term is used, there is a corresponding structure whose name includes the opposite term. For example, structures lying near the midsagittal plane are **medial** whereas those further away from the plane are **lateral**. The use of *lateral* in the naming of the lateral pterygoid muscle implies that there is probably another muscle lying nearer the midsagittal plane and indeed there is also a *medial* pterygoid muscle. **Superior** and **inferior** describe the position of structures relative to the horizontal plane; *superior* is nearer the head and *inferior* is nearer the feet. In descriptions of embryonic development and the nervous system, the terms **cranial** and **caudal** are also used in this context; *cranial* means nearer the head and *caudal* means towards the tail. The terms **anterior** and **posterior** relate structures to the coronal plane. *Anterior* structures lie in front of the plane and *posterior* ones lie behind it, although these terms are also used to describe the positions of structures relative to each other even if they both lie on the same side of the true coronal plane. For example, the anterior and posterior facial veins are both in the face which is anterior to the coronal plane; however, the anterior facial vein lies in front of the posterior facial vein. The terms **ventral** (nearer the anterior surface) and **dorsal** (nearer the posterior surface) are also used to denote the relationship of structures to the coronal plane and are synonymous with anterior and posterior respectively. When describing structures such as limbs or long nerves, the terms **proximal** and **distal** are often used to indicate the position of structures relative to the origin of structure. Thus the wrist lies distal to the elbow whereas the shoulder is proximal to it. Sometimes structures are described by virtue of their relationship to the body surface. Those lying near the body surface are **superficial** whereas those further away are **deep**. Even in the accepted anatomical terminology, **internal** and **external** are sometimes used synonymously with superficial and deep. This is not strictly correct and their literal usage is for description of structures which lie within a covering layer or tissue or lie outside the covering respectively. One set of terms referring to movement is also useful. If a part of the body is moved away from the mid-sagittal plane it is **abducted**, in the reverse movement it is **adducted**. Thus if you raise your arm from the anatomical position you are abducting it and when you lower your arm again it is adducted. Other descriptive terms are used in specific contexts and will be defined as they are encountered.

Two other terms which need definition to aid understanding of subsequent chapters are **somatic** and **visceral**. *Somatic* structures consist of the skin, the skeleton and muscles and the tissues which attach them to the bones whereas *visceral* structures are hollow organs such as the heart and blood vessels, the respiratory tract and the guts; these are known collectively as the viscera.

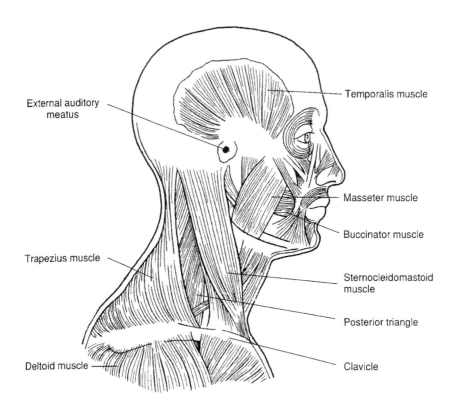

Figure 1.2 The use of anatomical terms illustrated by some muscles of the head and neck. The deltoid muscle lies *lateral* to the clavicle but the trapezius muscle lies *medial* to it. The temporal muscle lies *superior* (cranial) to the ear but the sternocleido-mastoid muscle lies *inferior* (caudal) to it. The sternocleidomastoid muscle forms the *anterior* (ventral) border of the posterior triangle of the neck and the trapezius muscle forms the *posterior* (dorsal) border. The buccinator muscle lies *deep* to the masseter muscle. Conversely, masseter is *superficial* to buccinator.

CHAPTER 2

How the body works – basic concepts of structure and function

This chapter introduces several basic concepts underlying the structure and function of the body. You may be familiar with many of these already in which case you can miss out this chapter. However, if in later chapters you encounter a general concept which you do not understand, refer back to the relevant section of this chapter. This chapter contains a lot of information and will be of particular relevance to those who are new to or returning to biology. There is almost certainly too much to take in at one reading so the advice is to read selectively from this chapter as the need arises.

The simplest forms of life are unicellular organisms, single cells which reproduce by dividing into two identical cells. Higher organisms are multicellular in which groups of similar cells specialized to carry out particular functions are organized into **tissues** for biological efficiency. In more complex higher organisms, tissues are organized still further into **organ systems** to carry out particular complex functions simultaneously. Organ systems and the individual cells are connected by highly sensitive communication systems to ensure that different functions occur in an integrated manner.

Cell chemistry

Cells are, in essence, bags of chemicals in an aqueous solution separated from their neighbours by a cell membrane. The chemicals are a mixture of organic and inorganic compounds. Cellular chemistry is dominated by **organic** carbon compounds which are capable of forming large complex molecules. Six chemical elements make up 99 per cent by weight of the cell: these are carbon, hydrogen, nitrogen, oxygen, phosphorus and sulphur. Cells use four basic types of carbon compound – **nucleotides**, **amino acids**, **fatty acids** and **sugars** – which can be joined together (polymerized) into larger **macromolecules**, to form the structural components of the cells. **Nucleic acids** are polymers of nucleotides, **proteins** are polymers of amino acids, **lipids** are polymers of fatty acids and **carbohydrates** or **polysaccharides** are polymers of sugars. Cells also contain many compounds which do not fall into these categories, but the simple molecules and their polymers listed above make up the majority.

Water, formed from hydrogen and oxygen, accounts for 75 per cent of the weight of each cell and therefore the weight of the body itself. Water is crucial: cellular reactions occur in an aqueous environment and cannot occur in the absence of water within which the substances used for these reaction can dissolve. Many cellular molecules are soluble in water including carbohydrates, nucleic acids and many proteins; these are called hydrophilic (water-loving) molecules. Water must be taken in to balance the loss which occurs in two main ways. A certain amount of water is lost by evaporation through the skin and in exhaled air. Water is also needed to dilute toxic substances excreted through the kidneys as urine.

The water in the body is far from pure. It contains all sorts of substances, gases like oxygen and carbon dioxide, nutrients and lots of **inorganic compounds** which do not contain carbon. The inorganic materials are often present as **ions**, that is the molecule carries an electrical charge. The charge can be positive or negative according to the substance in question and the type of charge is determined by the basic atomic structure of the element. Body water is present in cells but also surrounds cells as extracellular fluid; both contain ions. The most common ions in body water are sodium (represented by the chemical symbol Na), potassium (K), calcium (Ca), chlorine (Cl), bicarbonate (HCO_3) and phosphate (PO_4). Sodium, potassium and calcium are positively charged (**cations**), represented as Na^+, K^+ and Ca^{++} respectively; the value of the charge is also dependent on the atomic structure. Chloride, bicarbonate and phosphate ions are negatively charged (**anions**), represented by Cl^-, HCO_3^- and PO_4^- respectively. Like charges repel and unlike charges attract so cations will tend to bind with anions. A simple example of this is when a sodium cation binds with a chloride anion to form NaCl which is common salt. Essentially, because of the inorganic ions present in solution, body water is a dilute salt solution but contains chemicals other than just salt.

Cell structure

Each cell is separated from its external environment by an envelope known as the **cell membrane** (see Figure 2.1). In the same way that complex organisms are compartmentalized into organs, a similar division of functions is seen in cells. Cells are compartmentalized into the

nucleus, enclosing the genetic information in the form of chromosomes, and the **cytoplasm**, containing all other cellular components. The cytoplasm is separated into subcompartments by a set of internal membranes which separate the **organelles**. The division of cell cytoplasm into subcompartments enables cells to carry out several different, often mutually incompatible, functions simultaneously.

Cell compartmentalization enables thousands of different chemical reactions – some of which might be incompatible if they occurred next to each other – to proceed independently but to be coordinated with other functions to produce the desired end result. A cell making a particular product synthesizes that substance from the basic chemicals present in the cell and may have to synthesize several separate components of the final product which are put together at a later stage. The building blocks necessary for synthetic reactions are obtained from foodstuffs. Foodstuffs are broken down in the gut into components small enough to be absorbed into the body but these components may have to be broken down into further component parts within the cell. Many of the processes used to break down complex chemicals are nonspecific and would therefore break down any chemical of similar structure; to prevent breakdown of material so laboriously synthesized, breakdown occurs in compartments separate from those used for synthetic reactions. A cell can therefore break

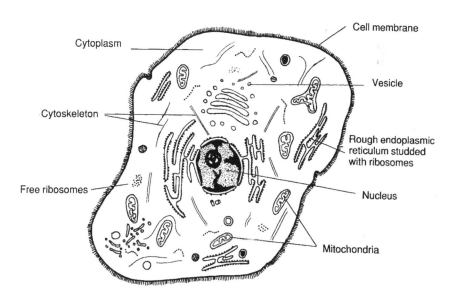

Figure 2.1 A diagrammatic representation of a typical cell.

down material, recycle the components and manufacture something new at the same time while producing energy to support all these processes by utilizing separate subcompartments for each process.

Energy production

All cells must carry out chemical reactions to sustain life. These reactions require two things, a source of fuel in the form of nutrients derived from food and a source of energy. All chemical reactions in the body are known as metabolic reactions or **metabolism**. Each metabolic reaction requires energy to drive it; energy production takes place within separate cytoplasmic organelles called **mitochondria** (Figure 2.1). The energy required by each cell when added together gives the overall energy requirement for the whole body. Energy is generated by burning fuel and requires oxygen. Because oxygen cannot be stored, it must be supplied continuously. Oxygen supply is therefore the paramount requirement of the body. Oxygen is obtained from the atmosphere by breathing air into the lungs through the system of tubes forming the **respiratory system**. Oxygen must be distributed continuously to all the cells within the body and this is achieved through the cardiovascular system. The **cardiovascular system** consists of a series of vessels carrying blood which is continuously pumped throughout the body and the lungs by the action of the heart. As blood passes through the lungs, it is oxygenated; oxygen diffuses from the air into the blood where it attaches to an oxygen-carrying molecule called **haemoglobin** in red blood cells. As blood passes through tissues, it diffuses from the blood into the cells of the body. Blood is not just an oxygen transport system; it carries waste products produced by cellular activity back to the lungs and to the kidneys. Carbon dioxide (CO_2), a waste gas generated by cellular activity, diffuses from the blood into the air in the lungs and is breathed out. Other waste products are removed from the blood by the **kidneys**, diluted with water and excreted as urine. The blood also carries many other compounds which act as signals to tell different cells in the body what to do.

Many organic compounds can be used to generate energy but the most common one is **glucose**, a simple sugar. Glucose is obtained from food directly or indirectly by breakdown of sugars in other food substances and their conversion into glucose. Glucose is broken down into a smaller sugar called pyruvate by a sequence of chemical reactions called **glycolysis**. Pyruvate is further broken down within mitochondria into carbon dioxide and water and this process releases a large amount of energy. When oxygen is required to produce energy, this is **aerobic metabolism** and most bodily processes rely on aerobic metabolism. Some tissues, such as muscle, can manage for a short time by using alternative biochemical reactions which do not require oxygen: this is **anaerobic metabolism**. In this case, pyruvate is not broken down but is converted into lactic acid. Anaerobic metabolism allows energy to be produced even when there is insufficient oxygen (an **oxygen debt**) to allow the complete breakdown of pyruvate. This only provides a temporary solution because lactic acid is toxic and must be broken down when oxygen becomes available again. The build up of lactic acid in muscles is one cause of muscle pain associated with heavy exercise. If the energy released from breakdown of sugars were allowed to escape, this would firstly be very wasteful and secondly would generate excess heat which would raise body temperature to dangerous levels. Instead pyruvate and oxygen are used by mitochondria to generate a molecule called adenosine triphosphate (**ATP**). When the third phosphate ion is added to form ATP, it is linked through a special sort of chemical bond called a **high energy bond**. When this bond is broken, the phosphate is released and so is the energy in the bond. ATP is reduced to adenosine diphosphate (**ADP**) which can be recycled to form another ATP molecule. Fats are the other major source of food that can be metabolized to produce energy using another series of chemical reactions.

In addition to taking in glucose from food, cells in some tissues and organs can also store glucose or fat as a reserve energy source. A certain amount of glucose is present in the blood but excess glucose is taken into certain cells in the body and converted into **glycogen** which can be stored. The liver is the main site for storage of glucose but many other tissues, such as muscle, can store a limited amount of glucose as glycogen. When blood glucose (blood sugar) levels are low, glycogen can be released either from reserves within the tissue or from the liver. The amount of stored glycogen determines how long a particular tissue or organ can survive without a blood supply. Some tissues in the body, such as the brain, are only able to use glucose; if the supply of glucose is insufficient, the brain fails to function correctly. As the brain cannot store glucose, it will use up supplies in about three minutes. After that, irreversible damage will occur. In contrast the heart has about 20 minutes' worth of stored glycogen. Many areas of the body can be rested if damaged so their energy requirements fall drastically and tissue damage is minimized. Excess fat which cannot be used by cells immediately is stored in specialized fat cells under the skin.

Diffusion

Why does oxygen move from air to blood and then blood to cells, and carbon dioxide move in the opposite direction? They move by **diffusion**.

If a particular substance is concentrated in a particular place, it will tend to spread out until it is evenly distributed. As the body is continually using oxygen, oxygen in the tissues is used up. Oxygen in the air is therefore much more concentrated than it is in the blood in the lungs. To achieve an even distribution, oxygen will move from the area of high concentration – the air – into the area of low concentration – blood – until the distribution is equal. This is **equilibrium**, which simply means a balanced state. When a substance is concentrated in a particular place and is diffusing to try to achieve equilibrium there is a gradient of the substance. Initially, it is very densely packed near the source and more thinly spread as it moves away from the source: this is described as a **concentration gradient**. You can demonstrate this very easily by placing a teabag in hot water and watching what happens. As the tea brews, tea diffuses from the tea bag into the water until eventually the water is evenly coloured brown. In the blood, oxygen concentration is high but it is low in the cells because it is being burned up so the concentration gradient will drive oxygen from the blood into cells which are depleted of oxygen. The concentration gradient for CO_2 is the reverse. Cells produce CO_2, but blood and air contain relatively little CO_2. Again, the concentration gradient will cause CO_2 to diffuse from cells into blood and from blood into the air in the lungs.

The cell membrane

This all seems quite straightforward until a complication is thrown in. The contents of all cells are enclosed by a **cell membrane** (Figure 2.2) to keep them separate from the surrounding environment and from other cells. The cell membrane is made of fats containing phosphate called **phospholipids**. All lipids are insoluble in water and therefore form a partition between the salt solution outside the cell, **extracellular fluid**, and the salt solution inside the cell. Ions in the salt solution will behave like other substances and will try to move to establish equilibrium on either side of the membrane. The complication is that inorganic ions and many other water-soluble substances cannot pass freely through the membrane by diffusion to establish equilibrium because, unlike oxygen and carbon dioxide, they are not soluble in lipids. Cells therefore require mechanisms to permit the transfer of such molecules between the inside and outside of cells. These mechanisms are provided by proteins embedded in and spanning the width of the cell membrane.

The two major classes of proteins are channel proteins and carrier proteins. Inorganic ions pass through membranes through small protein pores in the membrane called **ion channels**. Ion channels are specific for each ion and will only allow that ion to pass. When a membrane allows the

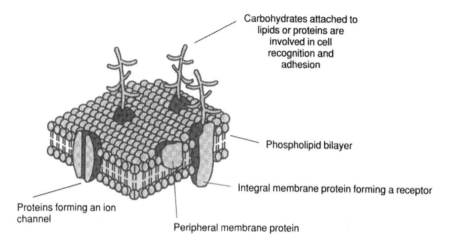

Carbohydrates attached to
lipids or proteins are
involved in cell
recognition and
adhesion

Phospholipid bilayer

Integral membrane protein forming a receptor

Proteins forming an ion
channel

Peripheral membrane protein

Figure 2.2 The structure of the cell membrane and associated receptors.

passage of some substances but not others it is called a **semi-permeable membrane** because it is only permeable to some materials. Ion channels are formed by proteins lodged in the phospholipids forming the cell membrane. The proteins are highly folded into a tubular configuration to form each channel. Most ion channels are not open all the time but open in response to specific signals.

Receptors

Most channels have receptors on the external surface of the cell membrane connected to the ion channel (Figure 2.2). Each **receptor** is specific for a particular substance which fits into the receptor like a piece of a jigsaw. When the substance, the **ligand**, binds to the receptor, the configuration of the proteins forming the ion channel is altered such that the channel opens and allows passage of the ions specific to that channel. Ion channels of this type are called **ligand-gated channels**. Other ion channels will open when the voltage across the cell membrane is altered; this again alters the protein configuration to open the channel, and this type of channel is described as a **voltage-gated channel**. Carrier proteins are the other form of protein involved in transfer of molecules across cell membranes. These transfer large molecules which cannot pass through the membrane directly or are too large for channels. They too have receptors that bind specific substances and the complex of receptor and ligand becomes soluble in the membrane and can pass through it. This is called **facilitated diffusion**.

If all the receptors are occupied by their ligand, no more ligands can enter the cell: the system is then described as **saturated**. Sometimes it is necessary to remove ions from cells when they become too concentrated. This requires the ions to move against the concentration gradient. Like trying to push something uphill, this requires energy. The energy to move molecules against the concentration gradient is provided by molecular pumps in the membrane which are often specific for a particular ion. Transport of ions against the concentration gradient is called **active transport**.

Receptors play other important roles in cell membranes. Many act as selective markers for different cell types and enable them to recognize each other. They can also act as receptors for signals originating in other cells.

Cell signalling

Many molecules act as signals. They are synthesized by one type of cell and exert their influence on other cells over short or long distances. Together they are called **first messengers**. Messengers may act on the cell that produces them, on cells in the immediate vicinity or at distant sites. Messengers acting on their own cells carry out **autocrine** signalling. The messenger is released then immediately binds to receptors on the surface of the cell; this is the equivalent of you writing a note to yourself to remind you to do something. Messengers acting on other cells in the vicinity are **paracrine**; this is the equivalent of someone putting a message on a noticeboard which will only be read by people to whom it is relevant. More distant signalling involves transport of the first messenger via the blood stream to distant organs and tissues. This is endocrine signalling using hormones (see below) and is the equivalent of putting an advertisement on billboards in public places.

First messengers can only affect cells anywhere if those cells have the appropriate receptors for the particular first messenger signalling molecule. More specific signalling and precise control can be achieved by sending a message directly to the recipient cells. This is achieved by the **nervous system**, which can transmit messages very quickly over long distances using electrical impulses but can route them to specific areas.

Some signal molecules, including certain hormones, are lipids and can dissolve in and pass through the cell membrane to exert a direct action on the cell. However, most signal molecules which do not enter cells directly still exert an influence on cell metabolism. They attach to specific receptors in the membrane and by doing so activate enzymes (see below) within the cell membrane coupled to the internal aspect of the receptor.

These enzymes in turn set off a chain of reactions within the cell which alter its metabolic activity. These are called **second messenger systems** because intermediate processes are necessary to translate receptor activation into metabolic activity within the cell.

Osmolarity and acid-base balance

The cell membranes of most cells are impermeable to most dissolved substances but are highly permeable to water. Consequently, if the ion concentration changes on either side of the cell membrane and the ions cannot move, then water in which they are dissolved will. The force responsible for movement of water is called the **osmotic pressure** of a solution and is dependent upon the number of ions in solution. If the concentration of an ion is unequal on either side of the membrane and the ions cannot move, water will flow from the lower concentration into the higher concentration until the concentrations are equalized. This achieves **osmotic balance** and ensures that ionic balance is maintained. If it is not maintained, too high an ionic concentration will attract water into the cell from extracellular fluid which will cause the cell to swell and possibly burst. If the concentration is too low, water will flow out of the cell and the cell into the extracellular fluid and the cell will shrink and possibly collapse. In some cells such as nerve cells (neurons), it is essential to maintain an unequal concentration of ions for them to conduct nerve impulses (see Chapter 6). This is achieved by ion pumps, which are carrier proteins using active transport to move some ions outside the cell against the concentration gradient. The number of ions needed to adjust the concentration is very small indeed; osmotic balance is preserved in such cases by the presence of other dissolved substances.

Most chemical reactions within cells operate optimally in a chemically neutral environment. If the environment becomes too acidic or alkaline, many processes will be halted with potentially serious consequences. The degree of acidity is measured by the concentration of hydrogen (H^+) ions, abbreviated to **pH**. A pH value of 7 is neutral, below 7 is acid and above 7 is alkaline. The value of pH is measured on a logarithmic scale, which means that for a change in value of 1 on the scale, the difference in hydrogen ion concentration is actually tenfold. The overall pH of the body is slightly alkaline and is about pH 7.4. The body can tolerate a pH ranging from 6.9 to 7.8; in effect the concentration of hydrogen ions can be doubled or halved.

Hydrogen ions are generated by many metabolic reactions within the body and would make the pH plummet into the acid range if not controlled. Control is achieved by **buffers**, present in the blood and extracellular fluid, which essentially mop up hydrogen ions. Bases are chemically negative ions which will combine with the positively charged hydrogen ions. Buffers will do this and the product formed will then dissociate into other substances containing the hydrogen ions. One of the most ubiquitous and important buffers in the body is bicarbonate (HCO_3^-). When H^+ binds with HCO_3^-, carbonic acid (H_2CO_3) is formed, which dissociates into water (H_2O) and carbon dioxide (CO_2). Carbon dioxide is breathed out and the water is added to the water already present thus rendering the hydrogen ions harmless and maintaining the pH.

Functions of proteins

The fuel burned up by oxygen is ultimately obtained from the food we eat. This provides all the basic nutrients, which can either be used directly or converted into other forms that can then be used to make other molecules. Manufacture of a new substance is **synthesis**. Certain substances are needed by all cells in the body to keep them alive and to repair parts of the cell when they are damaged or worn out. However, most cells in the body are specialized for particular functions and manufacture specific products as well as those needed by all cells. The type of cell depends upon the types of proteins it produces, which determine the cell type either directly or indirectly. Directly, many proteins are structural proteins and form parts of the cell or determine its shape. Indirectly, many proteins act as biological catalysts. A **catalyst** is a substance which enables a chemical reaction to occur but is not altered by the chemical reaction so can be used repeatedly to catalyse identical reactions. Biological catalysts are known as **enzymes** and the types of enzymes present will determine what a cell can make because each enzyme is specific for a given chemical reaction; if the enzyme is not synthesized, the corresponding reaction cannot take place. Proteins do not only function as structural proteins and enzymes as we have seen above. They are also involved in transport, storage, signalling and receptors.

Protein synthesis – from DNA to protein

We now need to consider how different proteins are made. This is determined by which genes in the genetic material present in cells are activated. All cells, with few exceptions, carry the complete genetic code in their nuclei as **chromosomes**. Thus, all cells are capable of making all the necessary materials required throughout the body, but they are not required to do so. During development (see Chapter 20), cells become more specialized to manufacture specific products by restricting the amount of genetic material which is translated to a subset of genes specific for the activity of that cell. A given cell will only express a small fraction of its genes. In much the same way as you translate combinations of letter symbols on this page into words, phrases and sentences and interpret their meaning, cells interpret the genetic code. Chromosomes are made of **deoxyribonucleic acid (DNA)**. This consists of repeated sequences of a sugar – deoxyribose – and phosphate coupled together to form a long molecular strand rather like a backbone. From this backbone, nucleic acids project. Only four nucleic acids (known as bases) are used to make DNA. They are adenine, cytosine, guanine and thymine. These have the remarkable property that they will pair with each other in strict register such that adenine pairs with thymine and guanine pairs with cytosine: this is called **complementary base pairing**. By complementary base pairing, a replica of each strand of DNA forms with the opposite of the pair of bases on the complementary strand. The base pairs are bonded together so that the two strands of DNA are linked and spiral round each other to form a **double helix**.

Each species has a characteristic number of chromosomes which in humans is 46: this is known as the **diploid** number and is kept constant during cell division (**mitosis**). In humans, the 46 chromosomes comprise 22 pairs of identical chromosomes known as **homologous pairs** and a pair of disparate sex chromosomes designated X (female) and Y (male). In males the remaining pair of chromosomes consist of an X and a Y chromosome, whereas in females there are two X chromosomes. During cell division, each coil of the double helix of DNA making up each chromosome is replicated by complementary base pairing to double the number of chromosomes. One of each replicated pair of chromosomes is donated to the two cells arising during cell division: the genetic material is thus passed on from one cell generation to the next.

The bases on each chromosome are not arranged at random but are grouped together in strict sequence into **genes**, each of which carries the code to manufacture a specific protein. Proteins are made by joining together amino acids in strict sequence and there are 20 amino acids which are used to make all the proteins in the body. The genetic code carries the coding to correctly sequence the amino acids. Bases are arranged in groups of three, each triplet **codon** coding for a particular amino acid. Each chromosome carries thousands of genes, and each gene comprises many hundreds or thousands of codons.

When a particular protein is required, the gene coding for that particular protein – and thus controlling its production – is exposed by unravelling of the relevant part of the DNA double helix. When the gene is revealed, a single strand of messenger RNA (**mRNA**) complementary in sequence to the exposed DNA is produced by complementary base pairing between the DNA and RNA nucleotides, by the process of **transcription** (Figure 2.3). **Ribonucleic acid** (**RNA**) is a single-stranded molecule and consists of nucleotides attached to a backbone of ribose and phosphate. As with DNA, only four nucleotides are used to form the RNA strand, with **uracil** substituting for thymine in RNA. Uracil, however, will still form a base pair with adenine. Thus an exact replica of the original gene is produced as a single strand of RNA. This type of RNA is called **messenger RNA** (mRNA) because it leaves the cell nucleus carrying a faithful copy of the message to make a particular protein. In the cytoplasm, the mRNA strand complexes with small particles called **ribosomes** (Figure 2.1). Ribosomes may be small aggregates within the cytoplasm or complex with membranes to form rough endoplasmic reticulum. Free ribosomes are used to make proteins for intracellular use and rough endoplasmic reticulum manufactures proteins for export from the cell. Ribosomes enable RNA to be **translated** into proteins by allowing carrier molecules called transfer RNA (**tRNA**) to align up on the mRNA. Each transfer RNA has a complementary codon at one end and a receptor for a given amino acid at the other to which that amino acid binds. Each tRNA base pairs with the appropriate codon on the mRNA so that the amino acids are aligning in the correct sequence. They are then assembled in the right order and polymerized into protein by the action of enzymes in the ribosome. The best way to remember this is that *DNA makes RNA makes protein*. The conversion of DNA into protein via RNA is called **gene expression**. The types of protein that a cell makes determine that cell's activities and its shape and structure.

Basic genetics

Genetic information encoded in the chromosomal DNA strands directs particular protein synthetic activities and is responsible for the enormous diversity of cell types within the body of any one individual of a species. This diversity is not just due to the expression of genes in the genetic make-up – the **genotype** – but is also the result of the effects of environmental factors. These interactions that produce the characteristic features of individual cells are referred to as the **phenotype** of an individual. Environmental factors thus direct the phenotypes which are produced from cells of identical genotype. In addition to the diversity of gene expression within individuals, there is also considerable variation between individuals resulting from variations in the genotype of individuals and differences in the environmental factors to which they are exposed.

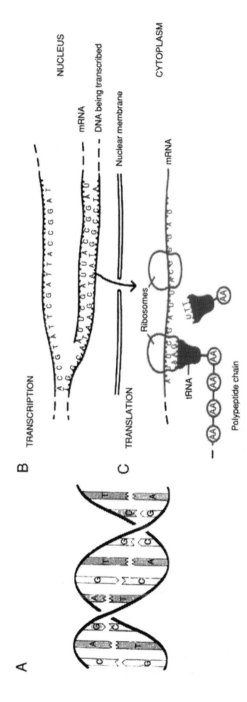

Figure 2.3 (A) The structure of DNA. (B) Transcription of mRNA from DNA. (C) Translation of protein from mRNA.

An important cause of genetic variation arises during the transition from diploid to haploid chromosome number during formation of the germ cells, the male spermatozoa and the female ova. The number of chromosomes is reduced by half by a special type of cell division called **meiosis**, so that each germ cell contains only 23 chromosomes (the **haploid number**). During meiosis, maternal and paternal genes are donated to each germ cell or gamete so that every gamete contains one copy of each chromosome and one of each pair of sex chromosomes. Donation of maternal and paternal genes occurs at random along any one chromosome resulting in the production of many gametes of differing genetic composition and ensuring considerable genetic variation when fertilization occurs. When an ovum is fertilized, the chromosomes from the male spermatozoon fuse with those of the ovum, the diploid number is restored, sex is determined and there has been a mixing of genes from the two parents within the resulting embryo. Thus the genotype of any individual is derived from both parents, each one contributing a varying proportion of genes along the length of one of each homologous chromosome pair and one sex chromosome. The genotype will differ from that of either parent because of the contribution from the other.

A particular gene is always located on a particular chromosome at the same site, known as the **gene locus**. Because the genome comprises 22 or, in the female, 23 homologous pairs, it follows that each gene locus is represented twice. They are, however, not always identical; if they are, they are referred to as **homozygous genes**, but if they differ, they are **heterozygous genes**. Variants at a single locus are known as **alleles** and they differ in their ability to be expressed. The allele of a heterozygous pair which is commonly expressed is the **dominant gene** whereas the one least likely to be expressed is the **recessive gene**. The gene controlling brown eye colour is dominant over the gene expressing blue eye colour. Thus, if an individual is heterozygotic at this locus and possesses a 'brown' and a 'blue' gene, the dominant gene will be expressed and their eyes will be brown. It is only when the individual has a pair of 'blue' genes that their eye colour will be blue. In some cases, both members of a heterozygous pair can be expressed equally and are **co-dominant**; for example, when an individual is heterozygous and possesses the genes determining the A and B blood groups, both are expressed and the individual will have the AB blood group. There are not necessarily just two copies of a gene in the genome; many genes have multiple copies at different gene loci. However, the number of copies bears no relationship to the importance of the gene; the gene coding for haemoglobin, the oxygen-carrying red pigment in erythrocytes, only has a single homologous gene locus.

By virtue of the ability of DNA to replicate by complementary base pairing, the hereditary information can be faithfully copied from generation to generation of cells during cell division and from parents to offspring during meiosis and sexual reproduction. However, if the exchange of genes between parents during meiosis is not perfect, then offspring can be produced with duplications in certain genes that are believed to be a major cause of genetic change in populations. There can also be mistakes in copying the DNA that occur spontaneously during cell division creating new genetic variants. Finally, certain external agents such as harmful ionizing radiation or certain chemicals can affect the DNA especially in rapidly dividing cells such as those in the immune system, the reproductive system, the lining of the gut and hair follicles. In the short term, cell division may be inhibited leading to hair loss, depression of the immune system and inability to digest food (radiation sickness) but it can have longer-term effects on the cells by altering the DNA. Whatever the cause, genes which differ from the originals are called **mutations**. Mutations may be major or minor and can produce a number of results by their effects on biochemical reactions within cells. A minor alteration in an unimportant gene sequence may produce no noticeable effect and is called a **silent mutation**. Alternatively a mutation in an important gene may affect cellular mechanisms so severely that the individual dies; this is a **lethal mutation**.

Each cell throughout the body has an identical genotype containing all the genes necessary to code for every protein in the body. As differentiation of cells takes place during development, cells become increasingly specialized until only a tiny fraction of the total gene pool is expressed, often only in response to demand. The expression of the majority of genes is repressed for most cells for most of the time. This is brought about by **gene regulatory proteins** which, in turn, are coded for by genes known as **regulator genes** to distinguish them from **structural genes** that encode structural proteins and enzymes.

The expression of genes does not take place in isolation but is the result of interactions between a developing individual and factors in the environment. This interaction produces the phenotype of an individual and is the reason why even individuals of a species with an identical genotype will not necessarily develop in the same way. Environmental factors generally do not affect the genes themselves, but the expression of the genes. For example, the drug thalidomide given to pregnant women caused limb malformations in their children. But for the administration of thalidomide, the environmental factor, these children would have had normal limbs. Genetic errors may remain dormant until the environmental factor is encountered. For example, one genetic abnormality leads to absence of a particular enzyme which goes largely unnoticed. This enzyme inactivates a harmful chemical found in certain vegetables which causes rapid breakdown of red blood cells. If the affected person eats broad beans, the chemical is not inactivated resulting in severe anaemia.

Cell growth and division

During development, new cells must be produced from the fertilized ovum to produce all the cells which make up the mature individual. In mature individuals, dead and dying cells need to be replaced as they are lost through wear and tear or injury; in general, the cells lost are replaced by a similar number of cells. The production of new cells in the body is carried out by cell division or **mitosis** to form two identical cells with identical genetic material.

Mechanisms of cell replacement

New differentiated cells are produced by two methods (see Figure 2.4). **Simple duplication** involves mitotic division of existing differentiated cells to generate two identical daughter cells. An example of cells which are replaced by simple duplication is liver cells. Replacement may also be effected by division of a more primitive cell type, a **stem cell**. Stem cells are **pluripotential**, that is they are able to differentiate into several different cell types. Stem cells are found in the early stages of embryonic development (see Chapter 20) and persist in some mature organs to enable replacement of damaged cells and repair of the organ. For example, bone marrow stem cells can produce all the blood cells. Different blood cell types are present in different numbers and have different lifespans and therefore each cell type must be produced at different rates to replace dying cells. When stem cells divide, two daughter cells are produced by mitotic division of the stem cell but one remains as a stem cell and can divide again whereas the other daughter cell undergoes a series of alterations to become a mature differentiated cell.

Stem cells are found in some tissues in which the fully differentiated cells are incapable of mitosis. An example is the epithelium forming the covering of the vocal folds. Such a tissue is arranged in layers with the stem cells at the base and the outermost cells forming a layer of dead cells on the surface. These dead cells are lost from the surface through wear and tear but homeostasis (see below) ensures that cell loss is balanced by production of new cells from the stem cells. The basal stem cells are **unipotent** and when they divide they can produce one stem cell and one epithelial cell. If the complete thickness of an area of epithelium is removed by injury, the denuded area is rapidly replaced by a monolayer

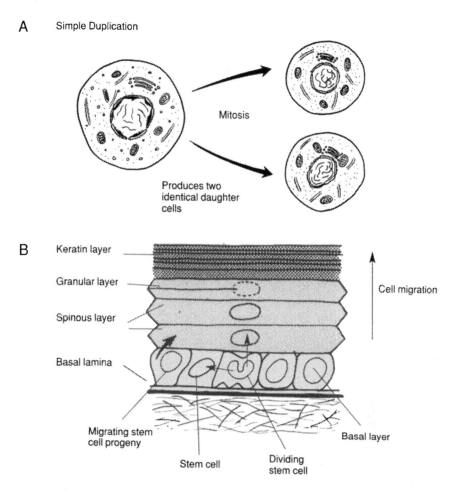

Figure 2.4 Mechanisms of cell replacement. (A) Simple duplication. (B) Stem cell renewal.

derived by simple duplication of adjacent undamaged basal stem cells. These cells spread until they meet and fill the deficit; it is only when confluence is achieved that the cells revert to normal stem cell activity and produce cells to form the normal multilayered epithelium. Some stem cells are pluripotential cells capable of producing several different phenotypes of daughter cells. For example, bone marrow stem cells can produce all the different types of blood cell (see Chapter 4).

Cell populations incapable of cell division are generated in appropriate numbers during embryonic development and have lifespans similar to that of the organism as a whole. These **non-renewing cells** include neurons of the central and peripheral nervous system and cardiac muscle cells in the heart. Although the cells cannot be replaced, their intracellular organelles are constantly replaced. Some non-renewing cells can respond to appropriate stimuli by growing in size (see below); for example, cardiac muscle cells will increase dramatically in size following various physiological or pathological stimuli which increase the work rate of the heart. However, if cardiac muscle cells or nerve cells are damaged, they will die and cannot be replaced, thus markedly impairing the efficiency of the heart or the nervous system.

Alterations in cell size, cell growth and differentiation

Various disease processes may affect cell size or interfere with cell growth and differentiation. **Hypertrophy** is an increase in cell size, which may ultimately affect the tissue or organ in which the cells lie. The effect of exercise on muscle is an obvious example. **Hyperplasia** is an increase in the size of a tissue or organ due to an increase in the number of cells present, for example, the thickening of the covering of the vocal folds if they are subject to constant vocal abuse. A hyperplastic tissue will return to its normal size if the causative stimulus is removed. **Atrophy** is a diminution in organ or tissue size due to a reduction in its constituent elements and may be physiological or pathological. Physiological atrophy is typified by diminution of the ovaries and uterus postmenopausally. Wasting of muscles and adipose tissue during starvation is an example of pathological atrophy. **Metaplasia** is a change in a differentiated tissue whereby it comes to resemble another tissue. For instance, the lining of the bronchi may change if continually irritated by cigarette smoke.

Cancer

Neoplasia literally means 'new growth', in which a mass of abnormal new tissue is produced and proliferates faster than the tissue from which it arises. Neoplasia is initiated by changes in gene expression and control which are passed on from one cell generation to the next. Neoplasms are classified on the basis of their destructive effects into **benign** or **malignant** neoplasms; malignant neoplasms are commonly referred to as **cancers**.

Benign neoplasms are sharply demarcated from adjacent normal tissues and are non-invasive. They are generally slow growing and their constituent cells resemble those of the tissue of origin and may be indistinguishable from them. Unlike hyperplastic tissue, neoplastic tissue will not return to its normal size if the causative agent is removed. They mainly cause damage by exerting pressure on adjacent tissues which often results in occlusion of their blood supply or the lumen of adjacent tubular structures. A benign lesion of the thyroid gland in the neck may cause constriction of the oesophagus with consequent difficulties in swallowing.

Malignant neoplasms, in contrast, divide and grow rapidly. Their constituent cells usually differ markedly in appearance from their normal counterparts. In many instances, they are so poorly differentiated and so irregular in shape and size that it is impossible to recognize their tissue of origin. They are very invasive and cause damage because normal tissue atrophies, by obstruction and destruction of adjacent tissues including nerves and blood vessels. In addition, cancer cells lose their normal intercellular junctions and also secrete enzymes which destroy the extracellular material surrounding them. These alterations render the cells more motile and the cancer cells are able to leave the primary neoplasm and invade adjacent or more distant normal tissues. This is **metastasis**: migrating cancer cells form secondary neoplasms (metastases) in distant sites where their proliferative and destructive effects continue. Treatment of cancer therefore involves not only destruction of the primary cancer by surgical removal, chemotherapy or radiotherapy, but also removal of secondary metastatic deposits or their potential sites of formation. Unfortunately, this is not easy and widespread dissemination of cancer is the cause of the high mortality rates of patients with malignant disease.

Disease

Disease is a state in which there is sufficient departure from normal structure and function to produce **symptoms**, which are the features of the disease reported by the patient, and **signs**, which are detectable by a clinician. For example, a client with a voice disorder may report that they experience a sore throat and that their voice is weak; the clinician may observe that the vocal cords are inflamed and enlarged. Disease may produce variations from normal structure, including alterations in biochemical pathways, which are known as **lesions**. Some diseases are characterized by a defined collection of lesions, signs and symptoms which taken together constitute a **syndrome**. The cause of a particular disease is known as its **aetiology**. Many diseases have no obvious aetiology and are said to be **idiopathic**, whereas others may be produced by the clinician, often inadvertently, and are classified as **iatrogenic**. An example of iatrogenic disease is inadvertent damage to the nerves supplying the larynx during thyroid or heart surgery.

The tissues of the body

All cells in the body share common structural and functional characteristics but most are specialized to perform specific functions which designate their individual character. Cells with particular functions are usually grouped together and are supported by extracellular materials made by cells to form the **tissues** of the body. Tissues are classified into four basic types, known as **epithelium, connective tissue, muscle** and **nervous tissue**. Epithelium covers external surfaces and lines internal surfaces of the body; it also forms aggregates of secretory tissue known as **glands**. Epithelium forms dense sheets of cells in intimate contact with no intervening extracellular material. Connective tissue consists of varying proportions of three components – cells, fibres and extracellular matrix; the cells produce and maintain the other two components. The number of fibres and the type of extracellular matrix determine their individual characteristics. For example, tendons connecting muscles to bone consist of dense bundles of fibres with little extracellular matrix. Some connective tissues have extra components in their extracellular matrix to make them more rigid; bone contains crystals of a calcium phosphate which makes it hard and cartilage contains many complex macromolecules which make it rigid but give it some pliability. Connective tissue is described more fully in Chapter 3. Muscle cells are specialized for contraction and contain contractile proteins which will slide across each other to effect contraction (see Chapter 3). Nervous tissue is specialized as a communication system by carrying electrical impulses over long distances to take messages from one part of the body to another, as described in Chapter 6.

Epithelial tissues

Epithelia form dense cellular sheets or glandular aggregates with individual cells attached to each other by desmosomes. They differ from the other basic tissues in that they do not contain blood vessels and rely on nutrients diffusing from blood vessels situated in adjacent connective tissue. Epithelia are therefore always supported by connective tissue. A **basal lamina complex** joins the epithelium to the connective tissue.

Epithelia are arranged in different ways in different organ systems to meet particular functional demands (see Figure 2.5). Epithelial cells may form a single layer with each cell in contact with the basal lamina or they may be arranged in two or more layers as a **stratified epithelium** with only the deepest or **basal** cells in contact with the basal lamina. A false impression of stratification may be given if an epithelium contains a number of different cell types whose nuclei are at different levels in the epithelium; such an epithelium is described as **pseudostratified**.

A

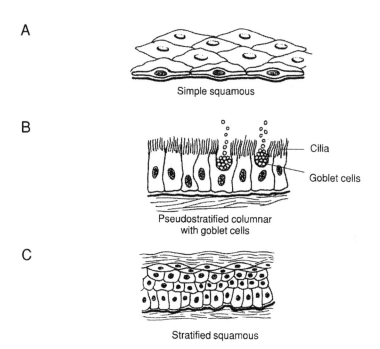

Simple squamous

B

Cilia

Goblet cells

Pseudostratified columnar
with goblet cells

C

Stratified squamous

Figure 2.5 The structure of epithelia. (A) Simple squamous epithelium. (B) Pseudostratified columnar epithelium with goblet cells (respiratory epithelium). (C) Stratified squamous epithelium.

Essentially, only three types of epithelium are significant to speech and language therapists: these are simple squamous epithelium, stratified squamous epithelium and pseudostratified columnar epithelium lining various parts of the respiratory system and vocal tract.

Simple squamous epithelium comprises a single layer of flattened (squamous) cells in a continuous sheet rather like floor tiles. This type of epithelium is very thin and delicate and is therefore an ideal lining for the alveoli of the lungs, where it provides a negligible barrier to diffusion of gases between blood and air.

Pseudostratified epithelium lines the respiratory tract for most of its length and is designed to entrap harmful particles breathed in to prevent damage to the delicate epithelium lining the lung alveoli. The columnar cells possess cilia – small hair-like projections – on their luminal surface, and mucus-secreting goblet cells are interspersed between the columnar cells. The mucus traps particles and the cilia are coordinated to beat in waves which move the particles away from the lungs into the pharynx, from where the particles may be swallowed. It is often called **respiratory epithelium**. Respiratory epithelium is only one cell thick and is not designed to withstand abrasion.

In areas subject to abrasion, a multilayered **stratified squamous epithelium** is found; it covers the whole surface of the skin, lines the oral cavity and covers the vocal folds. The **basal cells** adjacent to the basal lamina complex function as stem cells (see above). Their daughter cells enter a cycle of maturation, altering their shape as they pass successively higher through the layers until eventually they reach the surface where they become flattened and are shed. Such epithelia may be **non-keratinized** in which case the superficial surface cells are viable. Alternatively, the superficial cells may undergo **keratinization** by accumulation and concentration of cytokeratin intermediate filaments within the cell cytoplasm. This outer keratinized layer of dead cells is tough and protects underlying cells from physical forces.

In covering or lining epithelia, the rates of renewal vary according to functional demands. In all stratified epithelia, cell loss from the surface is matched by renewal from the basal cells. Because covering epithelia are stratified to provide protection, their turnover depends to a great extent on the frictional forces to which they are subject; the rate of turnover is fastest in areas subject to the greatest forces.

Glandular epithelia

Epithelia which have a secretory function may include goblet cells, but in many sites the number of secretory cells which can exist on a flat epithelial surface is grossly inadequate for functional demands. In such cases, glands are formed by differentiation from the epithelial cells. Glands are composed of epithelial cells which migrate beneath the surface epithelial layer and form aggregates of cells specialized to synthesize and secrete particular products.

Glands may be classified into two major groups. **Exocrine glands** pass their secretory products via a series of ducts to an internal or external body surface where the secretions act. **Endocrine glands** are ductless glands and secrete their hormone products directly into the blood stream, which transports them to their site of action.

Organ systems

The basic tissue types are combined in different proportions and with different degrees of specialization to form the **organs** of the body. In turn, the organs of the body are grouped into **organ systems** to carry out particular functions. As with individual cells, the body is capable of carrying out many functions simultaneously; this is achieved by having organ systems which can carry out a particular function while coordinating their activities with other systems. Each organ system does not operate alone but is dependent on other systems for efficient function and coordination.

- The **locomotor (musculoskeletal) system**, consisting of bones and cartilages connected by joints and muscles, supports and protects other organs, enables different parts of the body to move relative to one another and the body to move as a whole (see Chapter 3).
- Oxygen is required to support the activity of all tissues and organs and is distributed through **the circulatory system**. The circulatory system comprises the **cardiovascular** and **lymphoid systems**. The cardiovascular system consists of the heart, which pumps blood carrying oxygen and carbon dioxide through blood vessels to all tissues where gases are exchanged between blood and tissues. The lymphoid system is a series of small blind ending vessels which collect fluid leaking from blood vessels and return it to the cardiovascular system. It also has a crucial role to play in defending the body from attack by harmful microorganisms and other foreign material (see Chapter 4).
- The **respiratory system** transports air to and from the lungs where oxygen diffuses into the blood and waste gases, mainly carbon dioxide, diffuse out (see Chapter 5).
- The **digestive system** takes in food, breaks it down physically and chemically, absorbs the nutrients derived from food into the body, and reabsorbs useful material which it produces to assist the breakdown of food; finally, it excretes material in foodstuffs which cannot be broken down or absorbed.
- As water forms the major component of the body, it is vital that water levels are maintained and that water contains the correct balance of chemicals; as various chemical reactions take place in cells, tissues and organs, harmful waste products are formed which must be excreted from the body. The **urinary system** excretes these waste products and excess quantities of other material while ensuring that water levels and chemical balance are maintained.
- The **reproductive system** generates the cells necessary for reproduction and, in the female, nurtures the developing fetus prior to birth.
- The **nervous system** coordinates activities of the other systems as well as receiving and responding to external and internal stimuli. Highly specialized parts of the nervous system are responsible for reception of specific stimuli such as light and sound; the eyes, ears and nose are sometimes referred to as the organs of special sense. Other parts of the

nervous system control the movement of muscles including those involved in speech production. The nervous system also carries out more complex functions such as cognition, memory and production and interpretation of language. The nervous system is introduced in Chapter 6 and covered in detail in Chapters 8 to 13.

- The **endocrine system** is a series of glands scattered throughout the body which secrete **hormones**; these act as long range control systems influencing the activity of many of the components of other systems (Chapter 7).
- The **integumentary system** – the skin and its associated tissues and organs – is often overlooked but is, in fact, the largest system of all. The skin is not only vital for protection of the body and reception of external stimuli but also plays a role in temperature regulation.

It is almost impossible to describe the function of one particular system without referring to another system; their activities are all interdependent and coordinated for maximum efficiency. The coordinated efforts of all the systems also ensure that the internal environment is maintained at constant levels. The body is designed to function optimally within very narrow limits. If these limits are exceeded, the systems will coordinate their activity in an effort to return them to normal levels as soon as possible. The maintenance and correction of the internal environment is known as **homeostasis**. For example, body temperature must be maintained at about 37°C; a rise or fall in temperature of only 3°C can have fatal consequences.

Homeostasis

To see how everything acts together to maintain homeostasis, we will follow one example through. While sitting chatting to your colleagues in the tea-room, you suddenly realize that your next client is due in ten minutes and you have not read last session's case notes to prepare for the session. You run along the corridor, up two flights of stairs, along another corridor into the room, grab your notes, sit down and begin reading. You are now breathing heavily and rapidly, your heart is thumping and you are hot and flushed. Alarmingly, on the face of it, you have no control whatsoever over any of these events and these are the only ones you actually notice; many more have taken place which you are not even aware of. However, within the next few minutes your body will return to normal and you will present a picture of unflustered calm as your client walks through the door!

Within 20 seconds or so of leaving the tea-room at a run, you will have used up most of the energy sources in your muscles that can be used without oxygen. Your continued exertion demands oxygen and energy sources to keep your muscles going as you run upstairs. Waste products generated by muscle activity will make the blood vessels in the muscles dilate to increase blood flow. Muscular activity generates carbon dioxide and depletes oxygen; as CO_2 levels rise and O_2 levels fall in the blood, this will be sensed by special receptors in the cardiovascular system and the information will be conveyed to areas in the brain responsible for controlling respiratory rate. They will activate the muscles in your chest wall to increase the rate and depth of respiration to get more air into and out of your lungs. To make sure that the increased oxygen intake gets to the muscles, your heart rate and the amount of blood pumped from the heart at each beat will increase. Other signals from the brain will decrease blood flow to non-essential areas by narrowing blood vessels supplying these organs. Your muscles are demanding glucose, their main nutrient source, and as blood glucose levels fall as it is used up, the endocrine system will be activated to release stored forms of glucose to maintain the supply. As your muscles work, they generate heat which must be dissipated to prevent body temperature rising too much. Sensors in your brain monitoring blood temperature will send signals to dilate blood vessels in your skin (so that you become flushed); the hot blood flowing through these vessels will lose heat to the surrounding air and thus become cooled. The same signals will also make the sweat glands in your skin secrete sweat. To evaporate sweat from the body surface, water has to be turned into water vapour; this requires heat energy so heat is drawn off the dilated blood vessels in the skin thus adding to the cooling effect.

These cooling effects will continue until your blood temperature is back to normal. This will be sensed by the brain which will then send signals to narrow the blood vessels and stop sweat secretion. Most of your oxygen intake during exercise will have been used by the muscles so other structures will be in oxygen debt. This is why deep breathing continues even after exercise has ceased – to bring oxygen levels back to normal and clear any excess carbon dioxide. As these parameters return to normal, the signals will be generated to downregulate the activities recruited during exercise. Your heart rate and respiratory rate will return to normal. Now you do not need so much glucose, any excess in the blood will trigger off the release of another hormone which promotes the deposition of glucose in its storage form in the liver and some other organs.

Control of body systems

All the activities taking place in the example above are regulated unconsciously by **autonomic** (self-governing) mechanisms. Such systems monitor the internal environment and regulate activities of different systems to maintain homeostasis, the maintenance of the body in an optimal state. These mechanisms occur without us having to think about them and, moreover, they are beyond our conscious control. Many internal bodily functions are controlled by **negative feedback**. Essentially, the disturbance itself stimulates correction of the disturbance.

Particular levels of bodily activity are measured internally by sensors within the organ systems. For example, there are specialized receptors within the cardiovascular system which monitor the levels of oxygen and carbon dioxide in the blood. When blood carbon dioxide levels rise, this information is conveyed from the cardiovascular receptors to respiratory centres of the brain which regulate respiration. The rate and depth of respiration is increased by the respiratory centres until the carbon dioxide is cleared from the blood and levels are back to normal again.

Insulin provides another example. After a meal, blood sugar tends to rise as glucose and other carbohydrates are absorbed from the digestive tract into the blood. Increase in blood sugar stimulates release of a hormone called insulin from the pancreas. Insulin stimulates the transport of glucose into cells, where it can be used to generate energy if required or stored as glycogen, and therefore lowers blood glucose. As blood glucose falls, secretion of insulin is lowered until blood glucose levels are within normal limits. In insulin diabetes, clients cannot produce sufficient insulin and blood glucose remains high because cells cannot transport glucose across their cell membranes and therefore cannot generate energy. Eventually the client will succumb to a diabetic coma. If an insulin-dependent diabetic should take too much insulin, then blood glucose is lowered precipitously and there is not enough glucose to supply the brain; the client will fall into an insulin coma.

It is important to remember that negative feedback loops use two mechanisms to monitor function. Sometimes the absolute level of a particular substance or a particular measure in a given body fluid is important, but often the rate of change is measured rather than the absolute level. If the rate of change is too low or too high, the negative feedback loop will be activated to correct the rate of change to acceptable levels. This is rather like watching a pan of milk coming to the boil. We do not wait until the milk froths up and actually boils over to remove it from the heat, but monitor the rate at which bubbles form and froth begins to accumulate and act before danger levels are reached.

Chapter 3

The locomotor system

The next five chapters introduce the systems of the body pertinent to speech and language therapy. Each system is briefly described so that students without any biological background can appreciate the structure and function of each system, and so that students with some biological knowledge can obtain an overview and revise the salient features. The locomotor system interrelates to all other systems and regions, and detailed description of individual muscles and bones is placed in context in later chapters. The description of the endocrine and cardiovascular systems offered here should provide a sufficient working knowledge for clinical practice but certain points of clinical relevance are emphasized in context in other sections. A detailed understanding of the nervous and respiratory systems is fundamental to clinical practice and these topics are described comprehensively in Chapters 8 to 13 and 14 and 15 respectively.

The **locomotor system** comprises the bones of the skeleton, the joints between the bones, the muscles which move the joints, and the tissues connecting these structures. Synovial joints between bones are extremely mobile whereas other joints, typified by the sutures joining the bones of the skull, are designed for stability and allow little or no movement. Muscles are arranged to produce movement of bones at synovial joints in permitted directions and lie at variable distances from the joint to give a variety of leverages. These various components enable the body to move in its environment or parts of the body to move in relation to each other. The bones and their associated muscles also protect other bodily components and systems, including the central nervous system, the respiratory system, the heart and parts of the gastrointestinal and urinogenital systems.

The **axial skeleton** (Figure 3.1) consists of the skull and the **vertebral column** formed from the vertebrae as a flexible axis to which the **thoracic cage**, consisting of ribs and sternum, is attached. The appendicular skeleton comprises the limb bones attached through the shoulder and pelvic girdles to the axial skeleton.

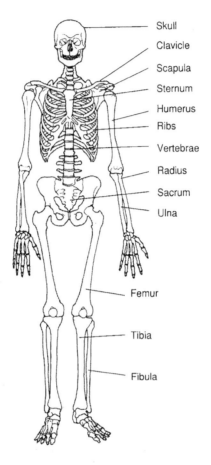

Skull
Clavicle
Scapula
Sternum
Humerus
Ribs
Vertebrae
Radius
Sacrum
Ulna
Femur
Tibia
Fibula

Figure 3.1 The skeleton.

The **skull** houses and protects the brain and special senses, and forms the entrance to the respiratory and gastrointestinal tract. It consists of a great number of bones united to form the **cranium** and the separate **mandible**. Functionally, the cranium can be subdivided into the **neuro-cranium**, enclosing the brain, the **facial skeleton** or **viscerocranium**, surrounding the respiratory and gastrointestinal tracts, and the **basicranium** (chondrocranium), linking the other two parts. With the mandible, the facial skeleton forms the masticatory apparatus at the entrance to the gastrointestinal tract.

The bones of the thoracic cage are described in Chapter 14 and the bones of the skull are considered in the appropriate context in Chapters 8, and 17 to 21.

Connective tissue

The locomotor system is composed of **connective tissue**, principally bone, cartilage and muscle. Connective tissue binds and packs the majority of the cells and tissues of the body and thus determines and maintains their form. Connective tissues have three components: cells, extracellular matrix and proteinaceous fibres embedded in the matrix. The extracellular matrix and fibres are formed by the cells. Connective tissues vary from other basic tissues in that they function principally through their **extracellular** rather than their cellular components: the extracellular components form the greater proportion of this tissue.

The **extracellular matrix** fills the spaces between connective tissue cells and fibres. Various components of the extracellular matrix are hydrophilic: they attract large amounts of water and form gels which make the extracellular matrix resistant to compression forces as well as serving as a medium through which tissue fluid diffuses to keep alive cells distant from blood vessels.

Distributed within the extracellular matrices of connective tissues are two main types of fibre – collagen and elastic fibres. **Collagen fibres** are found in all connective tissues in varying amounts. They have a high tensile strength and are inelastic. **Elastic fibres** are present in many connective tissues and are capable of stretching up to one and a half times their length and returning to their original lengths.

The cells of connective tissue can be divided into synthetic cells (**fibroblasts**), which produce the extracellular matrix and fibres, and defence cells, which participate in reactions to tissue damage and infection. **Adipocytes** (fat cells) are components of many connective tissues where fat is stored; for example, subcutaneous tissue under the skin contains many fat cells which also function as a thermal insulation layer. **Macrophages** are defence cells that can move about within connective tissue by amoeboid movement and, by a process known as phagocytosis, engulf foreign materials entering the body such as carbon particles inhaled into the lungs. They also converge on sites of infection where they phagocytose and destroy bacteria and other micro-organisms and also remove damaged body cells. White blood cells or **leucocytes** are present in small numbers in connective tissues in normal circumstances but appear in large numbers in infected or inflamed connective tissue.

Connective tissue with relatively few fibres is found in practically every site in the body, and supports and packs all organ systems. Connective tissue containing a preponderance of fibres is found in sites where tensional forces are exerted, for example, in tendons where muscles are attached to bones and in ligaments which strengthen and support joints. Where mechanical support is essential, the physical consistency of the extracellular matrix in connective tissue is altered to make it more rigid. Such specialized connective tissues are cartilage and bone.

Cartilage

Cartilage consists of cells embedded in a large volume of extracellular matrix which has additional components forming it into a solid gel (Figure 3.2). Cartilage is not as rigid or strong as bone but is more resilient and elastic. **Hyaline cartilage** has a blue-white glass-like appearance and is widely distributed. Hyaline cartilage covers the bones in most joints providing a low friction surface (see below), and forms extensions to some bones such as the ribs to confer a degree of extra flexibility such as that required during respiration. Cartilage also forms the major part of the skeleton of the larynx although this is strictly not part of the locomotor system but a modified part of the respiratory system. The respiratory tract is reinforced by cartilage throughout most of its length to prevent tubes collapsing under negative pressure and the laryngeal cartilages function in this way. However, the laryngeal cartilages differ from cartilage elsewhere in the respiratory tract, in that they articulate with each other through synovial joints which allows them to move relative to each other during phonation and articulation of speech.

    Elastic cartilage, a variant of hyaline cartilage with a high content of elastin fibres in the extracellular matrix, is found in areas where flexibility is a prime requirement such as in the external ears and some of the smaller cartilages in the larynx. **Fibrocartilage** contains a large amount of collagen fibres which gives it added strength.

    Cartilage also has the important property of being able to grow interstitially or throughout its mass. For this reason, cartilage is particularly abundant in the growing skeleton.

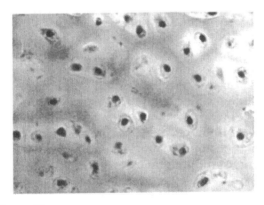

Figure 3.2 Hyaline cartilage.

Bone

Bone forms the majority of the human skeleton (Figure 3.3). The extracellular matrix of bone comprises two main components – collagen fibres and inorganic crystals formed from hydrated calcium phosphate. The collagen gives high strength and resilience to bone; removal of the collagen in various diseases of bone makes bone brittle and liable to fracture. Great rigidity and hardness is produced by **calcification**, the name given to the process of incorporation of crystalline inorganic salts into extracellular matrix. The inorganic components account for about 50% of the weight of bone. It is the combination of fibres and inorganic crystals which give bone its unique properties. Three cell types are associated with bone: **osteocytes** lie within the substance of the bone and maintain it; **osteoblasts** are bone-forming cells; and **osteoclasts** reabsorb bone. Unlike cartilage, bone can only grow by appositional growth on the

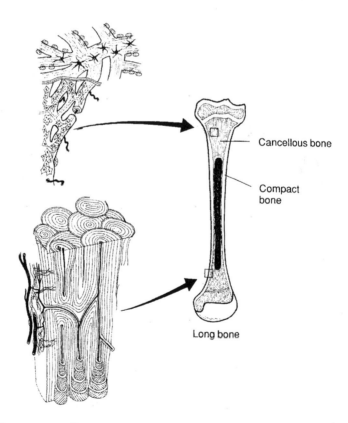

Cancellous bone

Compact bone

Long bone

Figure 3.3 The structure of bone.

ends or outer surfaces. Bone thus needs cells to form it but also cells that can remove bone so that the overall proportions of bones are preserved as they develop.

Bone is formed in two ways during development. It can be formed by osteoblasts directly laying down bone in connective tissue by a process called **intramembranous ossification**. Alternatively, bone may be formed by **endochondral ossification**: a cartilage replica of the bone is formed first and is gradually replaced by bone as the cartilage grows interstitially. The majority of bones in the skeleton are formed by endochondral ossification. Only the bones of the cranium, the facial skeleton and the clavicle are formed by intramembranous ossification.

When a bone is examined with the naked eye, its outer aspect appears smooth and dense. If a bone is split to reveal the internal aspects, the outer layer is made up of dense **compact bone** whereas the inside consists of a network of small spicules of **cancellous** (spongy) **bone** arranged along the lines of stress put upon an individual bone (Figure 3.3). This arrangement allows maximum strength for minimum weight. In living bones, the spaces between the spicules is filled with **bone marrow**. Living bone is not the dry brittle tissue which the study of anatomical skeletons suggests. It is an extremely dynamic living tissue, designed to provide maximum strength for minimum weight and is constantly changing to meet altered stresses and loading. Osteoblasts and osteoclasts add and remove cancellous bone thus remodelling the internal weight-bearing part of bone to meet changing functional demands.

Examination of individual bones can reveal a great deal about their function (Figure 3.4). In places where muscles, tendons or ligaments are attached to bone, the surface is either particularly rough or the surface is elevated. Linear elevations are usually called lines or ridges, sharp elevations are **processes** or spines and rounded elevations are tubercles. Sometimes there is a hollow where muscles attach, called a fossa or fovea. Some parts of the bone appear smoother than others: these are **articular facets** where joints are formed as bones **articulate** with each other. Where bone forms alongside other structures, these may make a groove in the bone. A **foramen** is a hole in bone through which blood vessels or nerves pass.

Muscle

Muscle is a connective tissue specialized for contraction. Individual muscle cells are bound together by connective tissue into distinct muscles, of which three structurally and functionally different types can be found in the body (Figure 3.5).

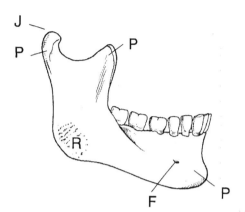

Figure 3.4 The mandible. Processes (P) and roughened areas (R) are for muscle attachment. Bone is smooth where a joint is formed (J). A foramen for transmission of nerves or blood vessels (F) is also visible.

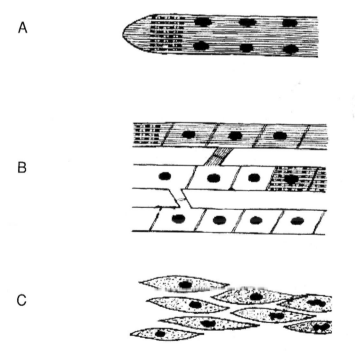

Figure 3.5 (A) Striated muscle. (B) Cardiac muscle. (C) Smooth muscle.

Striated (skeletal or **voluntary muscle**) is part of the locomotor system and produces body movements through interactions with the bones and joints. Striated muscle consists of highly elongated cells packed with fibrous proteins. The protein filaments are arranged in a regular pattern which produces a series of microscopically visible striations which lie perpendicular to the long axis of each cell. This type of muscle is capable of rapid forceful contraction and is under voluntary control.

Cardiac muscle is also striated and consists of elongated branched cells which meet branches of adjacent cells end to end at specialized zones of contact: these contact areas allow inorganic ions to pass from one cell to another during contraction so that muscle contraction initiated at one point can spread across the whole extent of the muscle (see Chapter 4). Cardiac muscle is only found in the heart and makes regular rhythmic contraction under autonomic control.

Smooth muscle consists of short contractile cells but the contractile filaments are not arranged in strict register and hence do not show striations. Smooth muscle is capable of a slow regular contraction, which can often be sustained for prolonged periods and is under autonomic control (see Chapter 12).

Striated muscle

The banded appearance of voluntary and cardiac muscle is produced by the regular arrangement of fibrous proteins within the cytoplasm of individual muscle cells in repetitive units. Each unit consists of a vertically stacked arrangement of proteins made up of actin and myosin (Figure 3.6). The thick filaments consist of **myosin** aligned in parallel rows

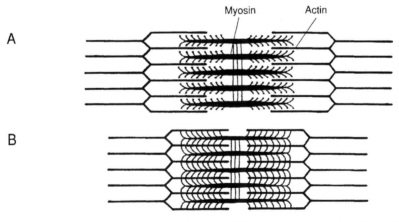

Figure 3.6 A diagrammatic representation of the structure of striated muscle: (A) relaxed, (B) contracted.

occupying the central region of each unit. The thin **actin** filaments lie between and parallel to the thick filaments and are attached to the boundary between adjacent units.

Myosin is a long, thin rod-like molecule. At one end is a globular projection, the head, with a specific binding site for ATP. Where thin and thick filaments overlap, a number of cross links, called cross bridges, form between the head end of the myosin molecule and parts of the actin filament. Contraction is produced by a **sliding filament mechanism**, in which there is a progressive overlap between thick and thin filaments. In resting muscle, ATP is bound to the myosin head region. Myosin cannot bind to the actin because molecular complexes obscure the myosin binding site on the actin filament. Following nervous stimulation of the muscle, calcium ions are released from intracellular stores which bind to this molecular complex and alter its spatial configuration to expose the myosin binding site on the actin filaments. The myosin head region breaks down ATP to ADP (see Chapter 2) at the same time, thus releasing energy which bends the myosin head and pulls the actin over the myosin filament. ATP and phosphate molecules detach from the myosin leaving it free to bind a new molecule. If the myosin head binds a new ATP molecule, the binding site is disrupted and the myosin head is prepared for attachment to another binding site further along the actin filament.

During a single muscular contraction, the making and breaking of actin–myosin binding numbers hundreds. However, because the formation of cross bridges occurs asynchronously, a continuous pull is maintained between the filaments. Contraction will continue until calcium ions are removed, when the myosin binding sites on the actin filament are once again obscured by molecular complexes. During contraction the length of each muscle unit is shortened as the actin filaments are pulled along the myosin heads, but the filaments retain their original length.

The nerve impulse which stimulates contraction of a muscle cell is conveyed by motor nerves (see Chapter 6) which terminate on muscle cells in a special type of junction known as the **motor end plate**. When a nerve impulse reaches the motor end plate, a neurotransmitter, **acetylcholine**, is released from the end of the nerve into the cleft between the nerve ending and the muscle fibre, where it binds to receptors on the muscle fibre. This opens small sodium channels in the muscle cell membrane. The influx of sodium ions results in a change in the membrane potential from negative to positive known as **depolarization**. Depolarization spreads from the end plate along the rest of the cell membrane but also penetrates deep into the muscle fibre and releases stored intracellular calcium ions which then initiate the contractile cycle described above. **Acetylcholinesterase** enzymes are present in the synaptic cleft which break down acetylcholine, thus preventing prolonged contraction.

Myasthenia gravis is a disease in which the body produces antibodies against its own acetylcholine receptors in neuromuscular junctions. This means that activity at neuromuscular junctions is reduced and the muscles feel 'heavy'. Although there is generalized muscular weakness and fatigue, it affects the muscles of the eye and eyelid, face and pharynx producing drooping eyelids, double vision, dysarthria and dysphagia. It can be relieved to some extent by administration of drugs which block the action of acetyl cholinesterase thus prolonging the action potential at the neuromuscular junction. Myasthenia gravis is an example of an **autoimmune disease** in which the immune system attacks components of its own body instead of foreign material (see Chapter 4).

Muscle actions

The majority of skeletal muscles are attached to bones, but some may attach to skin or to other muscles, often their opposite number from the other side of the body. The line of pull of a muscle between its attachments indicates which joints will be moved and in which direction. The arrangement of fibres and fibre bundles in the muscle also indicate something of the way it functions. Long, continuous fibres running the length of the muscle indicate that a great range of contraction is possible: shorter, oblique fibres attenuate range. Range of contraction is proportional to length of fibres, and muscles can contract to something like half their resting length if required. The strength of contraction is determined by the number of fibres contracting. Essentially, the force is proportional to the cross-sectional area of the muscle: the thicker the muscle, the more powerful it is. In many muscles, fibres do not run straight from one attachment to the other but run obliquely across the muscle to insert into intermediate tendons within the muscle. This increases the number of fibres, and hence power, at the expense of range of contraction. Force generated is maximal at the resting length of the muscle and decreases as length decreases.

Muscles differ in their chemical structure. Some operate using oxidative phosphorylation, while others use anaerobic glycolysis and can continue to contract even when an oxygen deficiency builds up. Muscles using oxygen are more resistant to fatigue and are capable of sustained contraction, whereas muscles using anaerobic glycolysis exert short, sharp actions, using up their metabolic reserves quickly. In many cases, of two muscles that apparently produce the same action, one is slow and the other fast, being used for postural maintenance and movement respectively.

The precise degree and force of contraction is modulated by **motor units**, which are the number of fibres in the muscle innervated by a single nerve fibre. If the ratio is low, the control is more precise than if the ratio is high. The laryngeal muscles have motor unit ratios of one nerve to between 6 and 12 muscle fibres, enabling minute regulation of movement. In contrast, large postural muscles in the shoulder or hip may have ratios of 1 nerve to 2000 muscle fibres.

About 60% of the nerves entering a muscle are motor nerves to produce muscle contraction and the other 40% are sensory nerves carrying information from the muscle. This may seem surprising at first until it is realized that, to perform accurate movement, sensory information on range, rate and force of contraction and position of muscles is essential. This information is gleaned from several sources, including sensory receptors in the muscle attachments and connective tissue surrounding the muscles, which convey information on stretch of muscle, and sensory receptors in the capsule and ligaments of joints, which provide information on joint position. Another mechanism is the **intrafusal fibre system**, which comprises atypical muscle fibres sparsely scattered through muscle. They have a motor supply distinct from the supply to the normal (extrafusal) fibres as well as a sensory supply and may play a part in comparing any actual movement achieved with what was intended. Sensory information of both types is known as **proprioception** and gives positional sense of bodily components.

Intrafusal fibres comprise a bundle of small specialized muscle cells surrounded by the larger extrafusal fibres. Each intrafusal fibre receives both motor and sensory nerves. Sensory nerves are attached to the central portion of each intrafusal fibre and the motor nerves innervate the contractile portions at each end of the fibre. The motor nerves supplying muscle spindles are called **gamma motorneurons** and arise from a group of motorneuron cell bodies in the spinal cord (see Chapter 6) separate from those from which the **alpha motorneurons** to the extrafusal fibres originate. The sensory nerves from muscle spindles are active all the time sending out a steady stream of impulses to the central nervous system. If the central portion of the intrafusal fibre is stretched, the sensory neurons increase the frequency of impulses they transmit. If the central portion is compressed, the frequency decreases. Sensory nerves synapse on to the alpha motorneurons controlling the extrafusal fibres but also send the information to the brain providing information about the state of each muscle. When a muscle spindle is stretched, the extrafusal fibres contract to increase muscle tone; this helps prevent damage to the muscle due to overstretching. Conversely when the spindle is compressed, the extrafusal fibres relax to decrease muscle tone and reduce the resistance to movement.

The brain can change the sensitivity of muscle spindles by stimulating contraction in the outer parts of the intrafusal fibres. This is important for voluntary movement which will alter the muscle length. As a muscle contracts, the intrafusal fibre thresholds are continuously reset so that any sudden change in muscle load can be detected and muscular contraction and tone can be adjusted to compensate. A good example of this compensation is during speech. As we breathe out to speak, the resistance in the airway is constantly changing as the larynx is closed for phonation (see Chapter 17) or other articulators are closed during articulation. If the muscle spindles in the respiratory muscles were not adjusted, then damage to the delicate lung tissue could ensue by increases in pressure as we try to breathe out against resistance.

So far the impression may have been given that contraction occurs uniformly throughout a muscle and that muscles act singly. Both ideas are categorically wrong. Contraction in a muscle is the sum of numerous rapid twitches of a motor unit interspersed by relaxations. Each twitch lasts just a few milliseconds, the result being a sort of oscillation. By recruitment of individual motor units at different times, the whole is smoothed into what is perceived as a steady contraction. When a muscle contracts the tendency is to shorten the length of each unit and, hence, the muscle moves its attachments closer (**isotonic contraction**). However, muscles can exert force without causing movement (**isometric contraction**).

Muscles rarely act alone. Movements are usually extremely complex, involving successive movement at different joints. Muscles act in an ordered pattern to produce group activity, although the obvious movement produced by a single muscle is often used to name the muscle. The brain controls muscles in terms of the compound movement rather than its individual components. In a complex movement, muscles may assume many roles in turn. The muscles used to produce an obvious movement are **prime movers**, and those which produce the opposite effect are **antagonists**. When the opposite movement is made, antagonists will be the prime movers and vice versa. Both may act together at certain times to produce **fixation** or immobilization of a joint in a specific position. Sometimes one movement will produce unwanted movement elsewhere; this is eliminated by **synergistic** muscles fixing the joint in question.

Joints

The other essential components in the locomotor system are joints, which allow movement of one bone relative to another. The term **joint** is very imprecise, meaning only a structure by which bones fit together. In many places, bones fit together not to move, but to provide a continuum of bones, for example in the skull, to form a protective shield. Essentially, joints are classified as **synovial joints**, which are freely mobile and what the layman would understand as a joint, or non-synovial joints where either slight movement occurs as a result of deformation of the soft tissue intervening between the bones or no movement occurs at all.

Synovial joints

Synovial joints are formed where two or more bones or cartilages come into contact. Although the bones are joined indirectly by various accessory structures, an apparent space separates the articular surfaces of the bones which move over each other (Figure 3.7). These areas are covered by cartilage, which provides a low-friction surface. Articular surfaces are lubricated by **synovial fluid** produced by a **synovial membrane** which lines the non-articular surfaces of the joint. Joints are enclosed by a **capsule** of fibrous tissue attached to each bone forming the joint. The capsule may be strengthened by bands of fibrous tissue known as **ligaments**, although ligaments may not actually fuse with the capsule. In some joints, cartilaginous wedges form **menisci** between the bones and, in one or two examples, the entire joint may be divided by a continuous **disc** of cartilage.

The stability and mobility of a joint is influenced by several factors. If the shape of both joint surfaces conform closely to each other, the joint is stable but if their fit is poor they tend to be very mobile. Usually one property is lost at the expense of the other. The hip joint in which the bones are a close fit is very stable whereas the shoulder joint in which the bones are poorly adapted is very mobile but comparatively unstable and easily dislocated. The range and axes of movement are also limited by the

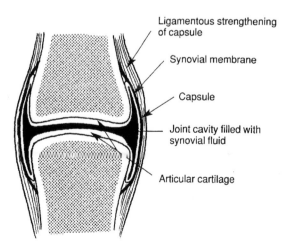

Figure 3.7 A typical synovial joint. The joint cavity is exaggerated for clarity.

degree of congruity and the shape of the articular surfaces. Menisci increase joint congruity by deepening one surface of the joint or by packing space when the joint is in an incongruous position. Ligaments limit the range of movement of a joint or help prevent unwanted movement in certain planes. They are often reinforced or replaced by muscle tendons. These are, however, purely physical restraints on a joint.

Joint capsules are richly innervated with receptors that detect change in joint position and the movements in the joint. Ligaments also have a rich supply of nerves that detect undue stress placed on the joint, and throughout the joint there are nerves that signal pain. Knowledge of joint position and movement is augmented by information from muscles acting on the joint. Sensory information (**proprioception**) received from these sources is extremely important in joint function. Joint innervation also has an important protective role. If a joint is overloaded or moved in an abnormal direction, proprioceptive information from the capsule and the disc will inform the relevant areas of the brain, which will formulate a response to prevent the overload by, for example, correcting balance. If this fails to prevent the strain, pain receptors will be activated as a more dramatic warning signal. If this is not heeded, only then do the mechanical constraints offered by ligaments being fully stretched come into play. Even these are unsuccessful in many cases and the joint will be sprained or dislocated.

Non-synovial joints

In these types of joint, the bones are connected by intervening soft tissue which may be fibrocartilage or fibrous tissue. The most obvious example of a cartilaginous joint is the joint between adjacent vertebrae where an intervertebral disc joins the two bones (Figure 14.4). The middle of the intervertebral disc is a thick fluid. The range of movement at any one intervertebral joint is quite small, but when this is summated over several joints, the cumulative effect is considerable movement. This is how we can touch our toes while keeping our legs straight.

Non-mobile joints in which the bones are united by fibrous tissue are exemplified by **sutures** between the bones of the neurocranium and the viscerocranium (Figure 8.2). In the mature skull, the bones forming the suture interdigitate with each other to form a rigid joint. However, the sutures in the neonatal skull are flat and the connective tissue is looser allowing bones to override slightly during childbirth. The sutures begin to interdigitate towards the end of the first year and are generally well integrated by the age of seven.

CHAPTER 4

The circulatory system

The cardiovascular and lymphoid systems

The main functions of the **circulatory system** are to distribute oxygen and nutrients to the tissues of the body and to collect waste products, including carbon dioxide, from the tissues. This system also transports metabolic products between different organ systems for signalling and control purposes. It comprises the **cardiovascular system**, through which blood circulates, and the **lymphoid system**, which returns excess fluid from the tissues back into the cardiovascular system.

The cardiovascular system consists of blood vessels through which **blood** is continuously circulated by means of a muscular pump, the **heart**. Blood vessels vary considerably in diameter and structure according to their position and function. Those carrying blood from the heart are known as **arteries**, and have thick muscular walls to withstand the pressure generated by the pumping action of the heart.

Very large arteries arising from or close to the heart where the pressure is highest have elastic fibres in their walls which stretch as the vessel receives the large volume of blood from the ventricles when they contract. These arteries smooth out the intermittent flow generated by the heart into a continuous flow required by tissues and organs. Smaller arteries lose their elastic tissue and have a greater proportion of smooth muscle in their walls, which enables their diameter to be regulated by the autonomic nervous system in response to changes in blood pressure, oxygen and carbon dioxide concentrations, and the concentration of other waste products in the tissues. A small degree of muscular contraction reduces their diameter and affects blood flow considerably, and hence the flow of blood to particular regions can be controlled.

Very small muscular arteries, **arterioles**, regulate blood flow through capillary beds thus controlling local blood flow. For example, when it is cold, contraction of arteries and arterioles in the skin directs blood away from the body surface where it would be cooled. Conversely when it is hot, blood is diverted through the skin to increase heat loss. Diffusion of nutrients and waste products to or from the tissues takes place through **capillaries** which have very thin walls only one cell thick.

Veins return blood from capillaries to the heart and are generally thin walled as they are not under so much pressure. Because the venous system is under low pressure, venous return is aided by muscular pumps, especially in the limbs. Contraction of muscles around the veins pumps blood. To prevent backflow of blood when pressure is reduced, most veins have a series of one-way **valves** at intervals along their walls to ensure blood flows only towards the heart.

During exchange of nutrients and waste products between the tissues and blood through capillaries, material will move from one to the other along concentration gradients. Some materials, particularly large protein molecules, cannot re-enter the blood because of osmotic and concentration gradients. There is also movement of water and solutes into the tissues from the capillaries as nutrients are exchanged. The net balance of osmotic and diffusion gradients means that some fluid accumulates in the tissues. If fluids were to remain in the tissues, they would cause water-logging or **oedema** and therefore must be drained away, since the fluid cannot return directly into the capillaries. A complementary network of thin-walled vessels called **lymphatics** returns excess tissue fluid to the cardiovascular system. The lymphoid system also plays a major role in the body's defence system. Very small lymphatic vessels pervade almost all tissues. They join to form large lymphatic vessels which often follow veins and eventually empty their contents into the venous circulation.

Blood

Blood itself consists of cells suspended in a straw-coloured fluid, the **plasma**. The plasma contains inorganic ions and various large molecular weight proteins. These proteins have several functions. Some act as carriers to transport various molecules, including hormones, between tissues, while others act as defence elements to remove harmful foreign material. Other soluble proteins can be converted to insoluble forms to form a framework during blood clotting and tissue repair.

Blood cells are classified into three major groups: **erythrocytes** (red blood cells); **leucocytes** (white blood cells); and **platelets**. Erythrocytes are the most numerous. They are small biconcave discs lacking a nucleus and contain the protein haemoglobin, which binds oxygen and carbon dioxide and carries the two gases around the body. The leucocytes are subdivided into neutrophils, lymphocytes, monocytes, eosinophils and basophils in order of numerical frequency in normal blood. **Neutrophils** are phagocytic cells which can remove harmful bacteria from the blood and sites of infection. **Lymphocytes** all look the same but are divided into several functional types according to the role they play in the bodily defence systems (see below). **Monocytes** are precursors of macrophages: in response to infection, monocytes leave the blood and enter tissues where they act as macrophages (see Chapter 3). **Eosinophils** appear in considerable numbers during parasitic infections of the blood such as malaria and **basophils** are prominent during allergic reactions. **Platelets** are very small anuclear cells which repair blood vessel walls after damage. All blood cells are produced in bone marrow.

The cardiovascular system

The cardiovascular system consists of the heart driving blood through arteries to capillary beds pervading the tissues. After passing through the capillaries, blood returns via increasingly larger veins to the heart (Figure 4.1). The heart is really two pumps lying side by side, conventionally referred to as the right and left sides of the heart. However, this terminology does not reflect accurately their relative anatomical positions. Each pump sends blood through one of the two separate circulations which make up the cardiovascular system. The **systemic circulation** passes oxygenated blood from the left side of the heart through virtually all the organs and tissues and returns deoxygenated blood from these tissues to the right side of the heart. The right side of the heart pumps deoxygenated blood through the **pulmonary circulation**, capillary beds in the lungs where it is oxygenated; oxygenated blood returns back to the left side of the heart.

The heart

The heart lies in the midline in the thorax and consists of four muscular chambers, two on the right side and two on the left side (Figure 4.2). The upper chambers on each side are the **atria**, which are thin-walled as they only have to pump blood into the lower chambers on each side, the thick-walled **ventricles**. Systemic blood returning from the tissues enters the **right atrium** and from there is forced into the **right ventricle** by contraction of the atrium. A one-way valve, the **tricuspid valve**, separates the right atrium and ventricle, preventing backflow as the right ventricle in its turn contracts. Blood is thus forced out of the right ventricle into the **pulmonary trunk**. Backflow into the relaxed ventricle is prevented by another valve, the **pulmonary valve**. The pulmonary trunk divides into the right and left **pulmonary arteries** supplying their respective lungs. The interface between air and blood in the lungs is very thin; oxygen

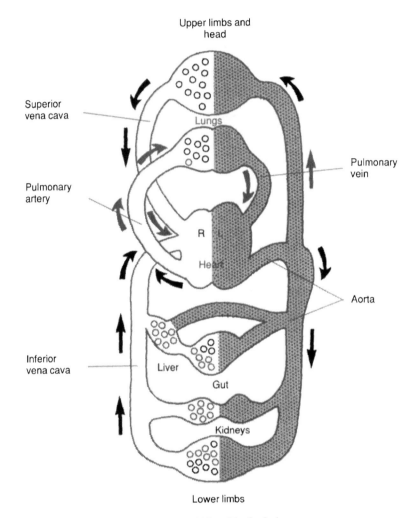

Figure 4.1 The circulation. Oxygenated blood is shaded.

diffuses efficiently across the alveolar walls into the deoxygenated blood and carbon dioxide diffuses the other way from the blood into the lung alveoli and is expired. The blood is then returned, now oxygenated, via pulmonary veins from each lung to the **left atrium**. The left atrium contracts and fills the left ventricle and another one-way valve, the **mitral valve**, prevents backflow from ventricle to atrium. The left ventricle then contracts forcing blood into the great systemic vessel, the **aorta**. As the ventricle relaxes, return of blood to the ventricle is prevented by the **aortic valve**. The two sides of the heart work in concert, the atria contracting simultaneously followed after a short delay by contraction of both ventricles. Control mechanisms ensure that the volume of blood pumped by each side of the heart is equal over time. Coordination of contraction is achieved through a network of specialized cells known collectively as **the conducting system** of the heart.

Major arteries and veins

The aorta has a short vertical part, the **ascending aorta**, before arching backwards as the **aortic arch** to become the **descending thoracic aorta**, which descends through the thorax to pass through the diaphragm into the abdomen. The **right** and **left coronary arteries** arise from the ascending aorta and supply the heart itself. From the arch of the aorta, large arteries branch off to supply each arm and the head and neck. The **brachiocephalic trunk** divides into the **right subclavian artery**

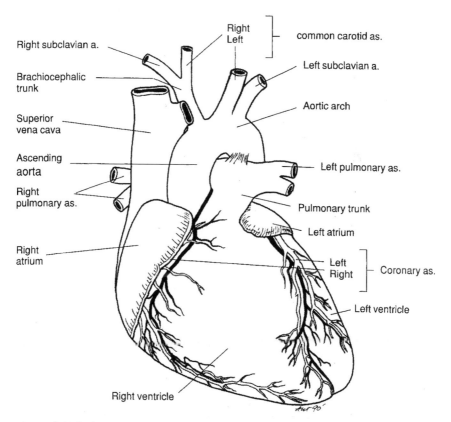

Figure 4.2 The heart and major arteries.

supplying the right arm and the **right common carotid artery** supplying the head and neck (see Figure 18.1). The **left common carotid** and **left subclavian arteries** arise independently from the aortic arch. The common carotid artery on each side divides high in the neck into an **internal carotid artery**, supplying most of the brain, and an **external carotid artery** supplying most of the other structures of the head and many in the neck. Each subclavian artery has important branches along its course; the **vertebral arteries** pass through the transverse foramina in the transverse processes of the cervical vertebrae to supply the brain, and the **thyrocervical trunks** supply the thyroid gland and some other structures of the neck including the larynx.

As it passes down through the thorax, the descending thoracic aorta gives off several paired **intercostal arteries** which supply the intercostal muscles and overlaying skin of the thoracic wall. It pierces the diaphragm to enter the abdomen as the abdominal aorta which gives off several branches to supply the abdominal organs including the kidneys. The abdominal aorta terminates by dividing into the two common iliac arteries which supply the pelvic organs before entering the lower limbs as the **femoral arteries**.

Veins draining different areas and tissues lie at two levels. **Superficial veins** drain the skin and superficial tissues and pursue an independent and highly variable course until they enter **deep veins**. It is very rare that the veins, usually clearly visible on the back of your hands actually have the same branching pattern in each hand. **Deep veins** generally follow the same course as the corresponding arteries and often have the same name. However, the veins draining the head, neck and brain do not always have the same name nor follow exactly the same course as the arteries (see Figure 18.2). These veins unite to form the **internal jugular veins**, which join with the **subclavian veins** to form the **superior vena cava** (**SVC**). This large venous channel opens into the right atrium of the heart (Figure 4.2). The veins of the lower limb and pelvis unite to form the **inferior vena cava** (**IVC**), which ascends through the abdomen before piercing the diaphragm and entering the right atrium almost immediately.

Functional aspects of the circulation

Most capillary beds have more than one artery feeding them to maintain the blood supply if one artery is damaged; this arrangement is known as an **anastomosis** (Figure 4.3). Very often the anastomosis consists of small diameter vessels and blood flow through them is minimal. It is only when one artery is occluded that blood flows in significant amounts through the connecting vessels. Following occlusion, it takes some time for the flow of blood through an anastomotic route to reach a sufficient volume for efficient tissue oxygenation. This is of little consequence if tissue function can be minimized, but is very serious if not: for instance, a leg can be rested but the heart cannot. The consequences are dependent upon the time the tissue can remain anoxic without incurring irreversible damage. For the heart, it is about fifteen minutes, but for the brain, only about three minutes. In the brain and retina of the eye there is no anastomotic circulation: each artery feeds its own capillary bed and is known as an **end artery** (Figure 4.3). In this case, if the artery is occluded there is no alternative supply route, thus the tissue will be deprived of blood and will die.

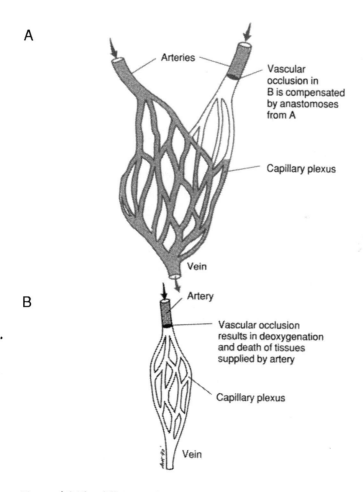

Figure 4.3 The differences between an anastomotic supply to a capillary bed (A) and an end artery supply to a capillary bed (B).

The heart beats at a rate of about 70 beats per minute, the **heart rate**, and the volume of blood, the **stroke volume**, ejected from the ventricles each beat is about 70 mls. **Cardiac output** is the amount of blood pumped by each ventricle in a minute and is given by heart rate × stroke volume. The heart rate and stroke volume and hence cardiac output can be adjusted to meet increased or decreased functional demands to maintain adequate perfusion of the tissues and organs. Stroke volume can double and heart rate can increase by two and half times under extreme circumstances.

The stroke volume depends upon heart rate because this determines how much time each chamber has to fill with blood: the faster the heart rate, the shorter time there is available to fill the chamber. This apparently simple relationship is, however, complicated by several factors. As a general principle, muscle acts optimally when the muscle length is long: the fibres can contract more forcefully and therefore eject more blood in the case of cardiac muscle. The effectiveness of heart contraction depends also on the peripheral resistance, which is determined by the state of the blood vessels through which the blood will be pumped: this is **peripheral resistance**. Peripheral resistance will be high if the blood vessels are constricted as a small change in vessel diameter has a marked effect in resistance. Heart rate can only increase a certain amount to match blood and oxygen demands before it becomes inefficient because the filling time decreases, at which point stroke volume also decreases.

Blood pressure, the pressure gradient driving blood through the circulation, is highest after ventricular contraction (ventricular **systole**) and lowest at the end of ventricular **diastole** when the ventricle is relaxed. Both are measured when blood pressure is recorded, and blood pressure is expressed as systolic pressure/diastolic pressure. A normal systolic blood pressure should be about 120 mmHg and diastolic pressure about 80 mmHg. This is expressed as 120/80.

The main regulator of heart rate is the autonomic nervous system which innervates the heart and blood vessels as well as most other tissues and organs (see Chapters 6 and 12). Sympathetic stimulation of the heart increases heart rate but also the amount and force of contraction, thus altering stroke volume. Parasympathetic stimulation of the heart has the opposite effects. The heart is also regulated by the action of certain hormones, including adrenalin (see Chapter 7), and intrinsic factors briefly mentioned above are also important.

The output from the autonomic nervous system is regulated by **cardiac centres** in the medulla oblongata of the brain. The input to the cardiac centres comes from **baroreceptors** which monitor blood pressure, and **chemoreceptors** which monitor blood chemistry, principally the levels of

CO_2 and O_2 and the blood pH. Baroreceptors are found in the **carotid sinuses**, dilatations of the common carotid arteries at their bifurcation into the external and internal carotid arteries. Chemoreceptors are located in the aorta just above the aortic valve and the carotid sinuses. As the cardiac centres receive information on blood pressure and chemistry, they regulate heart rate and cardiac output to maintain adequate circulation. A decrease in blood pressure or blood oxygen levels or a rise in blood carbon dioxide will stimulate the heart to try to increase the amount of blood and oxygen reaching the tissues or to clear the carbon dioxide by increasing blood flow through the lungs. In the case of oxygen deficiency, this effort will be useless unless the blood is carrying enough oxygen. To ensure this, information from baroreceptors and chemoreceptors is also transmitted to the respiratory centres in the brainstem which adjust respiratory rate to correct oxygen deficiencies (see Chapter 15).

The adjustment of the various factors determining output from the heart and blood flow is designed, above all, to maintain adequate levels of blood flow through and oxygenation of organs and tissues, and is another example of a homeostatic mechanism.

Clinical considerations

A common disease of the cardiovascular system is **hypertension**, a permanent abnormal high blood pressure. Blood pressure is usually considered abnormal if blood pressure is greater than 150/90. Treatment consists of giving drugs that dilate arteries and arterioles, thus reducing peripheral resistance and lowering blood pressure. High blood pressure in itself is not necessarily life threatening unless it is the result of other diseases. Sustained high blood pressure eventually causes hypertrophy of cardiac muscle, thickening of arterial walls to resist the pressure, and damage to the delicate filtration mechanisms in the kidneys, caused by the high pressure. Consequently, high blood pressure is a risk factor for cardiovascular disease. For example, the heart muscle may hypertrophy to a degree where the size of the muscle outstrips the coronary blood supply, thus predisposing to ischaemic heart disease (heart attack). Increased blood pressure also puts considerable strain on blood vessel walls which increase the risk of aneurysm (see below) and stroke (cerebrovascular accident).

Another common disease of blood vessels is **atherosclerosis**, especially in developed societies of the Western hemisphere. Changes occur in the walls of blood vessels causing them to thicken until they become partially or completely blocked. This is particularly dangerous when it occurs in the coronary vessels supplying cardiac muscle, as cessation of blood flow results in a heart attack. Reduction of blood supply preceding the heart attack is often accompanied by an agonizing vice-like pain (**angina**) across the chest.

Veins can become blocked by blood clots (**thrombi**). They are potentially very dangerous if they form in deep veins as portions of the clot may be detached and then come to lodge in another vessel as they are circulated through the cardiovascular system. If this happens in the lungs, heart or brain, it can be life-threatening. **Deep venous thrombosis** often occurs after long immobilization of the limbs, for example, during a long air flight or during postoperative immobilization. This is why passengers are encouraged to move about the aircraft cabin or perform exercises to stimulate the circulation, and why patients are encouraged to get out of bed as soon after an operation commensurate with their medical condition. Anticoagulant drugs are administered to minimize clot formation if such conditions occur.

Aneurysms are dilatations and thinning of artery walls. There are various reasons why this occurs but it can follow degeneration of layers of arterial walls in people with hypertension. Blood flow in the tiers between layers exacerbates the rip and causes the wall to bulge and dilate. The arterial wall is under great stress at the site of aneurysm and can suddenly burst often with fatal consequences. However, aneurysms can often be successfully surgically treated if detected.

The lymphoid system

The lymphoid system consists of a series of thin-walled vessels which begin within the tissues and carry excess fluid (**lymph**) back into the veins of the circulatory system. As well as returning excess tissue fluid into the cardiovascular system, the lymphoid system constitutes the most important defence system of the body, combating infection and removing foreign material. **Lymph nodes** are aggregates of lymphocytes, macrophages and connective tissue present along lymphatic vessels. Bacteria and other material present in lymph are filtered through and processed in these nodes. Any foreign material will stimulate the lymphocytes into a defensive **immune response**.

Lymphocytes respond to the foreign material in two ways. They may produce immunoglobulin proteins (**antibodies**) which bind specifically to foreign material (an **antigen**) and neutralize it by stimulating phagocytosis of the antigen–antibody complex by neutrophils. This is **humoral immunity** and typically occurs in response to bacterial infections. Alternatively, lymphocytes may proliferate and attack the foreign material directly: this occurs if the foreign material is tissue bound. The lymphocytes enter the cardiovascular system and leave capillaries at the appropriate site to destroy the foreign tissue, a response known as **cell-mediated immunity**. When grafted tissue is rejected, cell-mediated immunity is responsible for its destruction.

As well as lymph nodes spaced along the lymphatic vessels, there are other lymphoid organs. Patches of submucous lymphoid tissue are present in the small intestine and the appendix, and in the **tonsils** surrounding the entrance to the pharynx. The **spleen** is a large lymph node actually lying in the cardiovascular system in blood vessels in the abdomen. Many lymphocytes (B lymphocytes) enter the lymphoid organs directly from the bone marrow but some pass through the **thymus** in the thorax where they differentiate into T-lymphocytes before they enter other lymphoid tissues. The two types of lymphocyte play different roles in immune responses.

Generally, chemically inert but potentially physically harmful material, such as dust or carbon particles, is removed from the lymph by phagocytic **macrophages** in the lymph nodes. Macrophages are also widely scattered throughout the body forming a nonspecific defence mechanism. They are actively phagocytic and engulf particles of various sizes and composition, whether organic or inorganic. Macrophages are found in connective tissue in general, in lymphoid tissues, in the lungs and many other sites.

Lymphatic vessels draining skin and superficial tissues tend to follow the course of superficial veins which show considerable anatomical variation. The vessels draining deeper structures follow the course of corresponding arteries and are therefore more consistent in their course. Lymph nodes are relatively constant in position and form groups in specific locations. Superficial lymph nodes are found at junctional regions such as the axilla, groin and upper neck whereas deep nodes are often found at the branching points of major arteries.

The cellular changes in the lymph nodes producing immune responses can usually be detected clinically as enlargement of lymph nodes which become firmer in consistency (**lymphadenopathy**); superficially-placed lymph nodes therefore become palpable. Lymphadenopathy is often the first sign of infection in a particular area drained by those nodes.

The detailed course of individual lymphatic vessels is not clinically important. What is most significant is the area of the body which drains into each group of lymph nodes. The nodes draining each particular region or organ are known as the **regional lymph nodes**. The **lymphatic drainage** of a particular area or organ is described in terms of which regional lymph nodes it drains into.

Regional lymphatic drainage is also clinically important in the spread of cancer because as well as distributing immune cells, it can also distribute tumour cells. Primary malignant tumours usually begin in one organ or tissue but can spread by **metastasis** (see Chapter 2) to form secondary tumours in other areas. Lymphatic vessels are one route by which metastasis may occur and, as a consequence, secondary malignancies are often found in the regional lymph nodes from which further dissemination of malignant cells is also possible. Whenever a primary tumour is detected and treated, the regional lymph nodes into which the primary tumour would drain are also treated by surgical removal, chemotherapy or radiotherapy.

Tumour classification

There are several shorthand schemes for staging the spread of cancer in terms of extent of the primary tumour and the extent of metastasis in regional lymph nodes and distance sites. The scheme presented in Table 4.1 is one in common use.

Inflammation

Inflammation is a fundamental protective reaction of the body to prevent bacteria from proliferating, spreading and killing the host should they enter the body. The inflammatory response also initiates healing in damaged tissues. Although protective, inflammatory responses can also be destructive: loss of homeostatic controls in inflammation enhance tissue damage. Inflammation of a particular organ or tissue is indicated by adding the suffix '**-itis**' to the name. Thus laryngitis is inflammation of the larynx and tonsillitis is inflammation of the tonsils.

Together with loss of function, inflammation produces classical signs and symptoms of **heat**, **redness**, **swelling** and **pain** which are localized to the inflamed area and are produced by functional changes in the vasculature. Generalized symptoms include lassitude, malaise and fever. Heat and redness are produced by dilatation of small blood vessels and locally increased blood flow (**hyperaemia**). Swelling is mainly due to leakage of blood components into the extravascular spaces through increased permeability of blood vessel walls. Pain is due to pressure on nerve endings from swelling and release of factors from injured tissues which act on nerves to cause pain.

Inflammation is classified by the duration of the inflammatory process but is characterized by the type of blood cells which predominate in the inflamed tissue. The duration of **acute inflammation** is usually limited to a few days and neutrophils predominate. The duration of **chronic inflammation** is much longer and lymphocytes predominate.

Acute inflammation has several overlapping stages. Hyperaemia increases blood flow and allows blood cells and plasma to infiltrate the inflamed tissue. The plasma exudate contains antibacterial substances and

Table 4.1 Cancer staging

1. Extent of primary tumour

TX	primary tumour cannot be assessed
T0	no evidence of primary tumour
Tis	carcinoma in situ
T1	tumour 2 cm or less in greatest diameter
T2	tumour more than 2 cm but not more than 4 cm in greatest dimension
T3	tumour more than 4 cm in greatest dimension
T4	tumour invades adjacent structures

2. Absence or presence and extent of regional lymph node metastasis

NX	regional lymph node cannot be assessed
N0	no regional lymph node metastasis
N1	metastasis in a single ipsilateral lymph node, 3 cm or less in dimension
N2	metastasis in a single ipsilateral lymph node, more than 3 cm but not more than 6 cm in greatest dimension, or metastasis in multiple ipsilateral lymph nodes, more than 6 cm in greatest dimension, or metastasis bilaterally or in contralateral lymph nodes, more than 6 cm in greatest dimension
N3	metastasis in a lymph node more than 6 cm in greatest dimension

3. Absence or presence of distant metastasis (clinical and pathological categories)

MX	not assessed
M0	no distant metastasis
M1	distant metastasis present
R	residual tumour
R0	no residual tumour
R1	microscopic residual tumour
R2	macroscopic residual tumour

Thus, a report of a tumour in the tongue may be written in case notes as:
Stage III squamous cell carcinoma on left side of tongue anterior and ventral T2 N2 M0 indicating that the tumour is between 2 and 4 cm in diameter, that there is a large metastasis in the regional lymph node or multiple ipsilateral regional lymph nodes or metastases in contralateral regional lymph nodes but there is no distant metastasis.

antibodies and, as these act, neutrophils phagocytose the dead organisms and release enzymes which may damage host tissue as well as bacteria. The death of neutrophils, bacteria and enzymatic action produces liquefaction and pus formation. In the **demolition** phase, bacteria and tissue debris is removed by macrophages but host tissue is often damaged in the process: this phase proceeds more rapidly if pus drains naturally or is surgically removed. As demolition nears completion, the **resolution phase** begins as dead tissue is replaced by new tissue or scar tissue. Capillaries and fibroblasts differentiate from undifferentiated mesenchymal cells (see Chapter 20) to form **granulation tissue** and the tissue defect is reduced by contraction of newly formed collagen. Fibrous tissue will replace damaged non-renewable tissues such as muscle but regeneration by simple division or from stem cells occurs in renewing tissues.

If the cause of acute inflammation is not successfully removed during the demolition phase, the inflammation becomes chronic and the nature of the cellular infiltrate changes. Lymphocytes destroy cells and stimulate macrophage activity, and plasma cells, derived from lymphocytes in the regional lymph nodes, secrete antibodies from the node into the circulation and locally at the site of infection. Demolition and resolution may occur simultaneously. Full resolution does not occur until the source of infection is removed.

CHAPTER 5

The respiratory system

All cells in the body need a continuous supply of oxygen to carry out their functions. Air is inhaled into the lungs where oxygen diffuses into the blood by the process of **external respiration** and is circulated through the cardiovascular system. Inhalation and exhalation of air into and out of the lungs is the process of **ventilation**. Gaseous exchange between the blood and tissues in capillary beds by the process of **internal respiration** supplies cells with oxygen. As cells use oxygen to generate energy they produce metabolites which are eventually broken down into carbon dioxide. Dissolved carbon dioxide produces carbonic acid which is toxic if allowed to accumulate. Carbon dioxide dissolved in blood is returned to the lungs where the waste gas comes out of solution and is breathed out.

The respiratory system comprises a **conducting zone**, a system of tubes which conveys gases into and out of the body, and a **respiratory zone**, where gaseous exchange takes place between the air and the blood (Figure 5.1). The mouth and nose, pharynx, larynx, trachea and bronchial tree constitute the conducting portion; gaseous exchange occurs in the **alveolar sacs** within the lungs.

The conducting zone

The conducting zone must remain patent irrespective of the pressure inside it. Patency is maintained by reinforcement of the tubes with cartilage in most areas and bone in the nose. For most of its course, the conducting zone is lined by **respiratory mucosa** covered by pseudostratified ciliated columnar epithelium containing goblet cells (see Chapter 2). The mucus secreted by the goblet cells traps inhaled particles and the mucus is then moved by cilial action to the pharynx where it can be either swallowed or expectorated (spat out).

The first part of the conducting zone is the **nasal cavities**, which warm and humidify the incoming air. The mucosa lining the nasal cavities is very

63

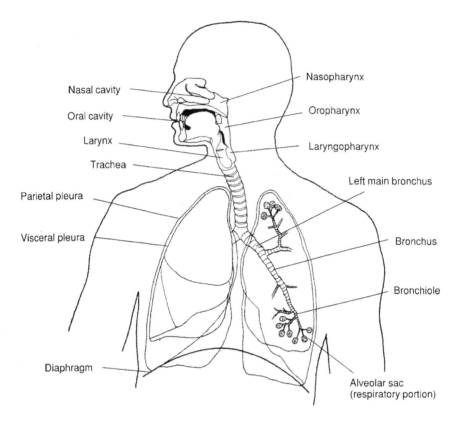

Figure 5.1 The respiratory system.

vascular to promote efficient heat exchange between the blood and the incoming air and also contains a large number of mucous cells and glands which humidify the air. The nasal cavities open on to the face via the nostrils and the area immediately superior to the nostrils is known as the vestibule which contains coarse hairs to trap large particles. The left and right nasal cavities are separated by a thin bony **nasal septum.** They are continuous posteriorly with the nasopharynx. The upper part of each nasal cavity is lined by an area of specialized **olfactory epithelium** for the sense of smell. The area of the lateral walls of each nasal cavity posterior to the vestibule is increased by three downwardly-curving bony structures known as **conchae**, which improve the efficiency of humidification and heat exchange by increasing surface area (Figure 5.2). Each concha overlies a passage running anteroposteriorly known as a **meatus.** Four paired, air-filled cavities within adjacent bones, the **paranasal air sinuses**, open into the nasal cavities. They are the **maxillary, sphenoid, ethmoidal** and **frontal** sinuses and are named after the bones in which they are located. The sinuses are lined by respiratory epithelium and provide a reservoir of mucus out of the direct air stream to maintain humidification when the air is dry and hot. They also add resonance to the voice, although since their shape is fixed, they play no active role in speech production.

The **pharynx** is a muscular tube attached to the base of the skull above and continuous below with the oesophagus. The muscles of the pharynx only make up its posterior and lateral walls; anteriorly, the pharynx is continuous with other cavities or tubes. The pharynx has three portions (Figure 5.1): the **nasopharynx** behind the nasal cavities, the **oropharynx** behind the mouth and the **laryngopharynx** behind and around the laryngeal inlet (see Chapter 16). Air enters the nasopharynx from the nose and passes through the oropharynx into the larynx. Food enters the oropharynx from the mouth and passes through the laryngopharynx into the oesophagus. Thus the digestive and respiratory systems share a common pathway in the oropharynx. Several protective mechanisms exclude food from the nasopharynx and larynx during swallowing: these are described in Chapters 16 and 21.

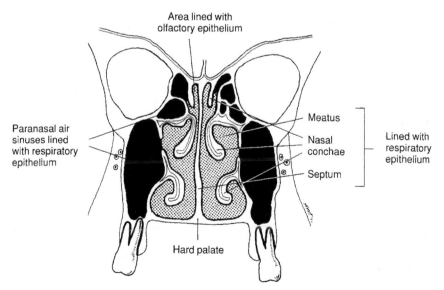

Figure 5.2 A coronal section through the maxillae and orbits showing the nasal cavities and paranasal air sinuses.

The **larynx** consists of several cartilages which articulate with each other by synovial joints and several muscles which move the cartilages. The **vocal folds** are bilateral folds of mucosa overlying muscles within the larynx. The folds function as a sphincter to close the larynx during swallowing, thus protecting the lower airway. However, their position and tension can be minutely regulated, and if the vocal cords are tensed and adducted into the exhaled air stream, they will vibrate producing sound: this is the **phonation** component of speech (see Chapter 17). The conducting zone as far down as the larynx is also known as the **upper respiratory tract**.

The lower respiratory tract commences at the lower border of the larynx at the **trachea** which passes down the neck into the thorax, where it bifurcates into left and right **main bronchi** at the level of the sternal angle (Figure 5.1). Its wall is reinforced by about 20 C-shaped rings of hyaline cartilage which are incomplete posteriorly; these keep the lumen patent and the posterior deficiency allows for dilation of the oesophagus during swallowing. The bronchi are similar in structure to the trachea.

As the main bronchi enter the substance of the lungs, they branch repeatedly and gradually lose their cartilaginous support as they get progressively smaller. Eventually their cartilage is replaced by smooth muscle and they are known as **bronchioles**. Smaller **terminal bronchioles** subdivide into **respiratory bronchioles** which are the transition between the conducting and respiratory portions of the tract.

The respiratory zone

From the respiratory bronchioles, numerous **alveolar ducts** lead into the **alveolar sacs**, which are small air-filled dilatations. It is in this region that gaseous exchange occurs between the air and the blood. The alveoli are lined by thin flattened epithelial cells immediately covering thin walled capillaries. The diffusion barrier in the lung thus comprises two very thin cells separated by a delicate intervening layer of supporting connective tissue. Oxygen passes across this barrier into the blood and carbon dioxide passes out of solution from the blood to the air.

Ventilation

Air is drawn into the lungs by **inspiration**. During inspiration, the lungs are inflated by increasing the volume of the thoracic cavity. This is achieved by actions of the diaphragm and the thoracic muscles. The **diaphragm** is a dome-like sheet of muscle which is attached to the lower ribs and separates the abdominal and thoracic cavities (Figure 5.2). When it contracts, it flattens and descends towards the abdominal cavity increasing the volume and reducing the pressure within the thoracic cavity. The **ribs** articulate posteriorly with the **thoracic vertebrae** and anteriorly with the **sternum** and are also connected to each other by **intercostal muscles**. If the first rib is fixed, contraction of the intercostal muscles pulls the ribs upwards and outwards, increasing the volume of the thoracic cavity and decreasing the pressure. The thoracic cavity is lined by the **parietal pleura** and the lungs are covered by the **visceral pleura** (Figure 5.1); the two pleural layers form a closed cavity which contains a thin layer of **pleural fluid** to lubricate the two layers as they move over each other, but also makes the two layers adhere. Thus as the thoracic wall expands in volume, the parietal pleura move with it and the visceral pleura also follow this movement pulling the lungs with them and thus increasing the lung volume. As the thoracic volume increases during inspiration, the elastic tissue in the lungs and the elasticity of the rib cage is stretched. During quiet **expiration**, the ribs descend to their original position by elastic recoil of the rib cage and the diaphragm relaxes, thus reducing the volume of the thorax. Expiration requires no muscular effort and occurs by **passive elastic recoil**. Each respiratory cycle of one inspiration and one expiration takes about the same time and the inspiratory and expiratory phases are equal.

During exercise or other activities which require an increased oxygen supply to the body, the volume of air entering and leaving the lungs is increased and the rate of respiration also increases considerably. **Accessory muscles of respiration**, muscles not normally used for respiratory movements, may also be brought into operation. During **forced inspiration,** the rib cage is raised more than in quiet inspiration by increased contraction of the intercostal muscles and the diaphragm. Accessory muscles attaching the arms and neck to the thoracic wall may also be used to increase the pull on the ribs, thus expanding the thoracic wall even further. **Forced expiration** involves contraction of the muscles of the anterior abdominal wall which exert pressure on the abdominal organs and thus push the diaphragm upwards; they also pull the rib cage down.

During **speech**, ventilation is modified considerably. The inspiratory phase is more rapid and deeper than that in quiet respiration and expiration no longer occurs by passive elastic recoil alone. The inspiratory muscles are used to counteract elastic recoil so that control of the force of expiration can be achieved. This is important for coordination of breathing with grammatical sense and for controlling loudness and emphasis.

Chapter 6

The nervous system

Imagine you have just sat down with a cup of coffee to do some serious study from this book when your next door neighbour starts to play some music. You may have several reactions. You could find you are tapping your foot to the rhythm without realizing you are doing so. You might be thinking that you know that tune so well and you are ready to sing along after the instrumental introduction as the singer comes in with 'Imagine . . .'. You might think, 'Oh, that's the music that is used in that advert for a certain make of jeans'. Your reaction might be more extreme. The music may be so loud and disturbing that you react by putting your hands over your ears, or get up and start banging on the wall to tell your neighbour to turn it down. Whatever your response, it is the nervous system which is carrying it out. It is receiving a signal that music is being heard from the sensory receptors in the ear and conveying this information to your brain. Your brain will decipher whether the noise is a string quartet or a rock band by detecting overtones and comparing these with your previous experience of different sorts of music. It will search your memory banks to see if you have heard it before. Other information will come into play. 'I wanted to do some study in peace' may trigger emotional responses such as anger which will make your heart beat faster and give you 'butterflies' in your stomach. If the music is loud and annoying, you may have clapped your hands over your ears almost without thinking about it. If your foot started tapping, your muscles will move your limbs and body to the rhythm of the music. Some responses are voluntary – such as putting your hands over your ears – and some involuntary – if the music is too loud, tiny muscles in your ear will contract to prevent damage to your eardrum as a reflex response outside your control.

All these potential scenarios demonstrate that the nervous system is an integrating system. The body receives stimuli from the external and its own internal environment and sends these along nerves connecting the specialized receptors which pick up the information to the central nervous system (your brain and spinal cord). The central nervous system then integrates the information with existing information and formulates appropriate responses. It then generates the signals to execute the response by coordinating the activity of the different body systems.

The nervous system achieves its integrating function by carrying messages as electrical impulses from receptors to the brain and spinal cord, between areas of the brain and from the brain and spinal cord to effector organs which may be muscles, both voluntary and involuntary, or glands. Electrical impulses need to travel considerable distances to effect communication throughout the body. It follows that the structure of neurons is rather different from most other cells so that they can reach long distances, and that they are physiologically specialized to convert various stimuli into electrical form and conduct the electrical impulses along their length.

The nervous system is divided into the **central nervous system (CNS)** and **peripheral nervous system (PNS)**. The central nervous system comprises the **brain** and **spinal cord**. The peripheral nervous system constitutes the connections between the CNS and the peripheral organs and tissues and carries out the integrative functions. The brain is incompletely divided into two **cerebral hemispheres** and the **brainstem**, which consists of the midbrain, pons and medulla oblongata. The medulla oblongata is continuous with the spinal cord and the **cerebellum** is attached to the brainstem posteriorly (see Figure 6.6). The peripheral nervous system comprises paired **cranial** and **spinal nerves**, from the brain and spinal cord respectively, which branch repeatedly to innervate the whole body. The nervous system is made up of billions of nerve cells called **neurons**. Nerve cells are surrounded by supporting cells called **neuroglia**, or more simply glia, which have several nutritive and supportive functions.

The structure of neurons

In most neurons, four parts can be recognized (Figure 6.1). The **cell body**, which is vital for the survival of the neuron, is where synthetic activity occurs and contains the nucleus and the majority of the cellular organelles. A variable number of thin branching **dendrites** arise from the cell body and constitute the main receptive area of the cell; these receive stimuli from other neurons and convey them to the cell body. A single neuron may thus establish contact with hundreds of other neurons. The **axon** is a single, and often very long, process which transmits the impulse either to other nerve cells or to other cell types such as muscles or glandular cells. The axon may branch, particularly in its peripheral part.

Nerve cells vary widely in size and shape according to their location and function in the CNS and PNS. In particular, axons may vary in length from a few thousandths of a millimetre to over a metre. Axons also differ in diameter from 1 to 20 thousandths of a millimetre. The diameter determines the speed of conduction of the nerve impulse: large diameter axons conduct rapidly whereas small diameter axons conduct more slowly (see below). It is axons which form peripheral nerves or tracts within the CNS. The fourth part of a neuron is the **axon terminal** forming the distal end of the axon. Generally, they are in close proximity to the dendrites or cell body of another neuron or adjacent to the target tissue innervated by a neuron. Often, the axon terminates a long way from the neuron itself. The axon terminal is separated from its target neuron or tissue by a narrow gap called the **synaptic cleft**. Communication between two neurons or a neuron and the target tissue is mediated by release of chemicals called neurotransmitters from axon terminals that diffuse across the synaptic cleft to the target (see below).

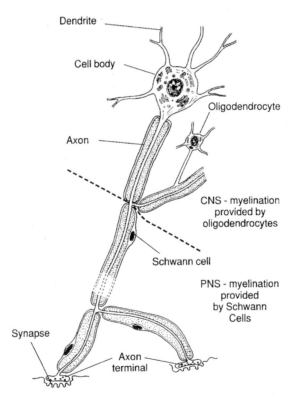

Figure 6.1 A diagram of a motor neuron. Note the differences in glial cells in the areas of the nerve in the central and peripheral nervous systems (shown by the dashed line).

CNS neurons can be classified into three main types. **Projection neurons** have long efferent axons that connect to other neurons at distant sites, usually in another part of the CNS. Within the CNS, neurons whose axons connect areas within the same hemisphere are called **association neurons** whereas those connecting left and right hemispheres are **commissural neurons**. **Interneurons** have short axons communicating with other neurons close by. PNS axons entering a particular region of the CNS from peripheral tissues synapse with interneurons or, in some cases, directly with projection neurons.

Neurons and their processes in both the PNS and the CNS are almost completely covered by **glial cells**; in the CNS there may be ten times as many glial cells as neurons. There are several different types of glia. **Astrocytes** have metabolic and supportive functions which are carried out through many radiating processes extending between neurons to contact the external surface of neurons and blood vessels within the CNS. They are also phagocytic and remove debris after CNS damage. Oligodendrocytes and Schwann cells electrically insulate many axons in the CNS and PNS respectively. Microglia are another type of glial cells and are involved in the response of the nervous system to injury.

One of the most important functions of glial cells is to ensheath neuronal axons to electrically insulate them from adjacent axons. Most large diameter axons have an insulating layer formed by the glial cells to ensure rapid conduction of nerve impulses without loss of charge. This layer is formed from the membrane of glial cells wrapping around the axon several times. The membrane contains a specialized form of lipid called **myelin** and axons enwrapped in a myelin sheath are **myelinated axons** (Figure 6.2). The myelin sheath is not continuous along the entire length of the axon but is interrupted by small gaps where the axonal membrane is uncovered. These bare areas are **nodes of Ranvier** and the length of myelinated axon between two nodes is the internode. In the PNS, the myelinating cells are known as **Schwann** cells; each Schwann cell produces myelin covering one internode of one axon. Some axons may be up to 1 metre in length and will therefore be enwrapped by many Schwann cells. Smaller axons, in the PNS are surrounded by only a single layer of Schwann cell membrane and are known as **unmyelinated** nerves. In contrast to myelinated axons it is usual for many unmyelinated axons to be ensheathed by a single Schwann cell (Figure 6.2). In the CNS, the structure and arrangement of the myelin sheath is similar to that of the PNS, but here **oligodendrocytes** are responsible for myelination. One oligodendrocyte may contribute to the myelin sheath of several different axons. In the CNS, unmyelinated nerves are not ensheathed but lie in direct continuity with and the cellular processes of other nerve cells and neuroglial processes. In both the CNS and PNS, myelinated axons will conduct nerve impulses faster than unmyelinated axons.

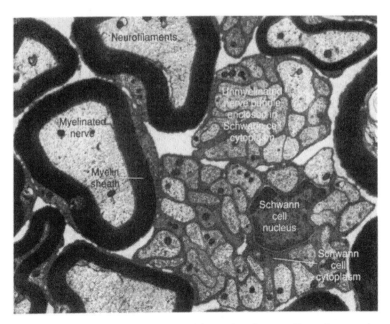

Figure 6.2 An electron micrograph of myelinated and unmyelinated nerves in cross section (courtesy of Dr P. Dockery).

Peripheral nerve axons vary considerably in diameter and degree of myelination and these differences are classified by letter or numerical designation. Motor axons to voluntary muscles and nerves from muscular and tendinous sensory receptors have large fast-conducting myelinated axons. Small myelinated axons are largely sensory nerves from cutaneous and visceral sensory receptors and motor axons to smooth muscles. Very small axons are unmyelinated and slow-conducting and originate from all types of sensory receptors. It was once thought that each type of axon carried a specific cutaneous sensory modality and for large axons this may be true; unmyelinated sensory axons are, however, **polymodal**, responding to a variety of stimuli. The classification of axons and their associated modalities is summarized in Table 6.1.

In peripheral nerves, individual axons with their Schwann cell sheaths are aggregated into small bundles by connective tissue called the **endoneurium** (Figure 6.3). Individual bundles are bound into fascicles by a denser layer of connective tissue called the **perineurium**. The fascicles are bound together to form a nerve by the **epineurium**. The epineurium holds the nerve together and the amount of damage to the epineurium in nerve injuries can have important consequences for the successful repair and regeneration of the nerve or otherwise (see below).

Table 6.1 Peripheral axon classification and function

Fibre type	Myelination	Diameter	Conduction velocity	Function
Aα	Thick	Up to 20 μm	c 80–100 m/s	Motor nerve axons. Proprioceptive and touch afferents.
Aβ	Thick	10–20 μm	c 25 m/s	Aα collaterals to intrafusal fibres.
Aγ	Thick	5–10 μm	c 20 m/s	Motor to intrafusal muscle fibres.
Aδ	Thin	< 5 μm	c 10 m/s	Pain, temperature afferents.
β	Thin	< 5 μm	c 10 m/s	Preganglionic autonomics.
C	None	0.1–2 μm	c 0.5–2 m/s	Polymodal afferents; postganglionic autonomics.

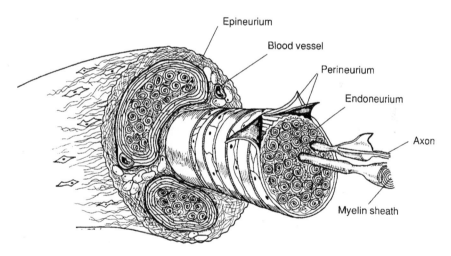

Figure 6.3 The connective tissue sheaths of peripheral nerves.

Synapses

Information is carried from dendrites through the cell body and along the axon of a neuron in the form of an electrical impulse. However, where the axon of one neuron meets the dendrites or cell body of another neuron, there is no direct continuity. The cell membranes of the two neurons in such regions are highly specialized and are separated by a small gap which effectively prevents the spread of electrical activity from one cell to another. This complex is known as a **synapse** (see Figure 6.1), a highly specialized intercellular junction which enables the nerve impulse from one neuron to activate another neuron by release of chemical **neurotransmitters**. Synapses are formed predominantly between the axon terminals of one nerve and the dendrites or the cell body of another but synapses between axons are also found. Transmission at synapses occurs *unidirectionally* across the gap between the closely apposed cell membranes of adjacent nerve processes. The electrical impulse travelling down the axon of one neuron (the **presynaptic cell**) causes the release of a chemical neurotransmitter from the specialized terminal region of the axon. The axonal termination of the presynaptic cell contains many **synaptic vesicles** concentrated adjacent to the presynaptic membrane, which contain the neurotransmitters. These are discharged into the intercellular space, the **synaptic cleft**, where the neurotransmitters interact with receptors on the membrane of the adjacent cell (the **postsynaptic cell**). Here they alter the flow of ions through the cell membrane causing a charge in membrane potential. If this change is large enough, a nerve impulse results (see below).

Electrical activity in neurons

In theory, nerve axons could act as passive wires rather like cables carrying electricity to conduct electrical activity around the nervous system. They could only function in this way over very short distances, however, because axonal membranes have a resistance to electrical flow which would allow current to leak from the axon into extracellular fluid. As the current progressed further along an axon, it would get less and less until it became negligible. Electrical conduction in neurons therefore has to be performed in another way to maintain the current over considerable distances. Neurons have the property, which they share with muscle fibres, of propagating waves of electrical activity, known as **action potentials**, along their length. In neurons, this results in the release of a neurotransmitter from the presynaptic terminal. Nerves possess this ability because of the structure of their plasma membrane and their metabolic activities, both of which contribute to maintaining a potential difference, the **membrane potential**, across the plasma membrane. This potential is maintained by unequal distribution of small inorganic ions inside and outside the cell (Figure 6.4) and, like a battery, provides the energy source to drive action potentials along the axon.

Ions are not free to move in and out of neurons, but have to enter or leave through ion channels specific for each ion. These channels are not

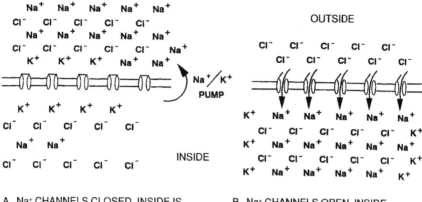

Figure 6.4 Propagation of action potentials by ionic movement across neuronal cell membranes. (A) When sodium channels are closed, the axon is negatively charged with respect to the extracellular fluid. (B) When sodium channels are open, the axon becomes positively charged with respect to the extracellular fluid.

constantly open but are **gated**, that is, their permeability to specific ions is regulated by the channel opening for a short interval in response to a specific stimulus. **Voltage-gated** channels open in response to voltage changes and **ligand-gated** channels are opened by extracellular chemical transmitters. In common with other cells, neurons also have a sodium/potassium ion pump to regulate cell volume and osmolarity by pumping sodium extracellularly and potassium intracellularly against their concentration gradients. The sodium/potassium pump also maintains the unequal distribution of sodium and potassium ions across the cell membrane. At rest, the concentration of potassium ions is high inside the cell and low outside whereas sodium concentration is high outside the neuron but low inside (Figure. 6.4). Despite the sodium/potassium pump and gated channels, potassium still tends to leak out through **leak channels** in the membrane, which is relatively impermeable to sodium. Potassium leaks out until the concentration gradient driving it out of the cell is balanced by the electrical gradient opposing potassium outflow. The **resting potential** of a neuron is reached when the net current flow across the membrane is zero (Figure 6.4). This results in an ionic imbalance making the resting potential negative with respect to the extracellular fluid. The actual value varies from neuron to neuron but is about –70 mV.

The ability to propagate action potentials depends upon the *selective* opening of ion channels to allow ionic movement, which will alter the potential to a point where it will become positive. This reversal of resting potential, or **depolarization**, is local at first but the current generated spreads in one direction along the axon activating adjacent voltage-gated channels as it does so. The current flows passively from one region to the next and changes the membrane potential just enough to cause voltage-gated sodium channels to open when the membrane is depolarized above a certain threshold. The opening of sodium channels allows an influx of sodium ions which counteract the negative resting potential and actually produce a positive overshoot. This causes current to flow into the next region starting the process all over again so that the action potential is constantly renewed. If current can spread along the axonal membrane as described, you may wonder why the action potential only travels in one direction. The reason is that sodium channels close again very swiftly and then remain in an unresponsive (refractory) state for a short while before they can be reactivated, thus terminating the generation of action potentials in their region of the membrane. The current can only pass in one direction because the region which has just conducted the action potential is refractory. At the same time as sodium channels close, potassium channels open allowing potassium out of the cell; these act more slowly so that potassium efflux only occurs as sodium influx falls off. This helps to restore the negative resting potential more rapidly by outward potassium movement (Figure 6.4). Thus a wave of depolarization will be self-propagating along the nerve and will stay at the same magnitude throughout. The self-propagation depends upon a ubiquitous distribution of sodium channels along the nerve which is found in unmyelinated nerves.

In myelinated nerves the myelin sheath forms an electrical insulating layer and covers the cell membrane so completely that there are no channels of any sort for long stretches. As described above, the myelin sheath is absent at **Nodes of Ranvier**, where sodium channels are extremely concentrated. Depolarization initiated at one node will pass current along the nerve to the next node without any current loss as the nerve is so well insulated. This allows passive currents to depolarize the axon over long stretches sufficient to cause sodium channels to open and propagation of the action potential to continue. The apparent leap of depolarization from one node to the other is known as **saltatory conduction**. Myelination provides for rapid conduction velocity because it is not necessary for ions to cross the membrane along its entire length; ion diffusion is slow compared to current flow. Saltatory conduction is also energy efficient in restoring the resting potential after depolarization because the sodium/potassium pump only needs to act at the nodes of Ranvier. Potassium channels are absent from myelinated nerves.

At the end of axons on the presynaptic side of synapses, the channels change in character and become voltage-gated **calcium channels**. The depolarization wave activates these channels which allows ingress of calcium ions. The increased intracellular calcium triggers release of neurotransmitter from **synaptic vesicles** into the synaptic cleft (see Figure 6.1). The neurotransmitters thus released activate ligand-gated channels on the post-synaptic neuron. These post-synaptic ligand-gated channels may be sodium channels which allow influx of sodium ions, causing a lowering of the post-synaptic potential towards zero. An **excitatory post-synaptic potential** is thus set up in the post-synaptic cell. Conversely, some neurotransmitters activate **chlorine channels** which allow influx of chloride ions, and which hyperpolarize the post-synaptic membrane by increasing the negative potential, producing an **inhibitory post-synaptic potential**. The state of the post-synaptic membrane depends therefore on the various inputs that a particular neuron receives and will become more or less likely to generate an action potential as the potential is decreased or increased. As the polarity changes spread across the cell membrane, they will instigate an action potential in the initial segment of the axon if the voltage changes reach a critical threshold level. Once instigated, it will be self-driving and propagation along the axon will ensue. In axons, excitation is an **all-or-nothing** phenomenon: either the threshold will be exceeded and an impulse will be propagated, or it will not be reached and consequently no impulse will occur. The incoming information to dendrites may be modified by other information which may alter the post-synaptic potential but an impulse propagated along axons cannot be altered until it reaches the next synapse. Post-synaptic inhibition is crucial in the functioning of the nervous system because it can prevent action potentials being generated in an axon when such actions would be inappropriate. The wave of depolarization along axons can be arrested by pharmacological agents which block ion channels to prevent further propagation of the action potential; this is the principal action of local anaesthetics.

In theory, the whole nervous system could work on synapses which are either excitatory or inhibitory and would thus require only two neurotransmitters. There are, however, many neurotransmitters in both the CNS and PNS including the catecholamines **noradrenalin** and **dopamine**. **Acetylcholine** is found at neuromuscular junctions as well as other sites in the peripheral and central nervous systems. These transmitters are used extensively in the PNS but very few synapses in the CNS use catecholamines or acetylcholine as transmitters. The neurotransmitters used by the vast majority of neurons in the CNS are still a matter for conjecture. The amino acids, **glutamate** and **aspartate,** are probably excitatory neurotransmitters and **gamma-aminobutyric acid (GABA)** is a ubiquitous inhibitory neurotransmitter.

The peripheral nervous system

The peripheral nervous system is divided into the **somatic** and **autonomic nervous systems** although these divisions are not always anatomically distinct. The somatic nervous system receives information from sensory receptors sensing information from the external environment and controls the action of voluntary muscles. The autonomic nervous system controls involuntary functions through the activation of smooth muscle in tissues and organs and glandular tissues.

The peripheral nervous system consists of 12 pairs of **cranial nerves** originating from the brain and 33 pairs of **spinal nerves** originating from the spinal cord. The autonomic system is superimposed on the somatic nerves but does have some distinct components. All spinal nerves have common components: they are **mixed nerves** formed from the axons of somatic **sensory** (afferent) nerves conveying information from the periphery to the spinal cord and brainstem and axons of **motor** (efferent) nerves controlling voluntary muscle. Some also contain elements of the autonomic nervous system. Cranial nerves cannot be categorized so simply. Some are mixed nerves whereas others are purely motor nerves, and some are specialized sensory nerves innervating the special sensory organs for olfaction, vision, hearing and balance. Various cranial nerves also have an autonomic component.

The spinal cord

Anatomically distinct spinal nerves consist of mixed sensory and motor axons bound together by the epineurium for most of their length. However, adjacent to the spinal cord the sensory and motor axons separate and connect with different parts of the spinal cord. This is the first level at which information of different kinds is segregated, a process which becomes much more refined at higher levels in the central nervous system.

The central nervous system contains distinct areas of **white matter** and **grey matter** based on their appearance in fresh tissue. White matter comprises axons; some of these are myelinated and it is the myelin which gives them their characteristic colour. Essentially, white matter is the cabling of the central nervous system connecting various parts together. Grey matter consists of cell bodies and their associated dendrites and synapses and the initial segment of axons adjacent to the cell body. Grey matter is the telephone exchange where connections can be made or broken, re-routed to different exchanges or sent between several exchanges so that your body can have its own teleconference.

Two important points follow from this division into white and grey matter. Firstly, nerves are not scattered at random in the central nervous system. The cell bodies are grouped together into clusters of cell bodies called **nuclei** or **bodies**. In the cerebral hemispheres and cerebellum cortex, cell bodies and synapses are clustered on the outside where they are known as the cerebral and cerebellar cortex. The axons arising from nuclei or cortex are bundled together into **tracts** or **fasciculi** in the white matter. Secondly, it was emphasized above that nerve impulses obey the 'all or none rule': once the nerve is depolarized sufficiently to conduct an impulse it will do so, and if it does not reach the requisite threshold no nerve impulse occurs. Once a nerve is conducting, the information cannot be stopped or modified by physiological means. This can only occur at synapses situated in the grey matter: therefore, nuclei and other areas of grey matter are important relay stations along nerve pathways.

The spinal cord is segregated into grey and white matter (Figure 6.5). The grey matter constitutes a central H-shaped area which is often likened to a butterfly. Bearing in mind that the H lies horizontally, the backward strokes of the H are the **dorsal horns** and the forward strokes are the **ventral horns**. The white matter surrounds the grey matter and is divided by the horns into anterior, lateral and posterior white matter. Sensory axons leave the mixed spinal nerve just after it enters the intervertebral foramen between adjacent vertebrae to form the **dorsal root** which enters the dorsal horn where many of the axons synapse. The axons of motor nerves arise from cell bodies clustered in the ventral horn and exit as the **ventral root** to join the sensory axons just before the intervertebral foramen. The cell bodies of sensory neurons actually lie outside the central nervous system on the dorsal root. As the cell bodies are larger than the processes emanating from them, they form swellings on the dorsal roots known as **dorsal root ganglia**. There are analogous structures on sensory cranial nerves adjacent to the brain.

During embryonic development, as the vertebrae and muscles form specific segments of the body, the spinal cord is also segregated functionally into spinal cord **segments**. Each segment gives rise to a pair of spinal nerves. Sensory information from a particular body segment enters the corresponding spinal cord segment through the corresponding spinal nerves and motor nerves supplying muscles of that segment leave at the same level. It follows therefore that for sensory information to reach higher areas of the central nervous system it must travel upwards through the spinal cord. Axons from cell bodies in the dorsal horn of the spinal

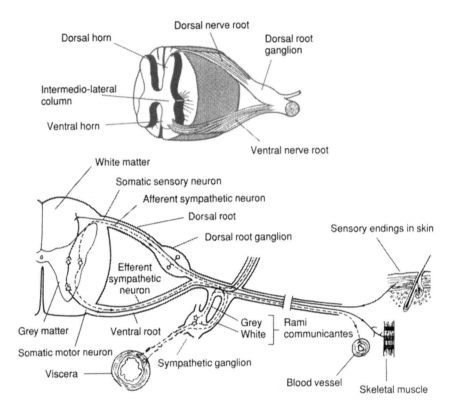

Figure 6.5 A spinal nerve from the thoracic region. (A) A three-dimensional view of the spinal cord and nerve roots. (B) A diagram of somatic motor and sensory and sympathetic nerves within the spinal nerve and spinal cord.

cord, on to which the incoming peripheral sensory nerves synapse, form **ascending tracts** in the white matter to do this. Likewise, the brain controls motor activity so information must be conveyed from the brain to motor neurons in the relevant segment of the spinal cord. **Descending tracts** in white matter link the brain and motor nerves.

Essentially, the integrative function of the CNS becomes more complex at progressively higher levels. Complex functions such as memory and learning take place in the cerebral hemispheres whereas function in the spinal cord is relatively simple.

Motor axons arising in the ventral horns of the spinal cord control movement of all voluntary muscles from the neck downwards. The dorsal horns receive sensory information from these muscles as well as the joints they act on and the overlying skin. Autonomic axons from the lateral horns control smooth muscle activity in the internal organs and blood vessel walls. The spinal cord also carries ascending tracts conveying sensory information to the brainstem and above and descending tracts carrying motor information from the higher regions of the CNS. The only integrative functions which take place in the spinal cord are those involved in reflex activity: a **reflex** is an invariable action generated as a response to a particular stimulus. A good example is the 'knee jerk reflex'. If the patellar tendon below the knee cap is lightly stretched by tapping it, the quadriceps muscles in the thigh will contract causing the knee to jerk. Receptors in the tendon responding to the stretch stimulus send impulses to the spinal cord along sensory nerves. Their axons pass straight through the dorsal horn without synapsing and instead form a direct synapse on to the motor neurons controlling the quadriceps muscles and thus stimulate them directly. The brain is not involved in processing this information at all. The knee jerk reflex is a **monosynaptic reflex** as only one synapse is involved. Most spinal reflexes are, however, **polysynaptic**: the incoming sensory nerves synapse in the dorsal horn with neurons which link the dorsal and ventral horns and convey the information on to the motor neurons via another synapse. The intervening neurons are known as **interneurons** and there may be several between the axon terminal of the sensory nerve and the dendrites of the motor neuron. These allow information to be disseminated to other areas or concentrated towards one location. Most spinal reflexes are concerned with regulation of posture. Reflex activity is not confined to the spinal cord. Other reflexes occur at all levels in the central nervous system and some very complex activities, such as swallowing, require an elaborate chain of reflexes which must be precisely sequenced and coordinated for the activity to be successful.

The brainstem

The brainstem links the cerebral hemispheres with the spinal cord through ascending and descending tracts but contains additional components with additional functions (Figure 6.6). The brainstem contains nuclei which control voluntary muscles in the head and neck and receive information from the same area. These include the lips, tongue, jaws, palate, larynx and pharynx, all of which have a vital role to play in speech. Other nuclei in the brainstem are involved in reception of special sensory information about hearing, balance and taste. There are, in addition, other nuclei with their own specialized functions.

The **medulla oblongata** is an upward continuation of the spinal cord and is the origin of the sixth to twelfth cranial nerves and thus contains

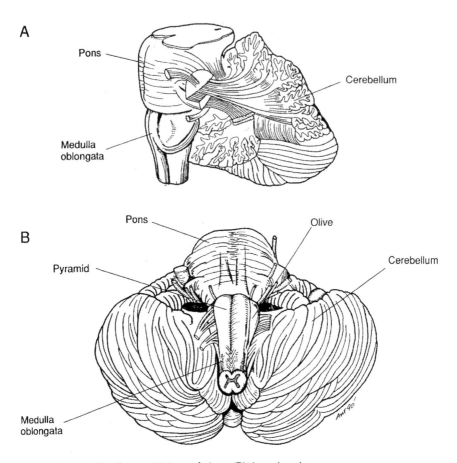

Figure 6.6 The hindbrain. (A) Lateral view. (B) Anterior view.

their nuclei where motor nerves originate and sensory nerves terminate. It also contains other groups of nuclei, the **respiratory** and **cardiovascular centres** which control respiratory and cardiovascular functions respectively. A diffuse network of neurons in the medulla, the **reticular system**, is involved in arousing the brain to prepare it to receive and interpret incoming sensory information. The reticular system is also involved in motor activity and continues upwards from the medulla into the pons. The **pons** forms a connecting bridge between the cerebellar hemispheres on each side (*pons* is Latin for 'bridge') and contains the nuclei of origin of the fifth and sixth cranial nerves and the upward continuation of the reticular system. It is also a major link between the cerebellum, the cerebral hemispheres and ascending and descending tracts. The pons and medulla seen together look like an inverted flower bulb and are sometimes referred to as the bulb: this terminology is formally used to designate corticobulbar tracts which connect the cerebral cortex to the pons and medulla. The medulla, pons and cerebellum constitute the **hindbrain**.

The **cerebellum** (Figure 6.6) on the posterior aspect of the brainstem receives sensory information from muscles and joints which give positional sense and information about the state of tension or contraction in individual muscles (proprioception). The cerebellum computes all this information and feeds it back into descending motor tracts so that muscles will contract at the appropriate rate, range and force to produce a given movement.

The **midbrain** is a short section about 2 cm long at the upper end of the brainstem. It is easy to overlook because it is so short and is well hidden by the cerebellum and cerebral hemispheres, but do not – because it is very important. It carries ascending and descending tracts to and from each cerebral hemisphere and these are arranged as two robust **cerebral peduncles** which lie anteriorly. The **red nuclei** are paired areas of grey matter in the peduncles although in a fresh brain they have a pink coloration, hence the name; they are the relay points where information from the cerebellum is fed into the descending pathways. The cerebral aqueduct, one of the conduits in the brain for cerebrospinal fluid, lies behind the cerebral peduncles and its roof is called the **tectum** from the Latin word for 'roof'. Two pairs of swellings project posteriorly from the tectum like four little hills. These are the colliculi (Latin for 'little hills'); the **superior colliculi** are involved in the coordination of eye movements and eye reflexes and the **inferior colliculi** with coordination of auditory reflexes such as turning the head towards the source of sound. Conveniently, the midbrain also contains the nuclei of the third and fourth cranial nerves which innervate some muscles of the eyes so they are near to the colliculi.

The forebrain

The forebrain consists of the left and right cerebral hemispheres which are incompletely separated by a median fissure. A thin strip of grey matter lies on the surface of each hemisphere, and the hemispheres are highly folded to increase their surface area. The convexity of each fold is a **gyrus** and the intervening cleft is a **sulcus**. Within the depth of the forebrain, there are two areas of grey matter. The **thalamus** immediately above the midbrain is a sensory relay area with all sensory pathways synapsing there. It also functions as a relay station between other areas of the cerebral hemispheres. The **hypothalamus** is a small area of grey matter below the thalamus which controls the activity of the pituitary gland and therefore regulates hormonal output. It is also involved in regulation of various basic bodily functions such as control of temperature, appetite and thirst and, in response to emotions, it plays a major role in the regulation of the autonomic nervous system (see Chapter 12). The thalamus and hypothalamus constitute the diencephalon. The **basal ganglia** lie laterally to the thalamus in each hemisphere and are involved in the regulation of movement. The two hemispheres are connected to each other by commissural neurons running transversely through the **corpus callosum**. A **commissure** is where nerves pass from one side of the CNS to the other.

Each cerebral hemisphere is divided into **frontal, parietal, occipital** and **temporal** lobes named according to the skull bones which overlie them although there is no correspondence exactly. The division between the frontal and parietal lobe is demarcated on the lateral surface of each hemisphere by the **central sulcus**. The prominent **lateral fissure** (sometimes called the Sylvian fissure) separates the temporal lobe below from the frontal and parietal lobes above. The temporal lobe is continuous with the occipital lobe and posterior part of the parietal lobe posteriorly. There is no obvious division of the parietal from the occipital lobe laterally but the parieto-occipital sulcus indicates the division medially.

Certain areas of each hemisphere are designated as primary areas because they deal exclusively with a particular function (Figure 6.7). Ascending and descending tracts from or to the spinal cord and brainstem or special sensory tracts from organs of special sense ultimately terminate or originate in the corresponding primary area. The **primary sensory area** lies in the **postcentral gyrus** immediately behind the central sulcus, and the **primary motor area** lies immediately anterior to the sulcus in the **precentral gyrus**. The **primary auditory cortex** is on the superior rim of the temporal lobe in the **transverse temporal gyri**, and the **primary visual cortex** is in the posterior pole of the occipital lobes. These areas are arranged in specific fashion which serve to introduce some important concepts about the organization of the nervous system.

The primary sensory and motor cortices are **somatopically** arranged, that is, the different areas of the body are represented sequentially in specific areas of each primary cortex. The representation is inverted so that the leg areas are superior and the head areas are inferior (Figure 6.8). The area devoted to a particular area of the body is not related to the actual size of that area, but to the density of innervation it receives from a given area or the quantity of motor output to muscles in a specific region. The hands, in particular the thumb, index and middle fingers, the lips and tongue are the most sensitive areas of the body and have a huge area of the primary sensory cortex devoted to them. The area for the thumb is bigger than the whole area for the trunk! Likewise in the motor cortex, large areas are devoted to parts of the body where fine movement is essential for

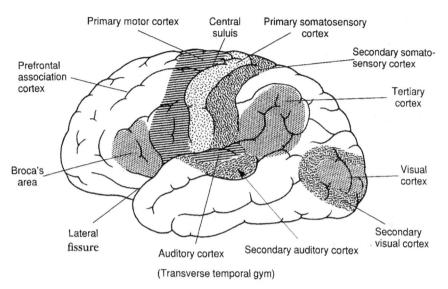

Primary motor cortex Central suluis Primary somatosensory cortex

Secondary somato-sensory cortex

Prefrontal association cortex

Tertiary cortex

Broca's area

Visual cortex

Lateral fissure

Auditory cortex Secondary auditory cortex Secondary visual cortex

(Transverse temporal gym)

Figure 6.7 A lateral view of the left cerebral hemisphere showing the primary cortical and association cortex areas and Broca's and Wernicke's areas.

function such as the hands, tongue and eyes. The primary auditory cortex is arranged **tonotopically** with different pitches represented in sequence across the cortex.

A very strange fact about the organization of the nervous system is that, generally, ascending and descending pathways cross (**decussate**) from one side to the other at some point in their course. This means that the right cerebral hemisphere receives information from and controls movement of the left side of the body and vice versa for the left hemisphere. It follows that damage to one half of the brain above the decussation point will result in dysfunction on the opposite side of the body. The control of one side of the body by the contralateral hemisphere is something which is often not appreciated by clients. In aphasia clinics, it is not unusual to be asked by the relatives of stroke clients or the clients themselves why the right side of the body is paralysed when the neurologist showed them an X-ray picture of the stroke in the left half of the brain.

The areas in each hemisphere not involved in primary function are known collectively as the **association cortex**. They do what their name implies and associate different primary functions by connecting primarily with other regions of the cerebral hemispheres through association and commissural axons. If someone kicks you on the shin, you will feel pain but you may want to know what your visual and auditory cortices are telling you at the same time. Did your assailant have an apologetic

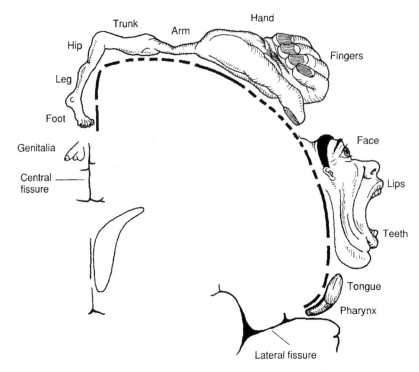

Figure 6.8 A diagram of the left somatosensory cortex showing the somatotopic representation of the body (the sensory homunculus).

expression and tone of voice or did they have a sadistic smile and curse you while they kicked you? Your immediate response and subsequent behaviour will depend on the associations you make at the time. These areas also control higher functions such as memory, learning and language recognition and use: **Broca's area** for linguistic encoding for speech is in the frontal association cortex, and **Wernicke's area** for language comprehension is in the temporo-parietal association cortex (Figure 6.7). As well as the representation of sensory and motor functions in the contralateral hemisphere resulting from decussation of motor and sensory tracts, the association cortex in each hemisphere deals with different functions and activities. This is lateralization of function, or **cerebral dominance**. The left hemisphere deals with abstract aspects such as language, logic and mathematics whereas the right hemisphere is more concerned with visuospatial function; artistic ability and facial recognition are examples of right-sided function. Brain damage to the association cortex can produce very subtle changes in behaviour and function depending upon which area in which hemisphere is injured.

Sensory pathways

Somatosensory pathways have a similar structure irrespective of function whereas those dealing with the special senses are more individual and complex. In somatosensory pathways dealing with sensations of temperature, pain and touch a minimum of only three neurons with two intervening relay stations in grey matter are required to convey the message that you have stubbed your toe all the way from the foot to the sensory cortex. At the two synaptic areas of grey matter, there are a variable and largely indeterminate number of interneurons. There are two main pathways conveying somatosensory information from the body to the cerebral cortex, the **dorsal column system** and the **anterolateral system**. The dorsal column system conveys discriminative touch, vibration and proprioception. The peripheral sensory receptors in this pathway are linked by **primary sensory neurons** to the spinal cord. When they enter the spinal cord, they send a branch to the dorsal horn but the major axons enter the dorsal white matter and ascend in the **dorsal columns** to the **dorsal column nuclei** in the medulla oblongata where they make their first synapse. The second set of neurons in the chain (the second order neuron) decussate at the level of the dorsal column nuclei and ascend in a pathway called the medial lemniscus to the thalamus. Here the second order neurons synapse with third order neurons which convey information to the primary somatosensory cortex (see Figure 9.1).

The anterolateral system conveys pain, temperature and certain kinds of touch sensation from the periphery to the somatosensory cortex. Primary sensory neurons in this system enter the dorsal horns of the spinal cord where they synapse with second order neurons, called thalamic projection neurons. The projection neurons decussate in the spinal cord at the level of entry of the primary sensory neurons and then ascend in the anterior and lateral white matter of the contralateral side, hence the name of this pathway. There are several pathways within the anterior and lateral white matter, each having a slightly different destination. Some axons form the **spinothalamic pathway**. (Incidentally, the nomenclature of pathways in the CNS is usually straightforward: the first part of the name tells you where the pathway starts and the second part indicates where it ends. Some pathways have compound names with the intermediate part of the name indicating intermediate relay stations: e.g. a spinoreticulothalamic pathway would start in the spinal cord, synapse in the reticular formation and then continue to the thalamus.) Axons in the spinothalamic neurons ascend all the way to the thalamus before they synapse with third order neurons conveying information from the thalamus to the primary sensory cortex. Other axons do not ascend directly to the thalamus, but make intermediate synapses in the reticular formation in the medulla and pons, forming the spinoreticular and spinomesencephalic pathways. From the intermediate relay stations, axons ascend to intralaminar nuclei in the thalamus which are believed to be involved in arousal. The primary sensory neurons from your toe give you some idea of how long axons can be: the axon carrying information to the spinal cord will be the length from your toe to the small of your back, and the axon carrying the information from the cell body in the dorsal root ganglion to the dorsal column nuclei will be the length from the small of your back to the base of your skull. In total the axons will be about 2 metres in length and will conduct the impulse in less than a millisecond!

Somatosensory pathways from the head follow a slightly different course to those from the body. The cell bodies of the majority of primary sensory neurons are in the trigeminal ganglia. The primary sensory axons pass from the periphery to the cell body, then axons travel into the brainstem. They synapse in the trigeminal sensory nucleus (see Chapter 11) and second order axons decussate, then join the medial lemniscus or anterolateral pathways as they ascend to the thalamus. The primary sensory neurons of other cranial nerves carrying somatosensory information also terminate in the trigeminal nuclei. Second order neurons end in a separate thalamic nucleus from those conveying sensation from the rest of the body. The third order neurons carrying sensory information from the head terminate in the primary sensory cortex.

Motor pathways

If you are about to play the piano, you will sit down and make yourself comfortable by getting your balance correct. You will then get your hands into position above the keyboard and your feet above the pedals and then you will move your fingers in fine elaborate movements to play your party piece. Of course, as your hands run up and down the eight octaves on your grand piano, you will have to adjust your balance so that you don't fall off the piano stool and move your arms so that your fingers can reach the upper and lower keys. Motor pathways are very complex to ensure that all these requirements are fulfilled and coordinated. To achieve all the necessary movements with skill and panache, there are several inputs on to each motor neuron in the spinal cord. Motor pathways are arranged hierarchically to control motor tasks of a complexity outlined above, or even apparently simple tasks like reaching out for an object, where a considerable degree of coordination is required.

Each level of the motor pathway hierarchy possesses circuitry that plays its part in the regulation of movement and is interconnected to other levels of the hierarchy. Furthermore, sensory information which is absolutely vital for the control of motor behaviour is processed in parallel and that information is distributed to several levels of the motor pathway hierarchy. The areas of the CNS that make up the motor system can be described simply as follows (see Figure 10.1). The first level of the hierarchy consists of the motor neurons in the spinal cord and brainstem connected to each muscle. They receive sensory information from the muscles themselves to form reflexes such as the knee jerk reflex. Reflexes constitute the basic building blocks of movement and many movements can be formed from these basic units. Motor neurons receive inputs from other regions of the CNS via descending pathways which form the next level of the hierarchy.

Descending pathways originate from the cerebral cortex and also from the brainstem. Pathways from the brainstem are divided into two categories, **dorsolateral** and **ventromedial descending systems**. Dorsolateral pathways include the **rubrospinal tracts** from the red nuclei in the midbrain which control fine movement in muscles of the hands and feet. Ventromedial pathways include the **vestibulospinal tracts** from the vestibular apparatus in the inner ear, the **reticulospinal pathways** from the reticular formation and **tectospinal pathways** from the superior colliculi in the midbrain which provides visual cues for movement. These pathways control posture, balance and proximal limb movement.

Pathways from the cortex include the **lateral and ventral corticospinal tracts** and **corticobulbar tracts** which pass directly to motor neurons or via interneurons in reflex circuits in the spinal cord and brainstem respectively. They control fine movement such as finger movement (lateral corticospinal tracts) and posture, balance and proximal steering movements of the limbs (ventral corticospinal tracts). The lateral tracts decussate in the pyramids on the anterior surface of the medulla whereas the ventral tracts remain on the same side. The cortex is also the source of indirect corticospinal pathways which follow a similar route to the direct pathways but have an intermediate synapse. Some form the rubrospinal tracts which relay in the red nuclei, others form corticopontine tracts synapsing in the pons on their way to the cerebellum whilst axons in the corticoreticular tract synapse in the reticular formation. These pathways control gross postural movements such as positioning your body or limbs. The direct corticospinal pathways travelling through the pyramids are sometimes called the pyramidal tracts whereas the other tracts which do not pass through the pyramids are referred to as the extrapyramidal system.

The **cerebral cortex** is the next level of the motor hierarchy and controls preplanning, programming and execution of movement. The areas of cortex involved include the **primary motor** and **sensory**

cortices, the **premotor** and **supplemental motor areas** and the prefrontal and posterior association areas. In addition to these cortical areas, the cerebellum and basal ganglia also influence motor activity. Both contribute to loop systems that receive information from the cerebral cortex, process the information and feed it back to cortical motor areas. The **cerebellum** receives proprioceptive information from the relevant ascending pathway and from the motor cortical areas via the pons. It acts as an error detector, correcting mistakes between the intended movement and the movement actually occurring. The cerebellum also plays a role in motor learning. The **basal ganglia** participate in complex loop systems linking sensory areas with motor areas of the brain. They initiate and stop movements and carry out motor programmes. It is somewhat easier to describe the actions of these loops in terms of what goes wrong if they are affected by disease or brain injury because it is still hazy as to what their precise actions are. Damage or disease of the basal ganglia produce movement disorders where there is either an excess or poverty of movement known as **dyskinesia**. An example of the former are the dance-like movements seen in Huntingdon's chorea and an example of the latter is the rigidity seen in Parkinson's disease.

Motor nerve injuries

Essentially, motor nerve injuries may occur at two levels. An **upper motor neuron lesion** disrupts descending tracts somewhere along their course in the central nervous system whereas a **lower motor neuron lesion** damages the peripheral motor spinal or cranial nerve between the spinal cord or brainstem and the muscles.

In **lower motor neuron lesions**, no information from any source can get to the muscles and they will exhibit **flaccid paralysis**, becoming floppy and non-contractile. Peripheral nerves can attempt to regenerate if their cell bodies are not injured. If a peripheral nerve is crushed by the injury, the axons are usually damaged but the epineurium and Schwann cell sheaths remain intact. The regenerating nerves therefore follow their established conduits and reach their target muscle and reinnervate it. If the nerve is cut, on the other hand, even if the two cut ends are surgically rejoined by microsurgical suturing of the epineurium of the two sections, it is unlikely that the hundreds of axons will be facing their own Schwann cell sheath. Regeneration in this instance is at best poor and at worst non-existent. If a muscle is not reinnervated within a few weeks, it will atrophy resulting in loss of contour in that part of the body which, if the muscle is superficial, may alter the appearance of the person. After a period of atrophy which may last several months, the muscle is replaced by fibrous tissue which contracts as it forms. This has the same effect as if the muscle was permanently contracted and reproduces the action of the muscle permanently. This can interfere with both function and aesthetic appearance.

Upper motor neuron lesions have a different effect and produce **spastic paralysis** of the affected muscles. Usually, all descending pathways are disrupted to some degree or other but the sensory information from the muscle entering through the spinal nerve is not affected. This is therefore the only information the muscle receives without any modification from the motor areas of the brain, eyes or vestibular apparatus. Unmodified muscle afferent information causes **hypertonicity**, over contraction, in the affected muscles. They therefore overcontract and become rigid. Reflexes involving these muscles are usually exaggerated, a condition known as **hyperreflexia**.

The autonomic nervous system

What is your reaction to an impending exam? Possibly your heart beats faster, your breathing becomes more rapid, you get a churning feeling in your stomach and you may sweat. When you have settled down and begun to write, your heart rate returns to normal, you stop sweating and that 'butterflies' feeling in your stomach goes. There is nothing you can do to prevent these 'panic' reactions in your body, and when you calm down again, you do not have to think, 'Slow down, heart' – it just does. This is what your autonomic nervous system (ANS) does. It controls internal bodily functions which are generally unconscious. The ANS usually acts locally to modify internal function to maintain the homeostasis of the body. However, in certain circumstances, it can act as a whole: your body is prepared for flight by increasing blood flow through muscles and increasing oxygen intake to power them while cutting down the activity in your gut and getting ready to dissipate all the heat extra muscle activity generates by sweating – this is sometimes called the '**flight or fight reaction**'.

The anatomically distinct parts of the ANS are the efferent (motor) components which largely control smooth muscle and glands. Visceral afferent (sensory) nerves which arise in the organs and tissues and monitor the internal environment travel with somatic sensory neurons to the spinal cord and brainstem and are indistinguishable from them. Higher centres in the brain, particularly the **limbic system** including the **hypothalamus**, regulate autonomic function in response to emotion. The efferent components of the ANS are subdivided into the **sympathetic** and **parasympathetic** systems. In the example about possible reaction to an exam in the previous paragraph, your sympathetic nervous system would have generated the responses to the imminent examination threat and the parasympathetic nervous system would have calmed you down again. The actions of these two subdivisions is thus largely antagonistic but they can also act synergistically.

Anatomically, both systems have two major neuronal pathways connecting the central nervous system to the peripheral effector organs or tissues. The two pathways synapse in peripherally located **autonomic ganglia; preganglionic neurons** connect the CNS and ganglia and **postganglionic neurons** connect the ganglia and peripheral tissues. The efferent parts of the ANS do not arise universally from the CNS. The sympathetic system exits from the CNS with the thoracic and upper lumbar spinal nerves (the **thoracolumbar outflow**) whereas the parasympathetic nervous system exits with certain cranial nerves and the sacral spinal nerves (the **craniosacral outflow**). This may seem peculiar at first but both systems have mechanisms to cover the areas to which there is no obvious distribution.

The sympathetic nervous system

The cell bodies of the sympathetic preganglionic nerves lie in the **intermediolateral horns** (or more simply the **lateral horns**) of the thoracic and upper lumbar spinal cord. These lie between the dorsal and ventral horns of the appropriate spinal segments (Figure 6.5). The short preganglionic nerves are myelinated and exit the spinal cord through the ventral roots in company with the motor neurons of the same segment. Shortly after exiting the intervertebral foramina, the preganglionic nerves leave the motor nerves as the **white rami communicantes** and these terminate by synapsing with the postganglionic neurons whose cell bodies lie in the sympathetic ganglia. There is a pair of sympathetic ganglia corresponding to each pair of spinal nerves with a sympathetic component. The ganglia lie on the bodies of the vertebrae. The ganglia are linked by both pre- and postganglionic neurons to form the **sympathetic chain**. The sympathetic chain is not restricted to the thoracolumbar region but is extended upwards as the **cervical sympathetic chain** which carries sympathetic nerves to the head and neck, and downwards as the pelvic sympathetic chain which supplies the lower abdomen, pelvis and legs. The long unmyelinated postganglionic nerves reach their effector organs by one of three routes. In the thoracolumbar region, they form a **grey ramus communicantes** which rejoins the corresponding spinal nerve and travels with it. Most commonly, the postganglionic neurons form plexuses around arteries and travel with them to the target tissues. In special cases, the autonomic nerves form separate nerves.

The parasympathetic nervous system

Parasympathetic preganglionic nerves exit the CNS with the third (**oculomotor**), seventh (**facial**), ninth (**glossopharyngeal**) and tenth (**vagus**) cranial nerves and the sacral spinal nerves. The third, seventh and ninth nerves supply structures in the head and the sacral nerves supply the pelvic organs. This pattern means that there is, potentially, a huge deficit in parasympathetic distribution in the thorax and abdomen. The gap is, however, bridged by the vagus nerves which travel down through the thorax and abdomen to supply the viscera in both areas. Parasympathetic preganglionic nerves are long and travel to the vicinity of their targets with the parent somatic nerve. Near their targets, the parasympathetic nerves branch off and enter the parasympathetic ganglia lying in or near the target where they synapse with the postganglionic nerves. The postganglionic nerves are generally quite short and exit the ganglia to ramify over the target tissue or join a convenient branch of a somatic nerve to innervate the target.

The two systems differ pharmacologically. **Acetylcholine** is the neurotransmitter at sympathetic and parasympathetic ganglia and at the synapses between parasympathetic nerves and their targets. In the sympathetic nervous system, **noradrenalin** is the transmitter at the postganglionic nerve terminals.

The actions of the autonomic nervous system on different organs and systems are outlined in Table 6.2. From the table, it will be appreciated that sympathetic innervation will affect the eyes and skin, signs which can be easily observed in an anxious or nervous client: their skin will be pale and sweaty and their pupils will be dilated. Signs and symptoms of autonomic nervous system activity are not, however, always due to its own activity. Many drugs have mimetic effects. Tricyclic antidepressants, for example, are **sympatheticomimetic** and emulate sympathetic activity but many adverse drug effects are due to inhibition of the parasympathetic nervous system allowing the sympathetic nervous system to act unopposed. Certain drugs given to relieve some of the symptoms of Alzheimer's disease are **parasympatheticomimetic** causing excess salivation. It is important therefore to obtain a full medical history of the client, including any drugs taken so that their intended pharmacological effects and unintended side effects can be anticipated.

Table 6.2 Actions of the autonomic nervous system

Target	Sympathetic	Parasympathetic
Heart	Increases heart rate Increases cardiac output Dilates coronary arteries	Decreases heart rate Decreases cardiac output Constricts coronary vessels
Lungs	Dilates bronchial tree and blood vessels	Constricts bronchial tree and blood vessels
Gastrointestinal tract	Inhibits secretion Decreases motility Increases sphincter tone Constricts blood vessels	Stimulates secretion Increases motility Relaxes sphincter No innervation
Salivary glands	Decreases secretion	Stimulates secretion
Skin	Stimulates secretion from sweat glands Constricts blood vessels Hair erection	No innervation No innervation No innervation
Eyes	Pupillary dilation No innervation of lens	Pupillary constriction Accommodation by contraction of lens
Muscle	Dilatation of blood vessels	Constriction of blood vessels

CHAPTER 7
The endocrine glands

While the nervous system regulates, coordinates and integrates the functions of the body by electrical connectivity and neurotransmitters, the endocrine glands regulate and integrate bodily activity by the production and secretion of chemical mediators, **hormones**, many of which act at long range. By definition, **endocrine glands** secrete their products directly into the circulation rather than into body cavities via ducts and thus their products are disseminated throughout the whole body. Hormones circulate to their appropriate targets which may be either specific tissues or organs or many different tissues. Despite the fact that hormones are circulated throughout the body, they only act on specific targets which have the corresponding receptors for the hormone in question.

The endocrine system is closely related to the autonomic nervous system although their modes of action differ. The autonomic nervous system uses the rapid conduction of action potentials and release of neurotransmitters to transmit information quickly. It acts in a localized fashion and its effects are usually of short duration. In contrast, the endocrine system releases hormones into the blood stream; their effects may be less localized but their actions are often prolonged. The activities of these two systems converge in the hypothalamus which is that part of the brain with an overall regulatory control of the autonomic nervous system; it also regulates the endocrine system largely by its effect upon the pituitary gland (see below). In functional terms, these two systems act together to produce homeostatic effects, controlling the internal environment of the body.

Various tissues throughout the body have an endocrine function. They may take the form of specific glandular aggregates which are entirely endocrine in function or be groups of cells within a tissue having other functions (Figure 7.1).

The **pituitary gland** in the head is closely related to the brain developmentally, anatomically and functionally and produces a range of

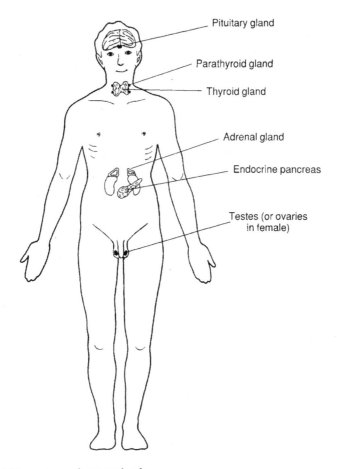

Figure 7.1 The major endocrine glands.

hormones, most of which are **trophic** in function: their hormones stimulate another tissue to produce, in turn, other hormones which exert a direct effect on the target tissue. Secretion of trophic hormones from the pituitary gland is regulated in turn by hormonal releasing factors formed in the **hypothalamus**. The **thyroid glands** in the neck produce hormones regulating metabolic rate and also a hormone involved in blood calcium regulation. The **parathyroid glands**, situated in the thyroid glands, are also involved in control of blood calcium levels. The **adrenal glands** lying adjacent to the kidneys produce a number of hormones controlling carbohydrate metabolism and electrolyte balance. A developmentally separate part of the adrenal gland produces hormones which produce a response similar to stimulation of the sympathetic nervous system. The other major endocrine tissues form part of other organs. The **ovaries** and **testes** both contain endocrine tissue secreting sex hormones which regulate the production of germ cells within these organs and effect secondary sexual characteristics. The **pancreas** also has an endocrine component producing hormones regulating carbohydrate metabolism.

The pituitary gland

The pituitary gland is a small pea-sized gland lying in the **pituitary fossa** of the middle cranial fossa (see Chapter 8). It is connected to the hypothalamus by the **pituitary stalk** or **infundibulum**. The gland is enclosed in bone anteriorly, posteriorly and inferiorly and by dura mater forming the cavernous sinuses laterally. The fossa is also roofed by dura mater so the gland is entirely enclosed except for its connection to the brain via the pituitary stalk.

The pituitary is divided into two lobes which are structurally and developmentally different and also have quite different functions. The **anterior pituitary (adenohypophysis)** develops from the roof of the oral cavity early in embryonic life and fuses with the **posterior pituitary (neurohypophysis)**, an outgrowth of the brain, to form the mature gland (Figure 7.2). The posterior lobe of the pituitary remains connected to the brain through neurons forming the pituitary stalk.

The anterior pituitary secretes six hormones, most of which are trophic hormones that regulate the release of other hormones from other endocrine glands. **Somatotrophin (growth hormone)** has an indirect effect on bone growth by stimulating the formation of **somatomedin** in the liver which exerts the direct effect on the growing bones. **Thyroid-stimulating hormone (TSH)** stimulates the thyroid gland to secrete its hormones. Two hormones, **follicle-stimulating hormone (FSH)** and **luteinising hormone (LH)**, affect secretion of hormones from the ovaries and testes. These are examples of gonadotrophic hormones which regulate the function of the gonads. In the female, FSH stimulates oestrogen secretion and development of the ova in the ovary during each menstrual cycle and in the male it regulates the formation and maturation of spermatozoa in the testes. LH promotes ovulation and secretion of progesterone from the ovary in the female and stimulates secretion of androgens by the endocrine cells in the testes of the male. **Adrenocorticotrophic hormone (ACTH)** stimulates the cortex of the adrenal gland to secrete some of its hormones. **Prolactin** is not a trophic hormone: it stimulates milk production in the mammary gland.

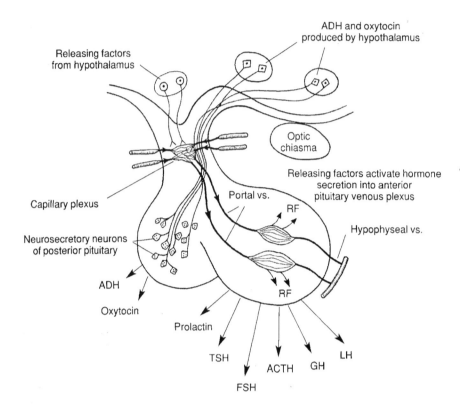

Figure 7.2 The hypophyseal portal system and neurosecretion from the posterior pituitary gland.

Release of anterior pituitary hormones is controlled by **releasing** and **inhibitory factors** corresponding to each hormone. These factors are synthesized in various hypothalamic nuclei and reach the anterior pituitary by an elaborate pathway (Figure 7.2). The neurons which synthesize releasing and inhibitory factors have relatively short axons which terminate adjacent to blood vessels at the junction of hypothalamus and infundibulum. In this area, the arteries supplying the pituitary gland form a dense capillary bed into which these factors are secreted. The capillaries unite to form the hypophyseal portal veins which break up into a second capillary plexus in the anterior lobe. The formation of two separate capillary plexuses within the course of a vein constitutes a **portal system** and restricts the transport of materials to a specific region rather than allowing them to enter the systemic venous system directly. Thus releasing and inhibiting factors synthesized in the hypothalamus are conveyed to the anterior pituitary by the hypophyseal portal system.

The trophic hormones secreted by the anterior pituitary prompt the release of hormones from other endocrine tissues. These in turn, as well as acting on their own target tissue, also reach the hypothalamus where they act on the nuclei synthesizing releasing and inhibitory factors. Thus a complete loop is formed of hypothalamus→anterior pituitary→target gland–hypothalamus. Generally the secretion of releasing factors increases as circulatory levels of a particular hormone fall and then decreases as the levels rise again, thus setting up a **negative feedback loop**.

The **posterior pituitary lobe** is structurally and functionally quite different from the anterior lobe. It consists of axons whose cell bodies lie in two hypothalamic nuclei where the two hormones secreted by the posterior pituitary gland are synthesized. They are transported down the axons in secretory granules and released into the circulation in the posterior pituitary (Figure 7.2). **Vasopressin** (or **antidiuretic hormone, ADH**) influences water reabsorption from urine in the kidneys. **Oxytocin** promotes milk ejection from the lactating mammary gland. It also causes uterine contraction during childbirth and this hormone may be administered to induce delivery.

Clinically, a deficiency of trophic pituitary hormones will lead to deficiency in hormone secretion from their target glands, the effects of which are discussed below. Because the cause of hormone deficiency is not due to disease of the target endocrine gland itself, such deficiencies are known as **secondary insufficiencies**. Deficiency of growth hormone stunts growth whereas excessive secretion leads to overgrowth or **pituitary gigantism**. In adults, excess growth hormone sometimes results from a pituitary tumour. Very few bones have any capacity for further growth in the adult with the exception of the fingers, toes and mandible. Excess growth hormone produces overgrowth of the mandible, large hands and feet as well as a heavy skeleton due to additional bone formation on the surface of bones. This condition is known as **acromegaly**.

The thyroid gland

The thyroid gland lies in the neck and consists of two large lobes lying on either side of the trachea connected by a narrow isthmus passing anterior to the trachea. The anatomy of the thyroid gland is described in Chapter 16.

When activated by pituitary TSH, the thyroid gland synthesizes **triiodothyronine (T3)** and **thyroxine (T4)** which are secreted into the circulation. Iodine is an essential trace element required for the synthesis of thyroid hormones. Both hormones have a general stimulatory effect on cellular metabolic rate, T3 acting immediately and T4 having a delayed action.

Thyroid gland disorders are of two main types: **hyperthyroidism** is overproduction and **hypothyroidism** is underproduction of thyroid hormones. Both conditions have widespread effects on the body, including speech production. Hyperthyroidism can result from a number of conditions, the commonest being an autoimmune disorder, **Grave's disease**. Overproduction of thyroid hormones leads to **thyrotoxicosis**, which is characterized by a large increase in metabolic rate resulting in weight loss and reduction in muscle bulk despite increased food intake. Overactivity, restlessness, intolerance of warmth due to increased heat production in the body, increase in heart rate, changes in breathing patterns and breathlessness, especially during exercise, are among other signs and symptoms. One form of thyrotoxicosis is accompanied by protrusion of the eyeballs known as **exophthalmic goitre**. Lack of thyroid hormone produces signs and symptoms essentially opposite to those of hyperthyroidism. Metabolic rate is low and there is weight gain unrelated to increased food consumption. Cold intolerance, reduced heart rate, drowsiness and lethargy usually occur. There is often striking fluid retention called **myxoedema** characterized by puffy features and fluid effusion into synovial joints and other spaces. In early infancy, thyroid hormone deficiency produces **cretinism**, with stunted physical growth, including retarded laryngeal development, and mental retardation. Cretinism is now very rare as thyroid hormone levels are regularly screened at birth; hormone replacement therapy is begun as soon as possible after detection of the deficit.

Both types of thyroid disorder can result in voice changes. Hyperthyroid clients may exhibit a high pitched, tremulous voice with uneven intonation. Increased respiratory rates, especially in Grave's disease, may cause vocal fatigue. Hypothyroidism can cause hoarseness of the voice due to oedema in the vocal folds with incomplete closure of the larynx during phonation (see Chapter 16) and atrophy of the laryngeal muscles. Fluid retention in the tongue and lips may interfere with articulation. In both hyperthyroidism and hypothyroidism, the gland enlarges considerably. In the former, the gland enlarges due to overactivity, and in the latter, the gland enlarges in a futile attempt to manufacture more hormones. Thyroid enlargement may compress the trachea but, because of the cartilaginous reinforcement of the trachea, it is often the oesophagus immediately behind the trachea which is compressed. This may cause dysphagia (see Chapter 21). Surgery for correction of thyroid diseases carries a risk of damage to the laryngeal nerves which adversely affects the motor and sensory functions of the larynx (see Chapter 16).

The parathyroid glands

The two pairs of parathyroid glands are usually embedded in the posterior aspect of the thyroid gland, one pair lying superiorly and the other pair inferiorly. They synthesize and secrete **parathyroid hormone (PTH)**. Parathyroid hormone regulates plasma calcium concentrations which are maintained within narrow levels of tolerance. Parathyroid hormone stimulates bone resorption and thus release of calcium into the blood. Excess secretion of PTH occurring in tumours of the gland causes widespread bone resorption and replacement of bone with fibrous connective tissue; the bone therefore becomes softer. Deficiency of parathyroid hormone, usually due to inadvertent removal during the surgical excision of the thyroid gland, leads to death as blood calcium levels fall rapidly causing tetanic spasm of muscle; tetany of the laryngeal muscle and respiratory muscles causes asphyxia. Replacement therapy by administration of PTH prevents tetany and death in such cases.

The endocrine pancreas

The pancreas is an accessory gland of the gastrointestinal tract secreting various digestive enzymes into the duodenum. Small clusters of endocrine cells known as the **islets of Langerhans** lie within the exocrine pancreatic tissue. The endocrine pancreas secretes two hormones, **insulin** and **glucagon**. Glucagon and insulin are often said to have antagonistic effects on blood glucose. Insulin promotes uptake of glucose by cells in general, particularly by muscle, and inhibits breakdown of glycogen and release of glucose into the circulation by the liver. These two effects lower blood sugar levels. Insulin deficiency gives rise to **diabetes mellitus** which, if left untreated, produces many symptoms all of which are a consequence of impaired glucose utilization and the necessity to depend upon other energy sources, principally the breakdown of fats and proteins. Fortunately, the majority of diabetic conditions can be controlled by insulin administration. In some cases, however, excess insulin administration rapidly depletes glucose to very low levels with consequent **hypoglycaemia** (low blood sugar). As glucose is the only energy source utilized by the brain, dizziness and confusion followed by an **insulin coma** may occur as the energy supply to the brain is decreased. **Glucagon** has apparently opposite effects to insulin on blood sugar levels by stimulating hepatic glycogenolysis converting glycogen into glucose. It has, however, been suggested that the two hormones cooperate, glucagon raising blood sugar levels and insulin facilitating its entry into cells. Glucagon is not thought to be an essential hormone as no disease states are directly attributable to glucagon deficiency. However, deficiency of glucagon may contribute to the pathogenesis of diabetes.

Glucose metabolism and control of blood sugar levels is a complex subject. The outline given here is simply intended to describe some of the more obvious features of the function of the endocrine pancreas.

The adrenal glands

The **adrenal** glands are two pyramidal glands lying on the superior pole of each kidney. Each gland consists of a **cortex** surrounding a small **medulla**. The cortex and medulla are functionally quite distinct (Figure 7.3).

The adrenal cortex

The adrenal cortex secretes **mineralocorticoids** and **glucocorticoids** as well as the male sex hormones, the **androgens**, and small quantities of female sex hormones. The major mineralocorticoid is **aldosterone**, which affects electrolyte and water balance by increasing sodium reabsorption and potassium excretion in the kidneys. The principal **glucocorticoid** hormones are **cortisol** and **corticosterone**. These increase blood levels of glucose, increase protein breakdown and lipid turnover, suppress inflammation and antagonize insulin by inhibiting uptake of glucose by tissues. Secretion of cortisol is also important in withstanding stress. Insufficiency leads to poor stress resistance but the mechanism of stress response is still poorly understood. Secretion of glucocorticoids is controlled by pituitary ACTH.

The adrenal cortex is essential to life and loss of secretion of its products produces **adrenocortical insufficiency (Addison's disease)** with increase in sodium excretion and increased water loss through the kidneys and hypoglycaemia due to impaired glucose uptake.

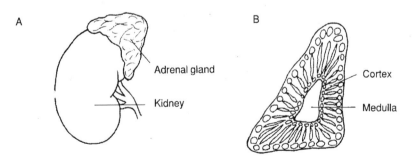

Figure 7.3 The adrenal gland.(A) The position of the gland in relation to the kidney. (B) The structure of the adrenal gland.

Cushing's syndrome is produced by increased secretion of cortisol and is often due to abnormalities of pituitary ACTH production. Since large quantities of glucocorticoids in the circulation exert mineralocorticoid effects as well as their normal functions, the symptoms in Cushing's syndrome are quite complex. A 'moonface' is characteristic of Cushing's syndrome and is probably caused by sodium retention and increase of extracellular fluid resulting in oedema. Loss of glucose uptake leads to increased protein catabolism as an alternative energy source with consequent muscular wasting. One of the commonest causes of Cushing's syndrome is long-term administration of glucocorticoids. They have anti-inflammatory properties and also suppress immune responses and are therefore used extensively in the treatment of autoimmune disorders such as rheumatoid arthritis; long-term administration can produce Cushing-like effects. When the levels of circulating cortisols are artificially maintained, pituitary ACTH production is switched off by negative feedback. The production of corticotrophin releasing factor by the hypothalamus and, in turn, the release of ACTH from the pituitary gland is profoundly depressed. If corticoid administration is rapidly withdrawn, the hypothalamus and pituitary cannot compensate rapidly enough to achieve the necessary levels of ACTH production, hence the production of adrenocortical hormones. This leads to the rapid onset of adrenocortical insufficiency, known as an **Addisonian crisis**. For this reason, patients on cortisol treatment must carry a card or wear a Medicalert bracelet detailing their treatment in case of accident. When corticosteroid treatment is withdrawn, the dose is decreased slowly over a number of weeks to allow compensatory pituitary ACTH secretion to build up again.

The adrenal medulla

The adrenal medulla is essentially a sympathetic ganglion without any axons arising from postganglionic neurons; instead the postganglionic cells synthesize 'neurotransmitter' for release directly into the blood rather than acting on target organs. The rich preganglionic sympathetic innervation of the medulla controls the activity of the postganglionic cells which produce two catecholamine hormones, **noradrenalin** and **adrenalin**. These are also the neurotransmitters at the synapses between the postganglionic sympathetic nerves and the effector organ. Their release therefore produces an effect comparable to simultaneous stimulation of the entire sympathetic nervous system (see Chapter 12). However, it is now thought that the adrenal medulla is of comparatively little importance in the 'flight or fight reaction'. The effects seen in response to emotional stress seem to be mediated by the sympathetic nervous system, which includes stimulation of the adrenal medulla.

Sex hormones

As described above, the secretion of sex hormones by the ovaries in females and testes in males is regulated by the hypothalamus which, in turn, regulates the production of gonadotrophic hormones from the anterior pituitary gland. This is a complex subject which is outside the scope of this book but there are some features which are pertinent to Speech and Language Therapy. Sex hormone secretion is at very low levels until **puberty** when increased activity of the hypothalamus and anterior pituitary produce a massive surge in sex hormone output. Ovum release during the menstrual cycle in females and sperm production in males is instigated at this time. The sex hormones also produce wide-ranging changes in the rest of the body at puberty. In both sexes, there is a **pubertal growth spurt** with height and weight gain and increased muscle bulk, which is more marked in males than females. Where the increased output has a differential effect in males and females, the resulting changes are known as **secondary sexual characteristics**. In both sexes there are marked, but obviously different, changes in the primary (ovaries and testes), secondary (internal and external genitalia) and accessory reproductive organs (the breasts, for example). One secondary sexual characteristic of particular relevance is that the pubertal growth spurt causes a large increase in the size of the thyroid cartilage of the larynx in relation to the other cartilages. This growth is more marked in males than females; the Adam's apple becomes more prominent and the vocal folds are elongated. As a result, the male voice breaks and pitch is lowered. This can cause temporary difficulties in control of the vocal folds with characteristic, and often embarrassing, pitch breaks (see also Chapter 16).

CHAPTER 8
The anatomy of the nervous system

The **nervous system** is divided into the **central nervous system (CNS)** comprising the brain and spinal cord, and the **peripheral nervous system (PNS)** comprising 12 pairs of **cranial nerves** and 31 pairs of **spinal nerves** and their associated ganglia, which connect the brain and the spinal cord respectively with peripheral structures and convey information between them.

The PNS is subdivided into **somatic** and **autonomic** components. **Somatic sensory (afferent)** nerves receive information from external sources impinging on the skin and mucosal surfaces of the body and visceral sensation derived from deeper structures in the body. They convey their information to the CNS. **Somatic motor (efferent)** nerves leave the CNS and carry information to striated voluntary muscles. Peripheral **autonomic** nerves control and monitor involuntary functions of the body carried out by the glands and smooth muscle. The peripheral autonomic system is also divided into **afferent** and **efferent** components. The afferent components run into the CNS with somatic afferent nerves but the efferent components often pursue a course independent of somatic motor nerves en route to the effector tissues. The cell bodies of somatic sensory and autonomic neurons are also located in the PNS where they are grouped together to form ganglia at particular points along the nerve.

The organization of the somatic and autonomic peripheral nervous systems is relatively straightforward anatomically. The nerves and ganglia can be dissected, visualized with the naked eye and followed to their destinations. Many structures in the CNS, on the other hand, cannot be visualized and can seem, therefore, very abstract. This is compounded to some extent by the naming of parts in the CNS. In the era of descriptive anatomy, when there was little idea of the functions of the different parts of the CNS, names were often based on their position or appearance. This nomenclature still exists, making it quite difficult to relate different structures to the functional organization of the CNS.

105

The CNS can be divided into two main regions, termed grey and white matter, based on their appearance in fresh tissue. **Grey matter** consists of cell bodies and their processes, synapses and glial cells. Myelin is absent but there is a profuse blood supply which accounts for the grey colouration. White matter comprises predominantly axons and glial cells, including those which produce myelin which gives it a white appearance. As a general principle of organization of the nervous system, the cell bodies of neurons tend to be grouped together. These groupings are known as **ganglia** in the PNS and **nuclei** or bodies in the CNS. In some regions, neurons are clustered together on the outside, the cerebral cortex and cerebellar cortex being the two main examples. The cortex and nuclei in the CNS are connected by bundles of axons forming pathways, usually in the white matter. These pathways have various names: the commonest being **tracts** or **fasciculi** but lemniscus, capsule and peduncle are also used.

The gross divisions of the CNS are the **brain** and **spinal cord**. The brain itself is divided into three main regions, the **forebrain**, **midbrain** and **hindbrain**, each of which has several components (Figure 8.1). The forebrain is subdivided into the cerebral hemispheres and the

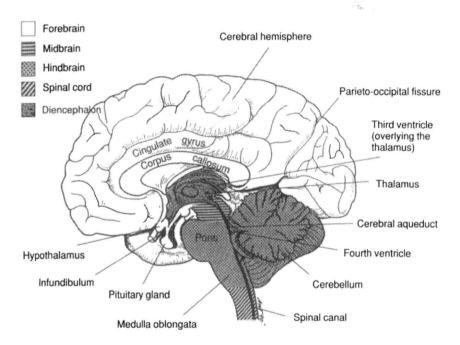

Figure 8.1 A hemisection of the human brain showing the major subdivisions.

diencephalon. The hindbrain comprises the pons, with the cerebellum attached to it, and the medulla oblongata. The medulla, pons and midbrain are grouped together as the brainstem. Within the CNS, there is a series of interconnected spaces, the **ventricles**, which are connected to the central canal of the spinal cord and the subarachnoid space in the meninges (see below). These spaces are filled with fluid known as **cerebrospinal fluid (CSF)**.

The cranial cavity and cranial fossae

The brain is contained within the cranial cavity of the skull. Viewed from above, the **roof** of the cranial cavity is formed by curved bones, the **frontal bone** anteriorly, the paired **parietal bones** laterally and the **occipital** bone posteriorly (Figure 8.2). Posteriorly, the cranium comprises the parietal and occipital bones. Laterally, the cranium is more complex. The frontal and parietal bones form a substantial part of the lateral walls but the squamous part of the temporal bones and the greater wing of the sphenoid also contribute to the lateral walls. The region where these bones meet is very thin. Internally, the **floor** of the cranial cavity has three fossae on progressively lower levels, known as the anterior, middle and posterior cranial fossae respectively (Figure 8.3).

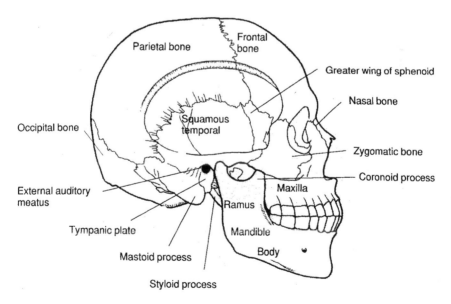

Figure 8.2 The main bones forming the cranium.

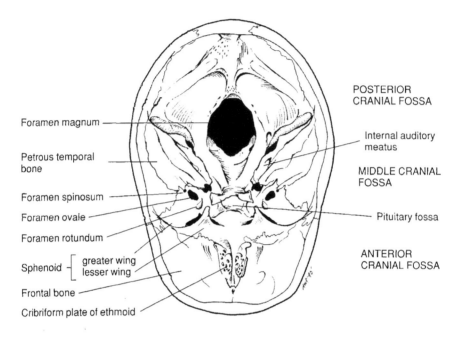

Foramen magnum

Petrous temporal
bone

Foramen spinosum

Foramen ovale

Foramen rotundum

Sphenoid ⎡ greater wing
        ⎣ lesser wing

Frontal bone

Cribriform plate of ethmoid

POSTERIOR
CRANIAL FOSSA

Internal auditory
meatus

MIDDLE CRANIAL
FOSSA

Pituitary fossa

ANTERIOR
CRANIAL FOSSA

Figure 8.3 The cranial fossae viewed from above with the cranial vault removed.

The **anterior cranial fossa** overlies the orbital and nasal cavities, the floor of the fossa and roof of orbit and nasal cavities being formed by the same bones. The floor of the anterior cranial fossa is formed by the frontal and ethmoid bones and its posterior margin is formed by the lesser wings of the sphenoid bone. The frontal lobes of the brain lie in the anterior cranial fossa. The **middle cranial fossa** lies below and behind the anterior fossa and contains the temporal lobes of the brain and the pituitary gland. The middle cranial fossa is formed by the sphenoid and temporal bones. The sphenoid bone forms a solid bar of bone running anteroposteriorly and has several extensions. The greater wings of the sphenoid bone project laterally and form the anterior wall and a substantial part of the floor of the middle cranial fossa. The lesser wings form part of the boundary with the anterior cranial fossa. The superior orbital fissure lies between the two wings on each side and is the main route for entry of nerves and blood vessels to the orbits. The floor is completed posteriorly by the petrous part of the temporal bone, a solid wedge of bone which houses the inner and middle ear. Several cranial nerves leave the cranial cavity through foramina in the middle cranial fossa and the internal carotid arteries enter the cranial cavity through this region. The pituitary gland is in the anterior midline enclosed by parts of the sphenoid bone forming the pituitary fossa. Most posteriorly, the **posterior cranial fossa** lies at the lowest level; this fossa partially surrounds the brainstem and cerebellum. Together with the sphenoid bone, the petrous temporal bones also form the anterior wall of the posterior cranial fossa. Its floor is formed by the occipital bone which is pierced by the **foramen magnum** through which the hindbrain is continuous with the spinal cord. Veins draining the brain converge on to the jugular foramen and pass through it to form the internal jugular vein on the outside. The ninth, tenth and eleventh cranial nerves also exit the skull through the same foramen.

The meninges

The brain is not in direct contact with the bones of the skull but is enclosed within three layers of membranes known as the **meninges**. The brain and spinal cord float in **cerebrospinal fluid** (**CSF**) enclosed by the meninges and are attached to surrounding tissue only by the blood vessels supplying and draining the brain and the cranial and spinal nerves. The meninges consist of a tough fibrous **dura mater** lining the cranial cavity, the thin membranous **pia mater** which adheres to the brain and spinal cord and the intervening **arachnoid mater** which lines the dura mater and sends thin strands of material across the subarachnoid space to the pia mater. CSF circulates between the arachnoid and pia mater in the **subarachnoid space** (Figure 8.4).

The **dura mater** consists of two layers during its development but these are fused in adult life except at points of folding from the bones, called dural reflections, that form sheets extending into the cranial cavity

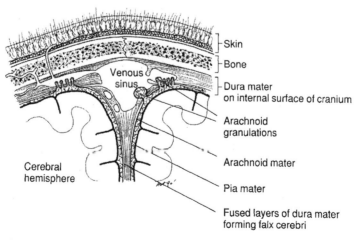

Figure 8.4 The meningeal layers.

between the major divisions of the brain. One reflection is formed along the line of the sagittal suture between the parietal bones, where a sickle-shaped double sheet, the **falx cerebri**, passes down between the two cerebral hemispheres ending in a free lower border above the corpus callosum (Figure 8.5). Another reflection is found along the upper border of the posterior cranial fossa and forms a sheet between the cerebral hemispheres and cerebellum, the **tentorium cerebelli**, roofing the posterior cranial fossa and pierced by the brainstem. The **venous sinuses** carrying venous blood from the brain are formed between the dural layers at the points of reflection and in the free border of the falx cerebri (Figure 8.5). The meningeal arteries lie between the dura mater and bone and mainly supply the bones. The **middle meningeal arteries** are the most prominent and produce grooves in the bones radiating from the foramen spinosum as they ramify across the walls of the middle cranial fossa. The **arachnoid mater** consists of very slender fibres adherent to the inner surface of the dura mater. Fine strands pass across the subarachnoid space to the **pia mater**, which also consists of delicate fibres (Figure 8.4). The arteries and veins enter and leave the brain through the pia and are surrounded by a covering of pia as they pierce the brain.

Any of the blood vessels within the cranial cavity can be damaged by head injuries or cerebrovascular disease. Bleeding inside the skull is potentially very serious requiring urgent medical treatment. The skull is rigid so any blood leakage will lead to raised **intracranial pressure** and compress the

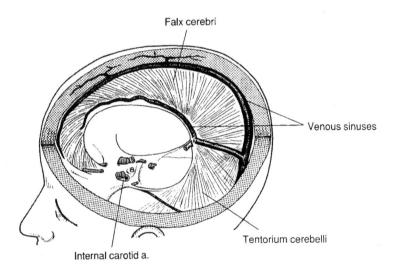

Figure 8.5 The dural reflections within the cranial cavity.

softer brain tissue which is usually fatal if left untreated. Intracranial haemorrhage is classified by the blood vessels which are damaged. In some areas, the skull bones are quite thin and blows to the head may damage the underlying meningeal arteries. This is **extradural haemorrhage** and the resultant blood loss is quite voluminous but has little room to spread because of the firm attachment of the dura to the bone. Local pressure at the site builds up, eventually producing coma and death. The onset of symptoms is usually very rapid and emergency treatment is required to relieve the pressure on the brain. This is achieved by drilling a hole through the skull above the middle meningeal artery at a site one thumb's breadth posterior to the lateral orbital margin and one thumb's breadth above the zygomatic arch. **Subdural haemorrhage** is due to damage to veins crossing from the surface of the brain to drain into the venous sinuses. It is commoner than extradural haemorrhage and may be the result of blows to the front or back of the head. Accumulation of blood can be acute or chronic, lasting several months. Again, raised intracranial pressure is relieved by drilling a hole in the skull. Blood loss into the subarachnoid space (**subarachnoid haemorrhage**) causes meningeal irritation and may present a variety of symptoms of rapid onset. It can be caused by rupture of an aneurysm (see Chapter 4) or by tearing of blood vessel walls after a fall. This is particularly so in elderly clients in which the walls of vessels lose some of their elasticity and are therefore more fragile. Loss of consciousness is a common sequel, but if not, vomiting occurs with severe headache and the patient becomes confused and irritable. In subarachnoid haemorrhage, blood is present in CSF. According to the exact location of the haemorrhage, local pressure on cranial nerves may produce specific symptoms (see Chapter 11). Cerebral haemorrhage is bleeding into the brain itself following rupture of arteries or veins penetrating the brain tissue. It produces a variety of symptoms depending upon the location of the damaged vessel.

The spinal cord and spinal nerves

The spinal cord is divided into segments with its corresponding pair of **spinal nerves** attached. Each spinal nerve is a mixed nerve containing sensory and motor axons. In addition, some spinal nerves contain autonomic axons. These all run along a common pathway in the peripheral course of the nerve but become partially segregated near the spinal cord. The incoming **afferent** sensory nerves form a **dorsal root** to enter the dorsal aspect of the corresponding spinal segment (Figures 6.5 and 8.6). The nerve cell bodies of these sensory neurons form a sensory **dorsal root ganglion** on the dorsal root. The outgoing **efferent** motor axons, together with any autonomic axons arising from that segment, form the **ventral root** leaving the ventral aspect of the corresponding segment. The ventral root joins the dorsal root to form the mixed spinal nerve, then leaves the spinal canal through the intervertebral foramen to innervate structures in the body. The **spinal cord** completes its growth before maturity is attained and as a result does not fill the whole of the spinal canal in the vertebral column. In the adult, it extends down about as far as the second lumbar vertebra. Consequently, the dorsal and ventral roots of the lower thoracic, lumbar and sacral spinal nerves pass down the canal for some distance to their corresponding intervertebral foramina. Below the third lumbar vertebra, the vertebral canal only contains the roots of the spinal nerves. A lumbar puncture to remove cerebrospinal fluid is often of diagnostic value and can be performed safely below this level. A needle is introduced between the fully flexed lumbar vertebrae through the dura lining the spinal canal into the subarachnoid space and fluid is withdrawn for analysis. As the spinal cord terminates above this level, there are only free-floating roots of the lower lumbar and sacral nerves present which will not be damaged. Epidural anaesthetics, often given to reduce pain in childbirth, are administered by the same route.

The 12 pairs of **cranial nerves** form the other major components of the PNS. The cranial nerves vary in the type of nerves they contain, some being purely motor nerves and others being mixed motor and sensory nerves, with or without an autonomic component. The cranial nerves are

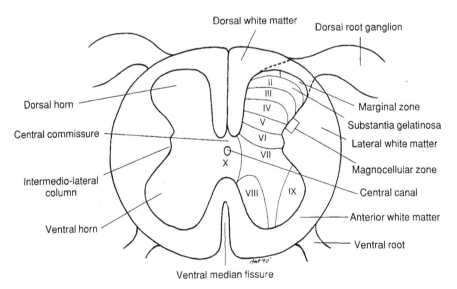

Figure 8.6 The spinal cord in cross section showing the subdivisions of grey and white matter.

connected to the brain and brainstem at various levels and are analogous in structure to spinal nerves. In some cranial nerves, the roots of the sensory fibres are less well segregated from the roots of the motor fibres than in spinal nerves but still have an aggregate of cell bodies at some point near the brain forming a cranial sensory ganglion.

The spinal cord

The internal structure of the spinal cord reflects the segregation of peripheral nerve function. Cut in cross-section, the spinal cord consists of a central H-shaped core of grey matter (Figure 8.6). The posterior arms of the H are the **dorsal horns** where the majority of sensory axons synapse and the anterior arms of the H are the **ventral horns** from which motor axons originate. The cross-piece of the H forms the **central commissure** where connections pass from one side of the spinal cord to the other. The **intermediolateral cell columns** (or more simply, the lateral horns) from which autonomic nerve fibres originate are found at the ends of the cross-piece of the H.

The grey matter is subdivided into a number of layers, the laminae of Rexed (Figure 8.6). Laminae I to VI are subdivisions of the dorsal horn and laminae VII to IX constitute the laminations of the ventral horn. Lamina IX contains the cell bodies of motor neurons innervating voluntary muscles. Lamina X forms the central commissure of the grey matter. An alternative and slightly simpler, older classification based upon the location, macroscopic and microscopic structure of the layers of cells in the dorsal horn is still used. The outer layer, corresponding to lamina I, is the **marginal zone** and beneath this is the **substantia gelatinosa**, the equivalent of lamina II. The deeper layers of the dorsal horn corresponding to laminae III to VI contain quite large cells and because of this are sometimes referred to collectively as the **magnocellular zone**. Some layers receive different types of nerves or different information from peripheral nerves or are the origins of motor nerves. Some laminae are the points of origin of tracts conveying information from the spinal cord to the brain or are the terminations of tracts bringing information to the spinal cord from the brain. These ascending and descending tracts travel in the white matter of the spinal cord which surrounds the H of grey matter (Figure 8.6). The white matter lying between the dorsal and ventral horns on each side is the **lateral white matter**. A deep **ventral median fissure** divides the **anterior white matter** lying between the ventral horns into two halves but the **dorsal white matter** lying between the dorsal horns is only incompletely divided anatomically. Functionally, however, it is divided into right and left dorsal white matter.

The hindbrain

The spinal cord is continuous above with the hindbrain through the foramen magnum in the base of the skull. The hindbrain itself comprises the **medulla oblongata**, an upward continuation of the spinal cord, the **pons** and the **cerebellum** (see Figure 6.6). Two prominent vertical ridges, the **pyramids**, lie on the ventral surface of the medulla oblongata near the midline. These demarcate the routes of the major motor pathways from the brain to the spinal cord; these pathways decussate at the **pyramidal decussation** just above the junction of the medulla and spinal cord. Lateral to the pyramids are two bulges, the **olives**, which enclose the superior and inferior olivary nuclei. The superior olivary nuclei are part of the auditory pathways from the ears to the brain (see Chapter 23) and the inferior olivary nuclei have connections to the cerebellum. The gracile and cuneate nuclei, important synaptic sites in the dorsal column pathways (see Chapter 9), form two bulges on either side of the dorsal midline of the medulla. The pons is a bulbous part of the hindbrain. The **cerebellum**, consisting of two incompletely separated lobes, is attached to the posterior aspect of the medulla, pons and midbrain which are known collectively as the **brainstem**. The cerebellum is connected to the brainstem through three pairs of **cerebellar peduncles** of white matter. The inferior peduncles carry pathways connecting the cerebellum to the lower brainstem and spinal cord, the middle peduncles connect the cerebellum with the pons and the superior peduncles run into the midbrain carrying connections between the cerebellum and cerebral hemispheres. The **fourth ventricle**, one of the spaces in the brain containing cerebrospinal fluid, lies on the posterior aspect of the medulla and pons and is bounded by the cerebellar peduncles and cerebellum to produce a pyramidal space with the base on the brainstem and apex on the cerebellum. The sixth to twelfth cranial nerves are attached to the medulla and the fifth nerve to the pons.

The midbrain

The **midbrain** is a small upward continuation of the brainstem connecting the pons to the forebrain (Figure 8.1). It is pierced longitudinally by the **cerebral aqueduct** which connects the fourth ventricle with the **third ventricle** in the forebrain. The aqueduct demarcates the junction between the posterior part of the midbrain known as the **tectum** and the larger anterior area, the **cerebral peduncles**. The tectum is unique to this part of the brain and has two pairs of bulges on its posterior surface, the **superior** and **inferior colliculi** which are involved in visual and auditory reflexes respectively (Figures 8.1 and 8.7). The cerebral peduncles are subdivided into the **basis pedunculi** (or crus cerebri) contains prominent tracts of descending white matter and the **tegmentum** which contains other fibre tracts. The basis pedunculi is separated from the tegmentum by the **substantia nigra**, a prominent area of darkly pigmented grey matter which is functionally part of the basal ganglia. The **red nuclei**, which have important connections with the cerebellum, lie within the tegmentum.

The **internal structure of the brainstem** is more complex than that of the spinal cord. The white matter tracts on the outside of the cord continue through the brainstem but do not necessarily retain their relative positions. The major change lies in the organization of the grey matter. It becomes discontinuous and is broken up into discrete **nuclei**. These nuclei of cell bodies and synapses have a variety of functions in the brainstem, such as providing the central connections for cranial nerve axons, connections to the cerebellum and relay nuclei on ascending and descending tracts through the brainstem for processing and transforming information. In the upper medulla and pons, a great number of transverse nerve tracts run between the nuclei of grey matter giving the whole area a net-like appearance; this is known as the **reticular formation,** which arouses the brain in response to incoming sensory information and is also an important relay station for ascending sensory pathways and descending motor tracts and is important in arousal.

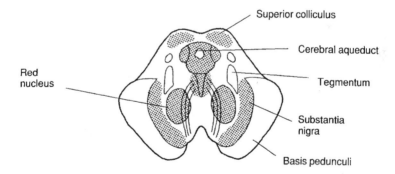

Figure 8.7 A cross section through the midbrain at the level of the superior colliculi.

The forebrain

The forebrain consists of the two cerebral hemispheres forming the **telen-cephalon** on either side of a region of grey matter immediately above the brainstem, known as the **diencephalon** (Figure 8.1). The diencephalon consists of the paired masses of the **thalamus** and **hypothalamus** with the slit-like **third ventricle** lying between them. The **hypothalamus** lies below and anterior to the thalamus and is connected to the pea-sized **pituitary gland**, an endocrine organ, by the **pituitary stalk** (Figure 8.1). The thalamus has several functions. All sensory pathways, except olfactory pathways, synapse in the thalamus en route to the cerebral cortex. Several pathways linking different parts of the cerebral hemispheres form circuits by passing through the thalamus. Similar circuits connect the cortex and the basal ganglia (see below). The hypothalamus regulates activity in the autonomic nervous system and the pituitary gland (see Chapter 7).

The **telencephalon** consists of the two cerebral hemispheres covered by a relatively thin strip of grey matter known as the **cerebral cortex** (Figure 8.8). The hemispheres have a convoluted surface to increase the area of the outer layer of the brain to about 2.5 m². The outward folds of cortex are **gyri** and the intervening clefts are **sulci**; very deep sulci are called **fissures**. For descriptive purposes, the hemispheres are divided into **lobes** corresponding approximately to the overlying bones. Viewed from the lateral aspect, there is a prominent **lateral fissure** between the **temporal lobe** below and the **frontal** and **parietal** lobes above. The frontal and parietal lobes are separated by the **central sulcus**, the frontal lobe lying anteriorly (Figure 8.1). The parietal lobe and **occipital lobe**, which forms the posterior pole of each hemisphere (or **cerebrum**), are not clearly distinguished laterally but on the medial surface of each

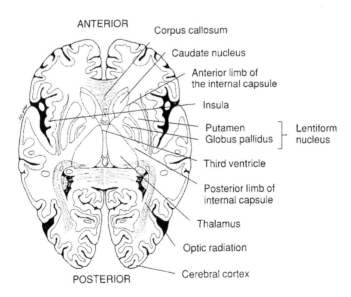

Figure 8.8 A horizontal section through the cerebral hemispheres to show the internal structures.

hemisphere, the **parieto-occipital fissure** forms the borderline between them. Another lobe in each hemisphere, the **insula**, is hidden beneath the other lobes and can only be seen by opening the lateral fissure. Sometimes, the area of the brain which encircles the diencephalon is distinguished as the cingulate lobe. It lies above the corpus callosum and the adjacent hemispheres above, separated from them by the cingulate sulcus. The two hemispheres are connected by a prominent band of transversely-oriented commissural nerve fibres, the **corpus callosum** which arches up over the thalamus.

Although most of the sulci and gyri are named, only a few of them need to be memorized as they are significant functional areas of clinical importance and will be met with again in subsequent chapters. The **cingulate gyri** lie immediately above the corpus callosum on the medial aspect of each hemisphere (Figure 8.1). On the lateral aspect of each hemisphere (Figure 6.7), the **precentral** and **postcentral gyri** lie anterior and posterior to the **central sulcus**. These are the primary motor and sensory areas respectively. Anterior to the inferior part of the precentral gyrus is a triangular gyrus known as the **frontal operculum** which forms part of **Broca's area**. On the superior surfaces of each temporal lobe, three prominent gyri, **the transverse temporal gyri**, run transversely into the lateral fissure: these are the location of the primary auditory cortex. The posterior end of the lateral fissure divides into two short sulci and the intervening triangular gyrus is the **angular gyrus** (Figure 13.1). Another prominent gyrus runs superior to the lateral fissure between the inferior part of the postcentral gyrus and the angular gyrus: this is the **supramarginal gyrus**. The angular and supramarginal gyri are both important in language processing (Figure 13.1).

Internally, the forebrain has other large areas of grey matter in addition to the thalamus and hypothalamus. The prominent **lentiform nucleus** lies lateral to the thalamus (Figure 8.8). In horizontal section, the lentiform nucleus lies anterolaterally to the thalamus. The nucleus has two subdivisions, the outer **putamen** and the inner paler area, the **globus pallidus**. An elongated C-shaped nucleus, the **caudate nucleus**, which is continuous with the anterior part of the lentiform nucleus, arches above the thalamus and descends behind it. These two nuclei are part of the system known as the **basal ganglia** which also include other structures (see Chapter 10). The lentiform nucleus is separated from the caudate nucleus and thalamus by a prominent band of white matter describing a shallow V with its apex pointing medially known as the **internal capsule** (Figure 8.8). The internal capsule carries fibre tracts between the cortex, the thalamus, the caudate and lentiform nuclei, the brainstem and spinal cord. The caudate and lentiform nuclei and the intervening white matter are known as the **striate cortex**.

The ventricular system and cerebrospinal fluid

Cerebrospinal fluid fills the ventricular system, spinal canal and surrounds the brain and spinal cord in the subarachnoid space. It is similar in some respects to blood plasma but has a very low concentration of proteins and few, if any, cells. It is produced by a combination of filtration of plasma and metabolic pumping of plasma constituents, particularly ions, by the **choroid plexus** in the ventricles of the brain. The choroid plexus consists of a delicate membrane of ependymal cells overlying a rich capillary network.

The **ventricles** are large cavities in the centre of the CNS lined with ependymal cells, a type of glial cell. The paired **lateral ventricles** lie in the cerebral hemispheres and are approximately C-shaped with the convex curvature posteriorly; the anterior part is in the frontal lobe and the inferior part loops down into the temporal lobe (Figure 8.9). An extension, the posterior horn, lies in the occipital lobe. The lateral ventricles communicate with the slit-like **third ventricle** through **interventricular foramina**. The third ventricle lies between the two halves of the thalamus and posteriorly the **cerebral aqueduct** passes from the third ventricle through the midbrain to open into the **fourth ventricle**. The fourth ventricle is a flattened pyramid with its base on the posterior surface of the medulla oblongata and pons and its roof and apex are formed by the cerebellum and cerebellar peduncles. The **central canal** of the spinal cord is the extension of the fourth ventricle into the spinal cord.

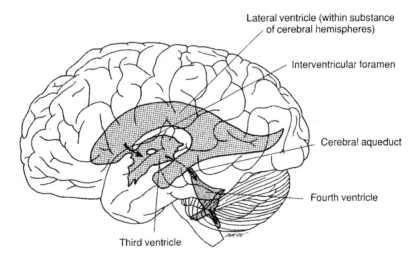

Lateral ventricle (within substance of cerebral hemispheres)

Interventricular foramen

Cerebral aqueduct

Fourth ventricle

Third ventricle

Figure 8.9 The ventricular system and circulation of cerebrospinal fluid.

The fourth ventricle communicates with the **subarachnoid space** through foramina in the pia mater (see above).

Cerebrospinal fluid is produced in the lateral and third ventricle although the fourth ventricle also makes a contribution. CSF flows backwards and downwards from the lateral ventricles into the third ventricle, the aqueduct and fourth ventricles and thence into the subarachnoid space. It is resorbed into the venous system through **arachnoid granulations** in the venous sinuses and along cranial and spinal nerves. CSF is produced at the rate of about 0.3–0.4 ml per minute but as the total CSF volume is only 100–150 ml, this is sufficient to effect a complete change three or four times a day. As well as providing a supportive and cushioning function, CSF also has a nutritive function and serves as a sink for various metabolic products of brain metabolism and may be a pathway for hormone-like messengers to reach the brain.

If circulation of CSF is impaired, continued CSF production leads to local accumulation above the level of the block. The most common site for blockage of the ventricular system is the cerebral aqueduct. The accumulation of CSF is known as **hydrocephalus** and often arises as a congenital condition frequently associated with a **spina bifida** defect. Spina bifida occurs when the separate ossicles forming the spinous processes of the vertebrae fail to fuse, most frequently in the lumbosacral region. As a result, the meninges surrounding the spinal cord and sometimes the cord itself protrude through the defect and become tethered to the adjacent tissue. The circulation of CSF around the spinal cord may thus be impaired. The resultant pressure increase consequent upon hydrocephalus will distort both the brain and the overlying skull and may cause mental subnormality. However, in some cases, distortion of the brain does not impair function but merely displaces structures so that the cortex exists as a thin rim around enlarged ventricles. Excess CSF may be removed by introducing a drain into the ventricles and running it subcutaneously into one of the superficial veins in the neck. Alternatively, the choroid plexus in the blocked parts of the system may be cauterized to stop fluid production.

The blood supply and venous drainage of the brain

The arterial supply of the brain is derived from two pairs of arteries, the internal carotid and the vertebral arteries. Arteries supplying the brain that arise from the **internal carotid arteries** are known collectively as the anterior circulation. Those arising from the **vertebral arteries** and their continuation, the **basilar artery**, are called the posterior (or **vertebrobasilar**) circulation. The internal carotid arteries branch from the common carotid arteries in the neck and enter the cranial cavity via the carotid canals in the petrous temporal bones. They emerge from the carotid canals and pass through the cavernous sinuses lying on either side of the pituitary fossa to terminate as the paired **anterior** and **middle cerebral** arteries on each side (Figure 8.10).

The **vertebral arteries** arise from the subclavian arteries in the neck and run through **transverse foramina** in the cervical vertebra. They leave this bony canal and then enter the cranial cavity through the **foramen magnum**. The vertebral arteries run up the anterior surface of the medulla and unite to form the single **basilar artery** at the cranial end of the medulla (Figure 8.10). Anterior and posterior spinal arteries branch from the vertebral arteries to supply the spinal cord. The cerebellum is supplied by three pairs of arteries (Figure 8.10). The **posterior** and **anterior inferior cerebellar arteries** supply its inferior surface and the **superior cerebellar arteries** supply its superior surface. All these arteries also supply the lateral medulla oblongata as do the small **medullary** and **pontine** arteries arising from the vertebral and basilar arteries. The basilar artery terminates at the level of the midbrain by dividing into the paired **posterior cerebral arteries**. Several smaller arteries arise from the

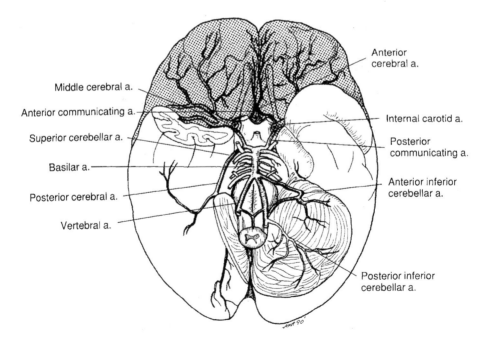

Figure 8.10 The arterial supply of the brain.

vertebral and basilar arteries to supply the spinal cord, brainstem and cerebellum (Figure 8.10).

An important principle underlies the organization of the blood supply to the brainstem. It is arranged in wedges from medial to lateral aspects. Close to the midline the brainstem is supplied by branches from the vertebral and basilar arteries, named according to the regions they supply, so there are medullary and pontine arteries. More laterally, the cerebellar arteries supply the brainstem. The lateral medulla is supplied by the posterior inferior cerebellar arteries, the pons by the anterior inferior cerebellar arteries and the midbrain by the superior cerebellar arteries. This arrangement is clinically significant because damage to these arteries gives a specific set of symptoms according to the structures underlying them and supplied by them. Lateral medullary syndrome (Wallenberg's syndrome) is described in Chapter 21.

The terminal branches of the internal carotid and basilar arteries are linked by communicating branches to form the **cerebral arterial circle of Willis** (Figure 8.10). The three terminal pairs of cerebral arteries supply the two cerebral hemispheres by ramifying across their surfaces. In addition, multiple small branches from the arteries pierce the brain substance on its undersurface through areas known as **perforated substance** to supply the deep structures of the brain.

The cerebral cortex itself is supplied by branches arising from the main distribution of the arteries as they ramify over the brain surface in the subarachnoid space (Figure 8.11). The **anterior cerebral arteries** supply the medial surface of the cerebral hemispheres as far back as the occipital lobes, and the **middle cerebral arteries** supply the corresponding lateral surface of each hemisphere. The occipital lobes and the inferior surfaces of the temporal lobes are supplied by the **posterior cerebral arteries** (Figure 8.11).

Once they have penetrated the brain itself, the arteries of the brain are true **end arteries** and there are comparatively few anastomoses between the arteries on the pial surface of the brain (see Chapter 4). Loss of blood supply to a given area, whether from occlusion or rupture of the blood vessel, will result in death of the brain tissue in that area in most cases. Because the actual cause of blood vessel dysfunction is often unknown, such lesions are referred to as a **cerebrovascular accident** (CVA) or, in lay terms, **stroke**. Extravasation of blood is accompanied by an inflammatory reaction which can cause additional tissue damage. The clotting, demolition and resolution phases of inflammation which remove extravasated blood (see Chapter 3) usually produce more severe widespread acute effects than those produced by chronic anoxic loss of brain tissue.

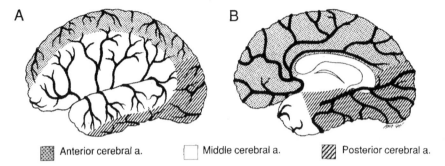

Anterior cerebral a.   Middle cerebral a.   Posterior cerebral a.

Figure 8.11 The distribution of the cerebral arteries to the cerebral hemispheres. (A) Lateral view. (B) Medial view.

The cerebral arterial circle of Willis

The cerebral arterial circle of Willis links the three major vessels supplying the brain by communicating arteries (Figure 8.10). The posterior cerebral arteries, the terminal branches of the basilar artery, are connected to the internal carotid arteries by the **posterior communicating arteries**, and the **anterior communicating artery** links the two anterior cerebral arteries. Thus the three major vessels supplying the cerebrum are linked either directly or indirectly. It has been claimed that the cerebral arterial circle functions as a collateral circulation if one of the major arteries supplying the brain is occluded. However, in the majority of cases, the circle is either anatomically incomplete or the communicating vessels are so narrow that doubts must be cast on the arterial circle functioning in this way. Furthermore, in normal individuals, the major arteries only supply their own terminal area, with no cross-flow between the vessels at the circle of Willis. The formation of the cerebral arterial circle is probably due to the embryonic formation and derivation of the cerebral arteries.

The **anterior cerebral arteries** from the internal carotid arteries pass forward between the two hemispheres and turn back over the corpus callosum to supply the medial surface of the frontal lobe of the hemispheres and a strip about 1 cm wide on the upper lateral surface (Figure 8.11). The primary somatosensory and somatomotor lower limb areas are included in its territory so that vascular accident would cause sensory and motor losses in the contralateral leg.

The **middle cerebral arteries** pass laterally into the lateral fissure where they run deeply between the frontal and temporal lobes before emerging on to the lateral surface of each hemisphere (Figure 8.11). The field of distribution of each middle cerebral artery includes most of the somatomotor and somatosensory areas, the auditory cortex and both

Broca's and Wernicke's speech areas, as well as much association cortex. The effects of damage to the middle cerebral artery are therefore far-reaching.

The **posterior cerebral arteries** wind around the midbrain to reach the medial and inferior surface of the temporal lobes and the occipital lobes (Figure 8.11). The most important area included in their field of supply is the visual cortex. Loss of blood supply therefore causes blindness in the contralateral temporal and ipsilateral nasal fields of vision, resulting in loss of vision on one side of the visual field.

Central (perforating) arteries

The deep parts of the cerebral hemispheres, the basal ganglia, thalamus and internal capsules are supplied by **central** (or **perforating**) arteries which arise from the major cerebral vessels in the region of the cerebral arterial circle of Willis. Several groups of central arteries can be identified. The **anterior group** from the anterior and middle cerebral arteries enter the brain through the **anterior perforated substance** which lies at the central end of the olfactory nerve, to supply the hypothalamus, basal ganglia and much of the internal capsule. The **posteromedial group** are branches of the posterior cerebral artery and enter the brain substance through the **posterior perforated substance** between the cerebral peduncles on the anterior surface of the midbrain. They supply the thalamus and hypothalamus. The **posterolateral** group supplies the posterior thalamus and the midbrain.

The central branches are relatively small and prone to rupture. It is often as a result of loss of blood supply to parts of the internal capsule that the classical upper motor neuron lesion of spastic paralysis is observed (see Chapter 6). This is due to loss of the many direct and indirect corticospinal tracts and loop systems of the motor pathways which pass through the internal capsule. The initial symptoms of a stroke are often very widespread but regress as extravascular blood is removed, leaving only those symptoms resulting from damage to a particular area of the brain.

The venous drainage of the brain

Veins from within the substance of the brain drain into veins on the surface which, in turn, drain into the **venous sinuses** lying at the lines of dural reflection and in the free border of the **falx cerebri** (Figure 8.5). They terminate at the jugular foramina from which the **internal jugular veins** continue extracranially. The inferior aspects of the brain drain into a complex of small sinuses around the pituitary fossa known as the

cavernous sinuses. These drain backwards into the internal jugular veins at the jugular foramen.

In old age, blood vessel walls become thinner and they are therefore more prone to rupture. The veins are prone to damage as they cross the subarachnoid space from the brain surface to the venous sinuses from head injuries or violent movement. Blood will leak into the subarachnoid space and produce a subarachnoid haemorrhage (see above).

Although most cerebral venous blood leaves the cranial cavity through the internal jugular veins, about 20 per cent leaves via a series of **emissary veins** which connect various venous sinuses with the superficial venous drainage of the scalp and face, especially round the orbital and nasal cavities (see Chapter 19) and through the major named foramina or minor foramina. All these veins lack valves and blood can flow in both directions according to the differences in venous pressure. The interconnections between the venous drainage of the face and the venous sinuses are a potential route for spread of infection into the sinuses and meninges.

Because of the structure of the cavernous sinuses, partitioned by septa of dura into many interconnected cavities, infected blood is prone to stasis and thrombosis here. As well as the high fever consequent on the infection, other structures passing through the cavernous sinus are damaged, in particular the nerves supplying the muscles moving the eye but, more importantly, the internal carotid artery.

Head injuries

The brain and spinal cord are completely enclosed by the meninges and surrounding bones of the skull and vertebral column. Anything which raises the intracranial pressure will therefore compress the brain as the pressure can neither escape nor be relieved by physiological means. Raised intracranial pressure may occur through inflammation of the brain, for example, after trauma producing cerebral oedema or inflammation of the meninges, through bacterial or viral infections leading to meningitis. Loss of blood from the arterial supply or venous drainage of the brain into the cranial cavity also increases intracranial pressure. Irrespective of the cause, the effect is the same: the brain is compressed and the medulla oblongata is pushed down through the foramen magnum into the spinal canal for which it is too wide. The medulla oblongata is therefore compressed and as it contains the respiratory and cardiovascular centres, these are depressed leading to coma and, if left untreated, death. This is known in medical jargon as 'coning'.

The weight of the brain is about 1500 g but because it is floating in cerebrospinal fluid the apparent weight is reduced considerably. The CSF has a cushioning effect on the brain in normal circumstances which is supplemented by the dural reflections, the falx cerebri and tentorium cerebelli. However, these systems are not fail-safe. Sudden violent acceleration or deceleration movements of the head can cause the brain to impinge on the bone and meninges. As an example, boxers' heads are continually subject to violent movement by blows to the head and the frontal and occipital lobes knock against the bones. Boxers often develop a disease known as 'punch drunkenness' long after their active boxing career has finished. Due to repeated trauma, small haemorrhages develop in the occipital and frontal lobes leading to blindness through their effects on the visual cortex and behavioural changes due to their effect on the frontal association cortex (see Chapter 10).

Most head injuries are usually the result of sudden violent impact. Head injuries are differentiated as **open head injuries**, if the cranial cavity is breached by the injury, and **closed head injuries** if the cranium remains intact. The short-term and long-term effects of the two types of injury may be quite different.

In **closed head injuries**, there may be little or no overt signs of injury; the scalp may not be damaged and bones may not be broken. However, the brain may still be damaged, particularly after fractures which cause depression of the skull bones. The damage may be diffuse or focal or a combination of both, and is dependent upon the force and extent of the impact and the shearing forces on the brain. Diffuse damage in its mildest form produces concussion with loss of consciousness, and with confusion and amnesia on recovery of consciousness. More severe injuries will cause compression and tearing of the brain and usually haemorrhage. Closed head injuries almost inevitably lead to some period of loss of consciousness. The client may have no memory of events leading to the trauma or of events in the recovery period: this is **post-traumatic amnesia**. Obviously, the specific effects resulting from closed head injuries depend on the area of the brain which is traumatized. The language areas are as vulnerable as any others and dysphasia may result, with or without other signs and symptoms. As injury is often diffuse, specific defects are often accompanied by memory loss and perceptual and behavioural problems, making this group of clients particularly challenging for the therapist. It has been said that clients with head injuries talk better than they communicate, there may be minimal disturbances of language and speech, but the other effects on memory and behaviour make communication bizarre; conversational skills, including such aspects as turn taking, are often disturbed and disturbing.

Open head injuries, from trauma or gunshot wounds, result in indriven bone fragments and haemorrhage but as the cranial cavity is opened, there is a likelihood of infection with oedema and abscess formation. Neurosurgical treatment aims to remove debris, blood clots, bone fragments and missile fragments if present. Post-traumatic epilepsy develops in about 50 per cent of open head injuries but is rarely a sequel to closed head injuries. Once again, the extent, severity and location of injury on the brain will determine the effects.

Imaging the brain

Until quite recently, much of the knowledge of the structure of the brain, its workings and the functional localization within the brain depended upon careful clinical observation followed by investigation of the brain after death to see which areas were affected. Many other techniques were used to supplement these neuropathological observations. Angiography of the cerebral blood supply by injection of radio-opaque dyes into the carotid or vertebral arteries, recording and stimulation of the brain during operation and recording of surface electrical activity of the brain by electroencephalograms all added to the understanding of the human brain. In addition, experimental studies on animals were used to trace pathways and connections by using special microscopical techniques to trace the destination of dyes injected at one end of a pathway. Although these experiments are performed on animals whose brains show the same overall pattern as the human brain, they do not compare in certain respects, especially in the complexity and extent of the cortex. Thus information on certain aspects of neuroanatomy and function is still sparse.

In the last two decades or so, there has been a major expansion in the methods available for study of the living brain. Non-invasive techniques have been developed which enable some of the functional aspects of the human nervous system to be studied in the living brain.

Computer assisted tomography (CAT), commonly referred to as brain scanning, is the technique of using a narrow beam of X-rays to examine a slice of tissue. As either the X-ray source and recording apparatus are moved across the patient, whole areas can be scanned. The resulting X-ray images are stored in a computer and individual slices through the brain can then be reconstructed on a display screen, using artificial colour graphics to enhance contrast (Figure 8.12). In this way, lesions can be precisely identified and their extent defined and correlated with clinical signs and symptoms. An example of the knowledge gained from CAT scanning is the correlation of location of brain lesions with different types of speech defects, the aphasias.

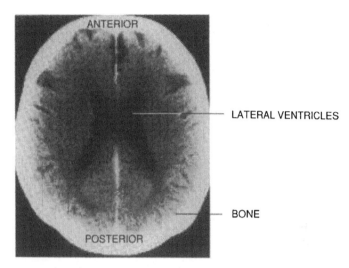

Figure 8.12 A CAT scan of the brain.

More recently, **magnetic resonance imaging (MRI)** has been applied to biological tissues (Figure 8.13). The spin of the millions of charged atomic nuclei making up the tissues are aligned by placing them in a magnetic field. A radio frequency impulse applied across the magnetic field causes the nuclei to behave like small gyroscopes and spin in a conical fashion. When the radio frequency is switched off, the gyrating atomic nuclei emit measurable electromagnetic radiation as they return back to their original alignment. Again, a slice principle linked to computers is used to obtain a record. MRI imaging has potential advantages over CAT, in that individual atomic nuclei behave quite differently and therefore some metabolic processes may be studied where specific elements or their isotopes are involved. MRI is available in most major hospitals.

Functional MRI imaging **(fMRI)** is an extension of this type of imaging and relies on the fact that molecules in different regions behave differently when exposed to magnetic fields. In particular, concentrations of iron-containing haemoglobin in the blood contrast with neural tissue. The local blood flow to specific areas of the brain increases when these regions are active so fMRI can be used to monitor local blood flow and detect brain areas involved in particular functions.

Positron emission tomography (PET scanning) can also be used to study the function of different areas of the living brain. The patient breathes in a very short-lived positron-emitting isotope of one of the inert gases and this is taken up in the functioning area of the brain as that area

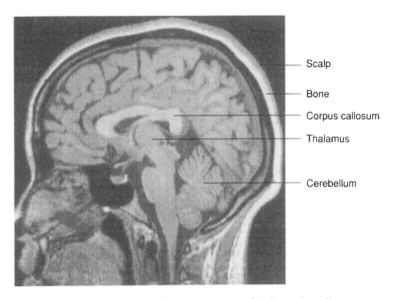

Figure 8.13 An MRI scan of the human brain. (Courtesy of Dr Patty Cowell.)

uses oxygen. The positrons cause secondary emission of X-rays which are detected using arrays of gamma cameras. The brain needs a constant supply of blood glucose and oxygen as it has virtually no metabolic reserves to fall back on. Blood flow to particular regions increases as they are used, so by administering appropriate isotopes, brain glucose and oxygen utilization and therefore the areas used for a particular activity can also be monitored using PET scanning (Figure 8.14). As the isotopes are short lived, only relatively simple tasks can be undertaken but these studies have increased our understanding of functional localization in the brain considerably (see Chapter 13).

Finally, **transcranial magnetic stimulation** can be used to determine the effect of stimulating nerve activity in superficial brain areas. Application of a magnetic field through a probe placed on the skin overlying the brain region of interest will stimulate nerve activity; the response can be monitored by observing muscular activity, for example. This method has considerably enhanced our understanding of some aspects of swallowing and dysphagia (see Chapter 21).

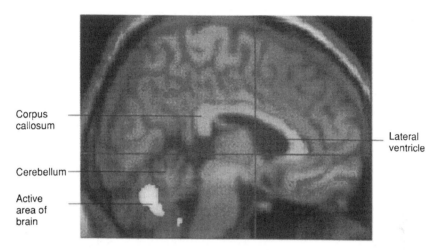

Corpus callosum

Cerebellum

Active area of brain

Lateral ventricle

Figure 8.14 A PET scan of the human brain. Activity in a brain region is indicated by intense white areas. In this example activity is in the cerebellum. (Courtesy of Prof. Rod Nicolson.)

CHAPTER 9

Sensory function and somatosensory pathways

The ways in which our CNS functions, the activity within it and the resultant actions are strongly, and sometimes solely, affected by the incoming sensory information we receive. Sensation occurs when the energy of a physical stimulus such as sound, pressure or light interacts with a specialized structure called a sensory receptor in such a way that the energy of that stimulus is converted (transduced) into activity within the nervous system. This activity is then relayed from the sensory receptor to the CNS by action potentials within the axons innervating those sensory receptors. The energy of a stimulus may excite a single receptor only, but more commonly many receptors are excited so that the CNS receives information from an array of receptors. Sensation may be received from a number of sources, including the skin, the mucosal lining of viscera, joints and muscles and specialized sensory organs for vision, hearing, balance, taste and olfaction. These sensations are used to perceive the external world and the internal state of our body, to keep us alert to changes within and outside our body and to control our movements and other aspects of motor function such as glandular secretion. This chapter deals with general aspects of the function of sensory systems and describes the pathways by which one group of sensations important for speech motor control, the somatosensory sensations, are relayed from the sensory receptors to the cerebral cortex. Another important sensation for speech control is hearing: the pathways relaying hearing to the cerebral cortex are described in Chapter 23.

There are many different kinds of physical energy to which we are exposed and no one group of animals is capable of detecting and responding to all the physical stimuli to which they are exposed. Man can hear vibrations in air as sounds over a frequency range of approximately 20–20 000 Hz but the hearing range of other animals extends to much higher frequencies. Similarly, we can detect light in our visible spectrum as a range of wavelengths that extends from red to purple: other animals, however, can see into the infrared or ultraviolet ranges. Different kinds of stimulus energies require different kinds of receptors. All sensory receptors are capable of responding to four basic features of a stimulus – its nature or **modality**, **location**, **intensity** and **duration** – and classification systems have been built on the first two of these properties.

Sensory receptors

Receptors may be classified into exteroceptors, proprioceptors and interoceptors. **Exteroceptors** respond to stimuli that originate from outside the body. They include both the receptors for the **special senses** of vision, hearing and balance and also the receptors that respond to touch and pressure on the skin. Touch is a broad term that is used to cover a range of stimuli from light pressure to dynamic touch – the ability to detect the direction and strength of a stimulus. **Proprioceptors** convey information from joints and muscles about the position of limbs in space, movement and muscle length and tension. **Interoceptors**, responding to **viscerosensation**, are located in internal organs and body cavities and monitor the state of the internal environment such as stretch or distension and painful stimuli from the viscera, as well as information from receptors specialized to monitor blood pressure or the chemical make up of the blood which is used to regulate the cardiovascular and respiratory systems. Sensations arising from the viscera are generally poorly localized: compare the accurate localization of the stimulus from touch or pain, such as a kick on the shin, with viscerosensation, for example, stomach ache.

Another way of classifying receptors depends on the nature of the stimulus and is now more commonly used than the classification system above. Receptors are classified into chemoreceptors, photoreceptors, thermoreceptors and mechanoreceptors. **Chemoreceptors** respond to a wide range of chemical stimuli, ranging from the senses of taste and smell to changes in blood oxygen or carbon dioxide concentrations or its pH. **Photoreceptors** detect light and are found in the eye. **Thermoreceptors** detect hot and cold stimuli. The most complex group are **mechanoreceptors** which detect physical deformation or change in shape or position of a structure. This category includes the touch and pressure receptors in the skin, **cutaneous receptors**, but extends to the cells in the ear and vestibular system that detect hearing and balance, receptors in muscles and joints that detect muscle length and joint position and even to the stretch receptors in the walls of certain major blood vessels that detect blood pressure. One group of receptors that are difficult to classify by either system are **nociceptors**, the pain receptors. Some stimuli are strong enough to damage tissues which release the products of that damage.

These products actually act as the stimulus for the pain receptor rather than the physical stimulus itself. Other pain receptors appear to respond to the physical stimuli of touch and heat but only at an intensity strong enough to be capable of causing damage rather than the stimuli of light touch or gentle warmth.

As described above, any stimulus has four fundamental characteristics: its nature or modality, its location, its duration and its intensity. The **modality** of a stimulus is signalled by the kind of receptor that is stimulated. Any receptor will only respond to a narrow range of stimulus energy and the nervous system is wired up in such a way that information from that receptor and the sensory neuron that innervates it is conveyed to the nervous system along a pathway specific for that type of stimulus. Furthermore, the stimuli are processed in particular regions of the brain and are generally segregated from different kinds of stimuli. These highly discrete specific wiring patterns are crucial in preserving information about the modality of individual stimuli but they are also important in conveying information about the location of a stimulus.

Any one sensory neuron that innervates a receptor or group of receptors responds not only to a particular type of stimulus, but also to stimuli from a particular location. This is easiest to understand in relation to receptors in the skin that respond to touch. A particular receptor responds to a stimulus that deforms the skin in a particular area. However, a single axon typically branches and supplies more than one sensory receptor so it will respond to a stimuli deforming a small patch of skin containing the receptors that it innervates. This is its **receptive field**. Other types of neuron have receptive fields: photoreceptors respond only to light in a particular part of space, and auditory receptors respond only to sound at particular frequencies. Again, this information is preserved by the way in which the nervous system is connected but the information can also be elaborated to enable the perception of complex stimuli. Information about the **intensity** and **duration** of a stimulus is conveyed by the fact that more intense and longer stimuli tend to produce more action potentials for longer periods of time. However, not all receptors respond to stimuli in exactly the same way. Some receptors respond to very weak stimuli, while other receptors require a more intense stimulus before they will fire an action potential. The magnitude of the stimulus that causes a neuron to generate action potentials is its **threshold**. Because thresholds vary, as the intensity of a stimulus increases, not only does the number of action potentials within any one axon rise, but the number of axons that respond also rises. This population effect is very important in signalling intensity. Some neurons respond to a long stimulus by showing a decline in the number of action potentials that they transmit. This is called **adaptation**. Neurons can be **slowly-adapting** or **fast-adapting**. Slowly-adapting receptors continue firing for a long time when the stimulus is applied but with a gradually declining rate. Fast-adapting receptors stop firing soon after a stimulus is applied but produce a further burst of action potentials when the stimulus ceases, thus responding to changes in stimulus intensity. Stimulus duration is coded by integrating the responses occurring in populations of neurons in just the same way as is done for intensity.

The way in which sensory receptors are activated is poorly understood. The mechanisms vary depending upon the nature of the stimulus responsible for exciting the receptor. In some chemoreceptors and photoreceptors of the special sensory organs, the receptors are attached to the nerves by synapses: the state of the receptor is signalled to the nerve by release of neurotransmitters from the receptor cell in response to biochemical changes induced by the stimulus. It is still not fully understood how mechanical stimuli cause nerve depolarization in mechanoreceptors. However, in those receptors where the mechanisms have been partly understood, transduction occurs because the stimulus changes the properties of ion channels within the membrane.

Sensory systems

The various sensory systems share a number of similarities in their organization, although the special senses show some distinctive features. In all cases, sensory information is processed in sequential stages in a series of relay nuclei throughout the central nervous system. The stimulus is conveyed from peripheral sensory receptors by **primary sensory neurons**, the sensory components of spinal and cranial nerves, to the spinal cord or brainstem where they synapse. The **second order neurons** or **thalamic projection neurons** carry the information to the thalamus where they synapse, but many have intermediate synapses in the reticular formation. Finally, information is conveyed to the cerebral cortex by **third order neurons**. This sequence of connections is called a **sensory pathway** which is the route taken by a group of axons of a particular function between two points in the CNS. Conventionally, pathways are illustrated by demonstrating the course taken within them by a representative axon or group of axons. The minimum number of neurons in a sensory pathway is three. However, this number may be increased by any number of intervening neurons, known as **interneurons**, found in the synaptic areas in the nuclei between the major neurons (Figure 9.1).

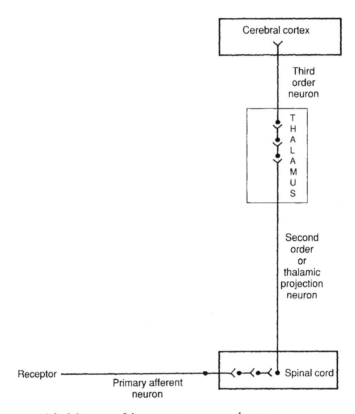

Figure 9.1 A simplified diagram of the somatosensory pathways.

Whatever the detailed arrangement of neurons in the spinal cord or brainstem, several general principles operate which also pertain to all synaptic areas. All the nuclei that are part of the ascending somatosensory pathways have much more complex functions than simple relay stations. These nuclei can keep information about modalities of sensation distinct or they can be combined. Depending on how important it is for the organism to discriminate each stimulus spatially, incoming information may converge or diverge. **Convergence** occurs when several primary afferent neurons send their information to one thalamic projection cell, thus losing some discrimination of the original source. **Divergence** is the converse: information is disseminated to a variety of neurons so that the effects are felt more widely. To accentuate the importance of information, **lateral inhibition** also occurs in many areas of the nervous system. The incoming axon, as well as passing on information to the next nerve in the pathway, has side-branches or **collaterals** which may inhibit adjacent cells thus cutting off potentially confusing information. Lateral inhibition sharpens the contrast between stimuli to increase the importance of particular signals. Nuclei frequently have mechanisms to screen out weak or intermittent signals. Taken together, these mechanisms ensure that only the strongest signals are transmitted and that they are clearly separated from background noise. All these mechanisms operate in the sensory areas of the spinal cord as well as other relay nuclei in ascending pathways.

Another important principle regarding organization of incoming information is that it is often arranged in a **somatotopic** fashion: neighbouring areas of the body are represented in neighbouring areas of the neural structure concerned. Thus, the information from discrete areas of the body is segregated. This arrangement is found to some extent in the spinal cord where information from a particular spinal nerve is arranged such that stimuli from the more distal part of the sensory field of the nerve lie most medially and more proximal areas lie most laterally within each segment of the spinal cord. Somatotopic projections are usually preserved throughout the whole of a particular nerve pathway.

The implications so far are that a given stimulus will activate a particular group of first order neurons which then transmit the information to the spinal cord. On a physiological level, this may be so, but psychologically, the perception and interpretation of a given stimulus depends not merely on simple all-or-none conduction in peripheral nerves, but on the threshold at which nerves fire, the intensity of firing, the time course and frequency of impulses and the area stimulated. All these variables are integrated in the spinal cord and, to some degree, are segregated to follow separate pathways within the central nervous system. This segregation may facilitate perception and interpretation when these signals reach the brain.

The remainder of this chapter describes the somatosensory pathways that convey somatic sensory information from the body and the head to the cerebral cortex. There are four modalities of somatic sensations:

- touch, including discriminative touch which is the ability to detect the direction and strength of a stimulus and is used to determine the size, shape and texture of objects;
- proprioception, which is sensations originating in muscles and joints;
- nociception, or the signalling of pain and tissue damage;
- temperature sensation.

These four sensations may be grouped together since the pathways that they take from the periphery to the cerebral cortex are, in part, common to all four modalities. As described in Chapter 6, there are two main pathways conveying somatic sensation from the body to the brain – the

dorsal column–medial lemniscal system and the **anterolateral system**. There are also pathways for proprioception from the body which partly overlap with and are partly separate from these other two. The pathways from the body are paralleled by similar pathways from the head. There is also a separate pathway for proprioception from the muscles and joints of the head. These somatosensory pathways from the head play a vital role in the motor control of speech. Touch sensation is vital for the control of articulation; anyone who has been to the dentist will have experienced the mild dysarthria that may accompany dental anaesthesia. In fact, the oral region possesses the highest concentration of mechanoreceptors anywhere in the body. These are vital in controlling articulation of any utterance in which two structures make contact and phonation whenever the vocal folds make contact. The production of open sounds, such as low vowels, requires proprioception to provide information about the state of muscle contraction and the position of joints; the muscles of the tongue and larynx have many proprioceptors. Perhaps less obviously, mechanoreception may be important during production of turbulence in the vocal tract such as fricatives when the additional air currents might be detected by this means. Somatic sensation from receptors in the thoracic cage, respiratory muscles and the lungs are vital in the control of ventilation, particularly that for speech.

Receptors and primary afferent neurons

The receptors for the cutaneous somatic sensation of touch, temperature and nociception are of two main structural types, encapsulated and unencapsulated. In **encapsulated endings**, the axons of sensory neurons are surrounded by some sort of connective tissue capsule. The capsule modifies the response of the receptors to mechanical stimuli in particular ways. Unencapsulated endings consist of free nerve endings ramifying through the skin, at their simplest, or endings which have accessory structures which do not actually surround the ending. Free nerve endings act as nociceptors, thermoreceptors in skin and some act as mechanoreceptors in muscles and joints.

Within muscle, there are also specialized proprioceptors called muscle spindles which are a particularly complex type of encapsulated ending. An outer capsule surrounds the middle of the spindle which contains specialized muscle fibres called **intrafusal fibres** to distinguish it from the **extrafusal muscle fibres** forming the bulk of the muscle. The intrafusal fibres are innervated by a special class of small **gamma motor neurons** so that contraction of intrafusal fibres can occur separately from that of the extrafusal fibres which are innervated by the larger **alpha motor neurons**. Large sensory afferent axons are wrapped around the centre of the intrafusal fibres and detect stretch of the fibres within the spindle. The ends of spindles are attached to extrafusal muscle fibres so that when the muscle contracts the spindles are stretched and the nerve endings excited. Contraction of gamma motor neurons can offload that stretch and so enable the sensitivity of the spindle to be varied. Muscle spindles are amongst the most complex of the receptors in the body. Their functions are still not fully understood but they appear to detect muscle length and tension. A second type of proprioceptor is the **Golgi tendon organ** which detects stretch in tendons produced by muscle contraction. Proprioceptors are also found in joints.

The cell bodies of the primary sensory neurons innervating somatosensory receptors are in the cranial sensory or dorsal root ganglia. A single short axon arises from each cell body, which soon divides into two axons. A peripheral axon terminates at a sensory receptor and a central axon terminates in the spinal cord or brainstem. The peripheral axons contribute to peripheral nerves and share a common pathway with motor and autonomic nerve axons originating from the same segment of the spinal cord. The central processes unite to form the dorsal root and enter the spinal cord or brainstem.

The spinal cord

The spinal cord is similar in structure throughout its length but functionally can be divided into 33 segments corresponding to the pairs of spinal nerves (see Chapter 8). Each spinal nerve supplies the myotomes and dermatomes corresponding to its segment (see Chapter 20).

The grey matter of the spinal cord is divided into different areas (the **laminae of Rexed**) on the basis of the density and size of the cells in each area. The central branches of the sensory axons enter the spinal cord and either terminate as segmental branches or form ascending or descending branches. The segmental branches terminate in the laminae which form the **marginal zone**, the **substantia gelatinosa** and **magnocellular zone** of the dorsal horn (see Figure 8.6). There is some segregation of axons carrying different modalities within these zones. Some segmental branches pass through the dorsal horn to end in the ventral horn by synapsing with interneurons or directly with motor neurons. Some segmental branches end directly on **thalamic projection** (second order) neurons located in the deeper laminae of the magnocellular zone, the marginal zone and laminae VII and VIII in the ventral horn; others, however, end on interneurons. Several interneurons may be found between the terminals of primary afferent neurons and thalamic projection neurons. Sensory information can therefore be modified at this level. Ascending branches carry sensory information superiorly either to the higher segments of the spinal cord or to the brainstem. Descending branches synapse on interneurons below their point of entry into the spinal cord.

Ascending sensory pathways

The segregation of particular sensory modalities found in the peripheral nerves and grey matter of the spinal cord is continued in the pathways which second order neurons take from the spinal cord to the brainstem and thalamus. The **dorsal column–medial lemniscal system** and **the anterolateral system** convey information from sensory receptors in the body to the cerebral cortex. The anterolateral system is not a single pathway, but consists of several pathways each with a different destination: these are the **spinothalamic tract**, the **spinoreticular tract** and the **spinomesencephalic tract** (Figure 9.2).

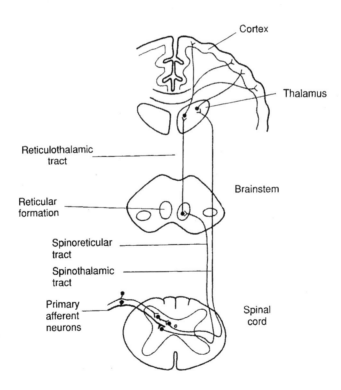

Figure 9.2 The anterolateral (spinoreticulothalamic and spinothalamic) pathways.

The dorsal column–medial lemniscal system

The **dorsal column–medial lemniscal system** conveys information about touch, particularly discriminative touch and vibratory sense, from the whole body and proprioception from the upper limb to the cerebral cortex. This pathway originates mostly from encapsulated receptors in the skin and proprioceptors including muscle spindles from the upper limb innervated mostly by large diameter myelinated axons with fast conduction velocities. The central processes of these axons enter the spinal cord in the dorsal roots. As these axons enter the spinal cord they divide into three branches. A segmental branch enters the dorsal horn and terminates either in the deeper laminae of the dorsal horn or in the ventral horn. A descending branch turns inferiorly to terminate in the dorsal horn of lower segments. An ascending branch enters the dorsal columns where it ascends to the medulla to synapse in the **dorsal column nuclei** (Figure 9.3).

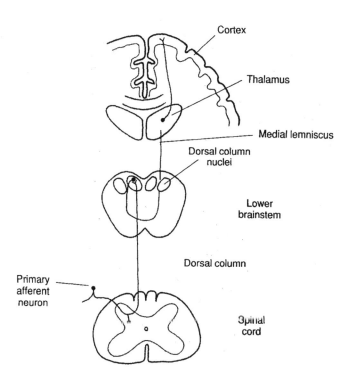

Figure 9.3 The dorsal column pathways.

There is a systematic relationship between the position of the ascending axons in the dorsal columns and the region of the body from which they originate. Each dorsal column is divided into two parts, the **gracile** and **cuneate fascicles**. The gracile fascicle contains axons originating from the lower half of the body while the cuneate fascicle contains axons originating from the upper half of the body. Within each fascicle, axons originating from progressively more superior parts of the body occupy a progressively more lateral location in the columns so that, when they reach the medulla, there is a representation of the entire body across the white matter with the sensory information from the leg being most medial and that from the neck being most lateral. This is an example of the somatotopic arrangement of pathways.

The **dorsal column nuclei** are located on the posterior aspect of the medulla oblongata and are somatotopically arranged. Axons within the gracile fascicle synapse in the medially situated gracile nucleus while those in the cuneate fascicle synapse in the cuneate nucleus. Much sensory processing is carried out within these nuclei including local synaptic inhibition producing lateral inhibition. Dorsal column axons synapse on second order neurons in the dorsal column nuclei and the axons of these neurons leave the nuclei, decussate and project to the thalamus. They join the **medial lemniscus** which is located medially in the medulla; axons from the gracile nucleus join the ventral part and axons from the cuneate nucleus join the dorsal part of the medial lemniscus, thus preserving the somatotopic arrangement of the pathway. The medial lemniscus ascends through the pons and midbrain to the **ventral posterior nucleus of the thalamus** where the axons within it synapse on third order neurons.

The classical view of the function of the dorsal column–medial lemniscal system was that it carried information of vibratory sensation, joint position and sensory discrimination. The modern view is that joint positional sense, at least for the lower limb, follows other complex routes in the spinal cord. Therefore, the main functional role of the dorsal column–medial lemniscal system is to enable complex discriminatory tasks to be carried out. Adjustment of grip when an object is slipping or discriminating the distance between two stimuli cannot be performed when the dorsal columns are damaged. Another function of the dorsal columns is to link together different regions of the spinal cord. In addition to the axons within the dorsal columns that ascend to the dorsal column nuclei, many other axons in the dorsal columns are **propriospinal**, linking different parts of the spinal cord and often travelling only a short distance. These mediate reflexes that coordinate upper and lower limb function and other tasks requiring integration of different regions of the spinal cord.

The anterolateral system

Information about pain, temperature and touch is carried to the cerebral cortex by the anterolateral system. The axons in this pathway ascend in the ventral and lateral white matter of the spinal cord. Axons in this pathway terminate in one of three destinations in the CNS, the thalamus, the reticular formation of the pons and medulla or the periaqueductal grey matter of the midbrain. This pathway originates mostly from unencapsulated receptors in skin and muscle. These receptors are innervated by small diameter myelinated and unmyelinated axons with slow conduction velocities. Axons from these receptors enter the dorsal horn and synapse predominantly with neurons in the dorsal horn. Different modalities of sensation terminate in specific laminae of the dorsal horn with pain and temperature axons terminating in the most superficial regions and touch afferents synapsing at deeper levels.

Unlike the dorsal column–medial lemniscal system, the second order neurons of the anterolateral system are located in the grey matter of the spinal cord. They are widely scattered but there is a relationship between the location of the second order neuron within the grey matter and the destination of its axon. Spinothalamic tract axons destined for the thalamus and spinomesencephalic tract neurons destined for the midbrain originate from the dorsal horn, while spinoreticular tract axons destined for the medulla and pons originate from the ventral horn. The axons of these neurons decussate in the spinal cord itself and enter the contralateral anterior and lateral white matter. There, axons in the pathway are somatotopically arranged, with information from progressively higher segments occupying a progressively more lateral location in the white matter. However, this somatotopic organization is not as precise as it is in the dorsal columns.

The spinothalamic tract axons end in the ventral posterior nucleus of the thalamus. Some axons also end in the intralaminar nuclei (see below). Spinoreticular axons terminate in the reticular formation of the medulla and pons and from here axons ascend to terminate in the intralaminar and posterior nuclei of the thalamus. The spinomesencephalic axons terminate in the periaqueductal grey that surrounds the cerebral aqueduct in the midbrain. The main function of the spinothalamic tract is the mediation of pain and temperature sensation. The spinoreticular pathways mediate arousal while the spinomesencephalic tract is involved in the descending control of sensation, particularly pain. There are a number of other pathways that relay sensory information. The most important of these are the **dorsal**

spinocerebellar tracts that relay proprioceptive information from the lower limb to the cerebellum.

Another way of looking at sensory pathways is in terms of the response they produce rather than the specific stimulus initiating the nervous impulse:

- Stimuli giving information about the environment (temperature, for example) travel by the spinothalamic pathways.
- Information demanding a response (such as pain) travels in the spinoreticular tracts.
- Information enabling analysis of stimuli (direction of movement, texture) travels in the dorsal columns.

Sensory pathways from the head

Sensory information from the head and neck is conveyed through the primary afferent neurons in various cranial nerves to the brainstem. Although several nerves have sensory components, irrespective of the nerve of origin, they all terminate on the trigeminal brainstem sensory nuclear complex (see Chapter 11). The trigeminal sensory nuclear complex is composed of three nuclei: the spinal nucleus of the trigeminal nerve extending from the upper cervical spinal cord to the pons, the main nucleus of the trigeminal nerve within the pons where the trigeminal nerve enters the brainstem and the mesencephalic nucleus in the midbrain. The main sensory nucleus receives discriminative touch information and the spinal nucleus receives pain, temperature and touch information. The mesencephalic nucleus is peculiar to the trigeminal nerve and receives proprioceptive information from structures supplied by the trigeminal nerve. Essentially, the main sensory nucleus is the equivalent of the dorsal column nuclei, the spinal nucleus is the equivalent of the dorsal horn of the spinal cord for sensory pathways from the rest of the body, and proprioception is the function of the mesencephalic nucleus.

The trigeminal lemniscal system is concerned with discriminative touch and vibration sense and originates from encapsulated receptors in the skin and mucosa of the head supplied by the trigeminal nerve. The cell bodies lie in the trigeminal ganglion in the middle cranial fossa and their central processes enter the pons to synapse within second order neurons in the main nucleus of the trigeminal nerve. The second order neuron axons decussate and join the contralateral trigeminal lemniscus, a medial extension of the medial lemniscus, which terminates in the **ventral posterior medial nucleus of the thalamus.**

The ventral trigeminothalamic tract is the pathway from the head that corresponds to the anterolateral pathway from the body. It conveys the sensations of pain, temperature and touch from the head to the cortex and originates from unencapsulated receptors in the skin and mucous membranes. These are innervated by the peripheral processes of axons in the trigeminal, glossopharyngeal and vagus nerves. The cell bodies of these neurons lie in the appropriate ganglion and the central processes of their axons enter the brainstem in the appropriate cranial nerve to enter the spinal trigeminal nucleus where they synapse with second order neurons. Second order neurons decussate to ascend with the other axons of the anterolateral system. These axons terminate in the ventral posterior lateral nucleus of the thalamus as well as the posterior and intralaminar nuclei.

The pathway for proprioception from the muscles and joint of the head is the spinomesencephalic pathway. It is unusual in that the cell bodies of the sensory neurons actually form the neurons of the trigeminal mesencephalic nucleus itself. The central processes of these neurons project to the motor nucleus of the trigeminal nerve to form a reflex arc controlling the muscles of mastication. They are also believed to project to the cerebellum.

The thalamus

All sensory information reaching the cerebral cortex, apart from the sense of smell, does so via synapses in the thalamus. The thalamus is thus a relay nucleus for all sensory information that passes to the cortex and therefore the next relay station in the ascending somatosensory pathways. The thalamus is also an important relay station between the basal ganglia and the cerebral cortex, particularly in relation to the function of the motor system (see Chapter 10). It consists of two bilaterally symmetrical groups of nuclei in the diencephalon separated by the third ventricle in the midline (see Figure 8.9). These nuclei are distinguished mainly by their afferent and efferent connections and are generally named by reference to their position in the thalamus. Although some nuclei have a major function attributed to them, they usually have several others. For example, the sensory thalamic nuclei are relay stations between the spinal cord and cerebral cortex. However, they interconnect with other thalamic nuclei and with areas of the cortex not primarily associated with sensory functions. Less than ten per cent of neurons in sensory thalamic nuclei actually participate in sensory function. Overall, the thalamus participates in a large number of pathways, not just sensory and motor pathways, and these various pathways each use a distinct portion of the thalamus.

The thalamus is divided by a thin internal plate of white matter into a lateral and a medial group of nuclei. The largest part of the thalamus is taken up by the lateral group nuclei. The lateral group includes the nuclei forming part of the ascending somatosensory pathways, the motor system, and the visual and auditory pathways. The intralaminar nuclei are located in the internal white matter.

The particular nuclei involved in handling sensory information are the **ventral posterior nuclei** and adjacent nuclei. The dorsal column–medial lemniscal system and spinothalamic tract end in the **ventral posterior lateral nucleus** (VPL), which together with the ventral posterior medial nucleus (VPM) constitutes the main sensory relay nucleus of the thalamus. The spinothalamic and spinoreticular tracts also project to the **intralaminar** and **posterior nuclei**. Sensory information from the head and neck is conveyed from the trigeminal sensory nuclei to the **ventral posterior medial nucleus** (VPM) of the thalamus and this is segregated from sensory information from the rest of the body. Axons from the VPM and VPL nuclei enter the internal capsule and travel to the sensory cortex. The intralaminar nuclei project diffusely all over the cortex and may have an arousal function. The posterior nuclei seem to have a specific role in pain transmission which is not yet fully understood.

The sensory cortex

The degree to which function is localized in the **cerebral cortex** is arguable, but some areas have been believed to mediate a specific function for many decades. However, in the light of modern research, ideas are changing and specific cortical areas are now regarded as having several functions. Two areas of the cortex are designated as **somatosensory cortex**, the **primary** area lying in the **postcentral gyrus** and the **secondary** area lying just below it in the upper bank of the lateral fissure. In the primary area, the body is somatotopically represented upside down on the contralateral cortex; the left side of the face is at the lowermost part of the right postcentral gyrus (see Figure 6.8). As well as being somatotopically arranged, the area of cortex assigned to a given area of the body is proportional to the importance of that area in sensory reception. The areas given to each finger or the lips are far bigger individually than the entire area attributed to the trunk. Stimulation of the appropriate area of the body can be recorded in the corresponding zone of the sensory cortex; conversely, stimulation of the somatosensory cortex will evoke apparent sensation from the corresponding body area. The function of the secondary sensory cortex is uncertain but may be involved in discrimination of texture and shape.

Interestingly, stimulation of the primary sensory cortex does not elicit pain and stimulation of a body area with a noxious stimulus does not elicit responses from the corresponding somatotopic area of the cortex. It appears that noxious stimuli travelling to the posterior and intralaminar thalamic nuclei in the spinoreticular pathway project diffusely to wide areas of the posterior cortex rather than to the somatosensory cortex.

Special sensory pathways

The special senses of olfaction, vision, hearing and balance have specific pathways which are quite separate from those conveying somatic and visceral sensation. The most important to speech and language therapists are the auditory pathways described in detail in Chapter 23. The visual and olfactory pathways are outlined in Chapter 11. They are important when testing of neurological function is carried out to determine, for example, the extent of head injuries.

Sensory association cortex

The primary auditory, sensory and visual areas in the temporal, parietal and occipital lobes receive raw incoming information and are modality specific. The adjacent areas of the cortex are necessary for interpretation and understanding of this information. These areas are known collectively as the **posterior association cortex** (see Figure 6.7). This may be divided into **secondary association cortex** in areas adjacent to the primary cortex and more remote **tertiary association** areas. The **secondary sensory cortex** lies posterior to the postcentral gyrus, the **secondary visual cortex** lateral to the visual cortex in the occipital lobe and the **secondary auditory cortex** inferior to the auditory cortex in the temporal lobe. Whereas the primary cortex is arranged very specifically – somatotopically in the sensory cortex – this arrangement is lost in the secondary cortices, although they are still specific for a given sensory modality. In their turn, the secondary association areas project to tertiary areas which lie around the posterior margin of the lateral fissure. This tertiary area is not specific for any sensation. As information passes from primary to secondary to tertiary areas there is convergence from different primary sensory areas and different sensory modalities interact.

The ascending somatosensory pathways all decussate at some level in their upward journey, thus the left side of the body is represented in the right primary somatosensory cortex and the right side in the left cortex. This is preserved within the association cortex but superimposed upon this pattern are the different functions of the two hemispheres.

Cerebral dominance

The left hemisphere is predominantly concerned with symbolic functions such as mathematics, logic, speech and mime. The right hemisphere is concerned with visuospatial functions – the ability to recognize faces, draw complex diagrams and solve spatial problems. Despite this functional segregation, the two cortices are connected via transversely running axons. The vast majority of these pass through the **corpus callosum** (see Figure 8.1) but there are other smaller commissural areas between the cerebral hemispheres. Sometimes the corpus callosum is divided to prevent epileptic foci in one hemisphere spreading into the other half of the brain. Generally, this 'split brain' can be used normally by ensuring that all the visual fields are examined by both eyes so that the requisite information reaches both halves of the brain. Experiments can be contrived which restrict the fields of vision and, in this case, an object presented to the left hemisphere can be named (the symbolic function) but not used (the visuospatial function). Conversely an object presented to the right hemisphere cannot be named but can be used correctly.

Like much of the brain, some functions of the posterior association cortex can be appreciated most easily by studying their malfunction. Damage to these areas results in various manifestations of agnosia and apraxia. **Agnosia** is the inability to interpret sensory information. For example, a key placed in the hand can be felt as cold, metallic and sharp-edged but it is not recognized as a key and it cannot be used correctly. **Apraxia** is the inability to make functional movements when the components of complex movements are intact. For example, a patient requested to salute would not be able to do so despite having normal movement of the arm and shoulder. It is surprising that the posterior cortex which appears to be essentially sensory should cause problems with motor activities but most motor activity is made in response to sensory inputs from various sources. The posterior association cortex turns raw sensory data into something one can perceive, interpret and act on through the motor areas of the brain.

Posterior association cortex defects

Lesions in the left auditory association cortex produce **pure word deafness**. The client is unable to understand or repeat spoken words, but can read and respond to environmental sounds. This is dealt with more fully in Chapters 13 and 23.

The parietal association cortex posterior to the primary sensory cortex has extensive connections with other association cortices, the limbic system and the frontal association cortex. Lesions in this area can lead to a wide variety of symptoms depending upon the location and extent of the lesion. There is sensory inattention to, and neglect of, the contralateral side of the environment following a unilateral lesion. In addition, left hemispheric lesions impair reading ability (**alexia**), writing ability (**agraphia**), naming of objects (**anomia**) and confusion between sides. Unilateral lesions of the right parietal association cortex are marked by **dressing apraxia**, the inability to dress correctly, which is particularly obvious when dressing the left side of the body, and **constructional apraxia**, the inability to draw simple figures and shapes. **Apraxia** is the loss of ability to perform movements in response to a stimulus which would normally elicit such movements when motor systems are intact. Apart from the special cases mentioned above, apraxia may take two forms. In **ideomotor apraxia**, actions can be performed automatically but not on command. In **ideotonal apraxia**, complex movements cannot be sequenced although individual movements can be carried out. Another aspect of posterior association cortex dysfunction is **agnosia**, the inability to comprehend stimuli in the context of past experience although the appropriate sensory modalities are functioning normally. In visual agnosia, objects cannot be recognized visually, but can be identified by touch. Tactile agnosia is the converse: things can be recognized visually but not by touch.

A summary of sensory function

Somatic sensation from the receptors in skin and mucosa and proprioception from muscle and joint receptors travel by primary afferent neurons from the periphery to the spinal cord or brainstem. Primary afferent neurons are the sensory components of peripheral nerves and have their cell bodies in the dorsal root ganglia. They enter the dorsal horn of the spinal cord via the dorsal roots. Nerves carrying different sensory modalities may terminate in different areas of the dorsal horn. Several interneurons are interposed between the primary afferent neurons and the second order or thalamic projection neurons which enable information to be inhibited, disseminated or concentrated. Sensory information then travels by one of three routes to the thalamus in the forebrain. The projection neurons carrying environmental information, such as temperature, cross to the opposite side of the spinal cord and ascend in the lateral white matter to the ventroposterolateral (VPL) nucleus of the thalamus. Reactional information, such as pain, also travels in crossed projection pathways to the reticular formation in the medulla oblongata and pons and thence to the intralaminar and posterior nuclei of the thalamus. Analytical information (touch, proprioception) is carried in primary afferent neurons which do not synapse directly in the dorsal horn of the spinal cord, but pass into the dorsal columns of white matter to reach the dorsal column nuclei in the medulla oblongata. Here they synapse and thalamic nuclei cross to the opposite side of the brainstem and ascend to the VPL nucleus of the thalamus. The VPL nucleus projects to the somatosensory cortex of the brain which lies in the postcentral gyrus. A somatotopic organization of sensory information is maintained at all levels in the spinal cord and cortex but the amount of brain area devoted to a given area of the body is directly proportional to the importance of that area in sensory reception. The area subserving information from one finger is therefore much larger than that subserving the whole of the skin of the trunk.

Sensation from the head and neck is conveyed to the CNS via some of the cranial nerves. The primary afferent neurons terminate in the trigeminal sensory nuclear complex; its different components are analogous to the spinal dorsal horn and dorsal column nuclei. The information from the head and neck projects to the ventroposteromedial (VPM) nucleus of the thalamus and thence to the somatosensory nucleus.

Noxious stimuli reach different nuclei in the thalamus from those used to process other somatosensory and proprioceptive information. These nuclei do not project to the somatosensory cortex and their site of projection is still uncertain. Some nerve pathways descend from areas of the brainstem to the dorsal horn of the spinal cord and may inhibit transmission of noxious stimuli at the spinal level.

CHAPTER 10

Motor function

The understanding of motor systems has traditionally lagged behind that of sensory systems. This is because even a relatively simple piece of motor behaviour, such as reaching for an object, consists of a considerable number of individual elements: defining a motor output in terms of the interaction of many muscles contracting for specific durations, with graded forces to produce movements of limbs through specific angles, can be a formidable task. It is much easier to test the capabilities of a sensory system in terms of giving a stimulus of a particular modality, intensity and duration, although that is a rather artificial event compared to the complexity of stimuli to which we are normally exposed. It can be argued that the function of sensory systems within the CNS is exactly opposite to that of motor systems, in that sensory systems set out to produce an internal representation of the outside world whereas motor systems make an internal map of the effect of an intended movement on that same outside world.

There are three broad classes of movement that can be recognized. In order from the most to the least automatic, they are **reflexes**, **rhythmic movements** and **voluntary movements**. Reflexes are simple pieces of involuntary, automatic behaviour in which a sequence of muscular contraction and relaxation is initiated by a particular sensory stimulation. The anatomy of a reflex has been described in Chapter 6. The most obvious example of rhythmic movement is walking, or locomotion, in which a sequence of alternating contractions of muscles extend and flex the two legs. Other kinds of movements that are rhythmic in nature include chewing and swallowing. Even speech with its pattern of opening and closing of the vocal tract could be viewed as a kind of rhythmic behaviour although that rhythm will be greatly modified during any one utterance. Voluntary movements are ones that are initiated to produce a particular outcome; they range enormously in complexity from simple reaching tasks to highly skilled acts. Voluntary movements, particularly complex tasks such as playing an instrument, are learned and improve with repetition and practice. Although it is convenient to regard the three types of movement as distinct categories, in practice any single movement requires the cooperative action of more than one type. For example, as you reach for an object, reflex circuits are activated in the lower and upper limbs to ensure that posture is maintained and you do not over-balance while, at the same time, circuits controlling rhythmic behaviour ensure an orderly sequence of contraction of muscles that flex and extend the limbs.

All movement is under continuous sensory control. Visual, auditory and cutaneous sensory stimuli from the outside of the body give information about the external environment. Information concerning the state of contraction of muscles and position of joints comes from the inside body from proprioceptors. This sensory information can be used to control movement in one of two ways. In feedback control, movements in progress are continuously monitored and the sensory information is used to make corrections or adjustments as the movement proceeds, for example, if you trip during walking or if the object you pick up is heavier than anticipated. In feed-forward control, there is anticipation about what is going to happen which is used to calculate an appropriate pattern of movement. An example of this is the act of catching a ball. Both mechanisms have advantages and disadvantages. Feedback control allows for adjustments to be made to an ongoing movement if changes occur after the initiation of that movement has begun. However, because of the neural circuitry involved, there can be significant delays in making adjustments so movements controlled this way tend to be slower. Feed-forward mechanisms are suitable for rapid movements but are inflexible. In speech, feedback mechanisms are particularly important for phonation and some phases of articulation; feed-forward mechanisms come into play during rapid utterances such as the release of stops.

All movements have to take account of the properties of muscles and joints. Muscles are not linear in their responses. The force of contraction of a muscle depends upon its initial length. As muscles are lengthened, their force of contraction increases to a maximum as more cross-bridges come into play but then this force declines as muscle length is increased further. Thus, the motor system needs information about initial muscle length in order to programme and control movements. The second peculiarity of skeletal muscles is that they are incapable of rapid contraction since, as the rate of stimulation increases, muscles go into a state of continuous contraction called **tetanus**. Therefore, rapid movements can only be achieved by muscles contracting in alternating patterns. This is of significance in speech to produce movements of the vocal folds during phonation (see Chapter 17). Finally, muscles can pull but not push and therefore movements in opposite directions at a particular joint can only occur as the result of muscles being organized in agonist–antagonist pairs in which one muscle, the **agonist**, moves the joint in one direction while another muscle, the **antagonist**, moves the joint in the opposite direction. All these aspects of muscle function have to be taken into account by the motor system in planning a movement.

An important feature of the motor system is that motor pathways are organized into a hierarchy that ranges from the most automatic to the least automatic. At each level of the hierarchy there are populations of neurons that regulate movement, and the production of complex movements is the result of interaction between the different levels of the hierarchy.

At the lowest level of the hierarchy are **motor neurons**. These are connected directly to the muscles and no muscle contraction occurs without their activation. At the next level of the hierarchy are the **descending pathways**. If the spinal cord is transected, no movement is possible below the level of injury, indicating that descending pathways from elsewhere in CNS are required for motor neuron activation. These pathways originate from the motor cortex and other areas of the cortex and brainstem and reach the motor neurons in the ventral horn of the spinal cord. Descending pathways also relay sensory information about balance and vision which affects motor neuron activation: this information reaches the spinal motor neurons by two other descending pathways (Figure 10.1). The next level of the hierarchy is the cerebral cortex itself. This includes the **primary motor cortex** which lies in the **precentral gyrus** anterior to the central sulcus (see Figure 6.7) but the motor cortex is much more extensive, encompassing premotor and supplementary motor areas anterior to the primary motor cortex. Although the motor areas of the brain are located principally in the frontal lobe, the sensory association cortex in the parietal lobe generates the idea of movement in response to sensory input (see Chapter 9). Transfer of information to the motor areas of the brain is achieved, in part, by two complex loop systems passing from the posterior association cortex to the motor areas of the brain. One loop passes through the **basal ganglia** and the other through the **cerebellum** en route for the motor cortex. Put as simply as possible, information enters the loop systems unrefined and leaves them refined. The loop systems project via the thalamus to the frontal cortex. These are involved in the conception and initiation of movement sequences whereas the primary motor cortex itself executes the movements.

Lower motor neurons

Motor neurons and interneurons in the spinal cord and brainstem are at the lowest level in the network of motor pathways. For the muscles of the

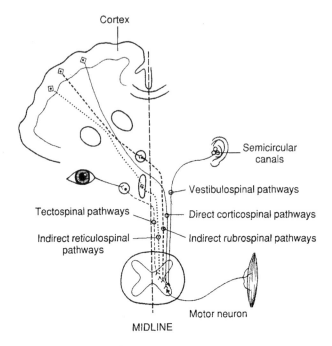

Figure 10.1 Descending motor pathways.

limbs and trunk, motor neurons and interneurons are found in the ventral horn and intermediate zone. For the muscles of the head, the neurons are located in the cranial motor nuclei and reticular formation. At this level, motor behaviour is largely in the form of reflexes and rhythmic behaviour. Motor neurons are often referred to as the **final common pathway** for movement because all other levels of the hierarchy can only generate movement through their effects upon the motor neurons. These parts of the motor system are responsible for the most automatic motor acts and can generate simple behaviours even when other parts of the motor system are damaged.

The **lower motor neurons** are the motor components of peripheral nerves. Their cell bodies are in the ventral horns of the spinal cord and the axons leave by the ventral roots to join the sensory fibres of the dorsal root to form the mixed peripheral nerve. There are two groups of motor neurons arranged as two columns in the ventral horn. The motor neurons in the medial motor column are present throughout the spinal cord and innervate muscles of the trunk. The motor neurons in the lateral motor column are only present in the cervical and lumbosacral enlargements (spinal segments C4–T1 and L2–S3 respectively) opposite the upper and lower limbs muscles which they innervate. There are two functional classes of motor neuron, **alpha motor neurons** and **gamma motor neurons**. Alpha motor neurons end on extrafusal muscle fibres at neuromuscular junctions where **acetylcholine** is used as an excitatory transmitter to cause depolarization of muscle and initiate contraction of the muscle as a whole (see Chapter 3). Gamma motor neurons end on intrafusal muscle fibres within muscle spindles and regulate the sensitivity of muscle spindles (see Chapter 9). The cranial motor neurons are found in the motor nuclei of the extraocular muscles, trigeminal, facial and hypoglossal motor nuclei and the nucleus ambiguus (see Chapter 11).

Motor neurons participate in reflexes which can be defined as simple acts of motor behaviour over which we can exert little or no voluntary control. Reflexes are initiated by sensory input from skin or muscle. An example of a reflex is the knee jerk reflex which is elicited when the leg is suspended in the air and a brief tap is applied to the patellar tendon connected to a muscle in the thigh. The brief tap stretches its tendon and the muscle responds with a brisk contraction that straightens the leg. This reflex has a relatively simple anatomy: the sensory axons innervating the muscle spindles that detect the stretch form the **afferent limb** of the reflex and enter the spinal cord to synapse directly upon the motor neurons, to form a **monosynaptic reflex**. The motor neurons respond by an excitation that results in action potentials passing down the motor axons which form the **efferent limb** of the reflex. The two limbs of the reflex are connected together by a single **synaptic connection** directly onto the motor neuron.

This type of reflex is called a **stretch reflex** and is unusual in that the synaptic connection is direct. More commonly, one or more interneurons are interposed between the afferent and efferent limbs. Afferent axons not only pass directly onto the motor neurons of the same muscle whose tendon is stretched, but make connections via interneurons with antagonist muscles to inhibit the motor neurons of those muscles: this ensures that they do not interfere with the muscle contraction in progress. Interneurons may also excite synergist muscles with the same action as the stretched muscle to ensure they cooperate with the contraction initiated by the reflex. One of the properties of stretch reflexes is that they may be important in maintaining muscle length in response to stretch, a property called **muscle tone**.

Tendon reflexes originate from Golgi tendon organs and these reflexes, when activated, inhibit the muscle whose tendon organs have been excited together with its synergists, while exciting the antagonist muscles. This reflex is sometimes called the **inverse myotactic reflex** to distinguish it from the stretch reflex which is also known as the **myotactic** reflex. One function of inverse myotactic reflexes is thought to be in reaching tasks when objects are grasped, muscles are inhibited at the point of contact to reduce the likelihood of an object being crushed.

Reflexes can also originate from skin and one well-known example is the **flexor reflex** in which a limb is suddenly withdrawn from a painful stimulus such as a hot surface or a sharp object impaling a foot. The flexors of the affected limb contract briskly while the extensors are inhibited. At the same time, the extensors on the opposite side contract to ensure posture is maintained. It is easy to see in principle how such reflexes could be combined to produce rhythmic or other movements involving alternating patterns of muscle contraction. In practice, it has proved quite difficult to elucidate how this is achieved.

As well as being involved in patterning of movement, reflexes are also vital in controlling force of contraction and, again, it has proved difficult to elucidate in detail how this is achieved. Cranial nerve motor neurons also participate in reflexes such as the jaw jerk reflex which is a monosynaptic reflex in which the loosely open jaw responds to a brief tap by forceful closure. A knowledge of reflexes is important because following brain injury, such as a stroke, characteristic changes in reflexes are observed. There are increases in the force and range of certain reflexes, termed **hyperreflexia**. These reflexes would normally be inhibited by the intact brain region before damage. The jaw jerk reflex is one such example: it is not normally elicited in healthy individuals with an intact nervous system.

Each lower motor neuron has six inputs influencing its activity:

• direct corticospinal pathways
• rubrospinal and reticulospinal tracts
• the vestibulospinal and tectospinal tracts
• sensory fibres including those from its own stretch receptors from intrafusal fibres which form the reflex arcs with the motor neurons.

Division of the peripheral nerve produces a **lower motor neuron lesion** characterized by **flaccid paralysis** and **wasting** of the muscles innervated by the affected nerve. The muscle is paralysed because no information reaches it at all. If no reinnervation occurs, the muscle atrophies in a matter of weeks, eventually being replaced by fibrous connective tissue. As fibrosis occurs, the fibrous tissue shrinks causing a permanent **contracture** which has the same effect on the joints as the muscle would have had except the effects are permanent and irreversible.

An **upper motor neuron lesion** occurs when several descending pathways or loops are affected at the same time, often by a lesion in the internal capsule, causing degeneration of cortical efferent axons and axons passing between the corpus striatum and thalamus. Voluntary movement of the muscles on the opposite side of the body from the lesion is lost or becomes severely weakened but atrophy does not occur since the muscle is not denervated. The overriding symptom of this lesion is **spasticity** of the muscle due to increase in the muscle tone. Muscle tone is normally modulated by descending tract activity. In an upper motor neuron lesion, only the sensory input from stretch receptors in and around the muscle is conveyed to the motor neuron without modification, hence the spasticity. There may also be exaggerated reflexes such as withdrawal reflexes which might be initiated by the lightest touch.

Although the individual contributions of different loops and tracts can be determined on the basis of experimental and clinical studies, movement is the summation of all these effects. The brain does not think in terms of movement of individual muscles but probably in terms of movements of whole joints and quite complex functional movements. There is evidence that final position is predetermined by the brain as a balance between the tension–length settings of agonist and antagonistic muscles. Under experimental circumstances, a final position can be achieved without vestibular or visual cues but these cues are extremely significant if position is disturbed. Likewise, sensory feedback is applied during movement. In other words, the motor control areas of the brain are pre-programmed but the programme may be modified during its execution by relevant sensory information.

Major descending pathways

The next level of the hierarchy is the brainstem which contributes descending pathways that control motor neurons and reflex circuits. This region integrates afferent input, input from special senses and from cerebral cortex and subcortical regions as well. It is the site of origin of all but one of the descending pathways. There are two systems of descending pathways that originate from the brainstem. The **ventromedial descending systems** control predominantly proximal and axial extensor muscles, balance and posture and guide the limbs into place prior to completion of movements such as grasping. The **dorsomedial systems** control predominantly the distal flexor muscles of the limb and fine voluntary movements, especially of the forearm and hand. These two groups of pathways cooperate in the production of complex movements. These pathways either end directly on the motor neurons in the ventral horn or brainstem or on interneurons that form part of the reflex circuits within the spinal cord or brainstem Often there can be several interneurons between the descending neurons and motor neurons.

The dorsomedial pathway originating from the brainstem is the **rubrospinal pathway** (Figure 10.2). This originates from the **red nucleus** in the midbrain and decussates to end on interneurons in the spinal cord that connect to motor neurons. The function of this pathway is not known in man. The main ventromedial pathways originating in the brainstem are the vestibulospinal, reticulospinal and tectospinal pathways. The **vestibulospinal pathways** from the vestibular apparatus in the inner ear monitoring balance also have an input on to motor neurons via interneurons; these pathways are one of the few which do not decussate. The vestibular apparatus gives information on angular and linear acceleration of the head. Rotation (**angular acceleration**) of the head causes movement of fluid in the semicircular canals in the inner ear which stimulates the cilia on hair cells projecting into the fluid. To compensate for rotation, the eyes and head move accordingly and the nuclei controlling the relevant muscles (see Chapter 11) receive direct projections from the vestibular nuclei. The vestibular apparatus also monitors information on the relationship of the head to the ground and the plane in which the head is held. Crystals of calcium carbonate press on hair cells under the influence of gravity and when the angulation of the head is altered (**linear acceleration**), deforming the hairs and initiating a series of impulses. The information is conveyed by the vestibulocochlear nerves from the inner ear to the vestibular nuclei in the medulla oblongata from where the vestibulospinal pathway originates. The tracts conveying linear acceleration information project ipsilaterally through the anterior white matter of the spinal cord to stimulate extensor muscles and inhibit flexor muscles to maintain an upright posture. The **reticulospinal pathway** originates from groups of neurons in both the medulla and the pons from a region called the reticular formation. The predominantly ipsilateral reticulospinal pathway ends on motor neurons, again via interneurons, but also has a contralateral component. The reticulospinal pathways constitute the main motor route to the trunk; they are complex with some axons decussating and others remaining uncrossed. One peculiarity of the reticulospinal pathways is that one descending axon will often give off several collateral branches to motor neurons in different levels of the spinal cord. These may be involved in synchronization of complex movement involving the upper and lower limbs, such as swinging the arms during walking. **Tectospinal pathways** carry information from the superior colliculi in the tectum of the midbrain to the ventral horn of the spinal cord. Visual cues are important for correct movement and it is these pathways which provide this information. The tectospinal pathways are short tracts from the tectal area of the midbrain to the cranial nerve motor nuclei in the brainstem and the ventral horn of the cervical spinal cord (Figure 10.2).

The main inputs to the tectum are from various parts of the visual pathway, the auditory cortex and somatosensory information from the neck and shoulder. These pathways are involved in orientating the body to aural, tactile or visual stimuli by turning the head and eyes towards the source of stimulus.

The other source of descending pathways onto the motor neurons originates from the next level of the hierarchy of motor pathways from within the **primary motor cortex**, together with the **premotor** and **supplementary motor areas**. This is the point where motor commands from other parts of the cortex converge and from which direct commands to the brainstem and spinal cord are issued. There are four major efferent pathways from the cerebral cortex to the spinal cord, two of which pass directly to the cord and the other two of which pass through intermediate nuclei. This is also the other source of descending input onto motor neurons and also of descending pathways that influence the brainstem and thus other descending pathways indirectly. There are two groups of **direct corticospinal pathways** that originate from the motor cortex. The first are known as the **lateral corticospinal tracts** and arise from the

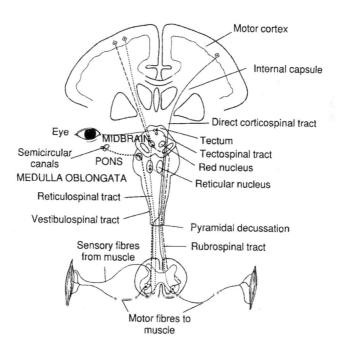

Figure 10.2 The pathways affecting activity of motorneurons in the ventral horn of the spinal cord.

primary and supplementary motor cortex in each hemisphere with lesser contributions from the premotor area and the somatosensory cortex. They pass through the internal capsule and cerebral peduncles to the ventral surface of the brainstem where they produce two longitudinal ridges, the **pyramids**. The majority of axons decussate in the medulla oblongata (the **pyramidal decussation**) and descend the spinal cord in the lateral white matter. The direct corticospinal tracts control precision and speed of fine movement; the major effect of damage is loss of fine movement of the individual fingers and toes. Other axons in this pathway end in the brainstem and control muscles of the tongue, face and jaw. These are the **lateral corticobulbar axons**. The other direct corticospinal pathways are called the **ventral corticospinal tract**. Axons in this pathway remain uncrossed and they initially follow a similar course in the brainstem but do not decussate in the medulla oblongata, remaining ipsilateral and descending anteriorly. At the appropriate level in the spinal cord, the descending axons terminate in the deeper parts of the dorsal horn and upper parts of the ventral horn. These pathways control mainly postural muscles in the neck, shoulder and trunk. Some of the axons in this pathway also end in the brainstem. These are **the ventral corticobulbar axons** and they terminate in the extraocular motor nuclei, nucleus ambiguus and reticular formation.

The motor cortical areas are also the source of **indirect cortical pathways** that control the other brainstem pathways and the cerebellum. Some other cortical neurons follow the direct corticospinal tracts as far as the **red nucleus** in the midbrain where they synapse. These are the **corticorubrospinal tracts.** The other major input to the red nucleus is the cerebellum. The efferent fibres from the red nucleus, which has a pinkish tinge in the living brain, are the origin of the rubrospinal tracts as described above. The corticorubrospinal tracts are thought to influence flexor muscle motor neurons through interneurons, although this is difficult to verify as there is no place on the pathway where the axons do not mingle with those forming other tracts, making it impossible to achieve experimental or clinical section of these tracts alone. The second major indirect tract is the **cortico-reticulo-spinal tract**. This tract probably controls movements which require little dexterity. The major inputs to this pathway are descending axons from the motor cortex, cerebellum and ascending spinoreticular fibres which all converge in the reticular area of the pons and medulla. The third pathways from the cortex are the **corticopontine pathways.** These pathways terminate in the **pontine nuclei** within the pons through which the corticospinal and corticobulbar fibres pass as they travel to the medulla. The output from the pontine nuclei then passes to the cerebellum after decussation.

This division of descending motor pathways into ventrolateral and dorsomedial systems from the brainstem and pathways originating from the motor regions of the cortex replaces an older classification of pathways into **pyramidal** and **extrapyramidal** systems. The pyramidal system referred to the cortical pathways that were located in the pyramids. The descending pathways that did not pass through the pyramids were then referred to as the **extrapyramidal system**. It was thought that the pyramidal system had primacy in movement control. It is now believed that motor control is carried out through the cooperation of the two systems. The older classification may be encountered in older literature and textbooks and is sometimes still in clinical usage.

Motor pathways to the cranial nerves

The cranial nerves are peripheral nerves originating from the brain itself (see Chapter 11). Descending inputs enter their motor nuclei, which are the equivalent of the ventral horn of the spinal cord, via **corticobulbar** pathways. These are equivalent to the tracts described above. They only have a sparse input from the red nucleus but they do, however, have a significant input from the tectum. The components of the direct corticospinal tract supplying these nuclei are known as lateral and ventral **corticobulbar tracts**.

Most of the cranial nerve nuclei lie superior to the pyramidal decussation, and many also lie at the level of the reticular nuclei. Thus, by this stage, many of the descending tracts have *not* crossed. Most of the motor nuclei in fact receive an input from both crossed and uncrossed pathways. Interruption of these pathways therefore produces characteristic weakness (**paresis**) of the many muscles in the head and neck controlled by the cranial nerves because some input is usually preserved which maintains some innervation to the muscles. Only the contralateral lower facial muscles and tongue muscles are paralysed by a unilateral upper motor neuron lesion: the former due to an anatomical peculiarity and the latter because the nerve to the muscles of the tongue lies below the level at which all the fibres have crossed (see Chapter 11).

Suprabulbar or **pseudobulbar palsy** is the condition resulting from lesions in the corticonuclear pathways. The lesion must be bilateral, affecting pathways on both sides, otherwise paresis is seen. The major clinical features of suprabulbar palsy are **dysarthria**, **dysphonia** and **dysphagia**. Speech is slow, there is inappropriate use of pitch and phonation, and speech tends to be hypernasal. Intervals between words and sentences and even individual phonemes are prolonged and phrasing is therefore disturbed. The usual cause of suprabulbar palsy is CVA in the brainstem.

Cortical control of movement

The functions of this level of the hierarchy are to control movement directly and to plan movement. The motor cortex and certain premotor areas including the lateral premotor supplementary motor areas can affect movement directly through the corticospinal and other pathways. Other premotor areas including the prefrontal association cortex are important for the planning of movement and motor programmes. These regions receive input from other cortical regions including the prefrontal association cortex and posterior parietal area.

The **primary motor cortex** is somatotopically arranged in the **precentral gyrus** in each frontal lobe (Figure 10.3). Like the arrangement of the primary sensory cortex, the area controlling the legs is situated at the superior aspect of the cortex overlapping on to the medial surface of each hemisphere whereas the area controlling muscles of the head are on the inferior lateral part of the precentral gyrus. The area representing different muscles is not proportional to the size of the muscles but to the intricacy of potential movement such that large postural muscles have relatively small areas whereas muscles of the fingers, lips, tongue and eyes have huge areas.

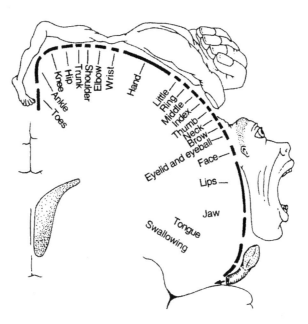

Figure 10.3 The somatotopic representation of muscles in different areas of the body (the motor homunculus).

Two other parts of the frontal cortex are essential for movement. The lateral **premotor cortex** is immediately anterior to the primary motor cortex on the lateral aspect of each hemisphere and the **supplementary motor cortex** is on the upper part of the lateral surface but overlaps on to the medial surface (Figure 10.4). The lateral premotor area is poorly understood. Its main inputs are from the parietal association cortex and its major outputs are via the reticulospinal system. Essentially, this area prepares for movement and damage affects the design of movement strategies. The supplementary motor cortex is involved in sequencing complex movements and blood flow increases when movement is thought about prior to execution. It is important in achieving gross posture prior to fine movement, for example, correct positioning of the arm prior to playing the piano. Lesions in the supplementary motor cortex impair the orientation for fine movement and coordination of both hands. There is an additional area in the cingulate gyrus which is activated prior to motor activity. This may be the motivational input into motor activity.

The frontal association cortex

The frontal lobe anterior to the motor areas is known as the **prefrontal cortex** or **anterior association areas** and is responsible for behavioural organization (see Figure 6.7). Its main inputs are from the thalamus and posterior association cortex. The effects of prefrontal cortex damage can produce a wide variety of symptoms. **Unilateral lesions** lead to neglect of contralateral extrapersonal space. With more widespread lesions, concentration spans are reduced and there tends to be extreme rigidity and

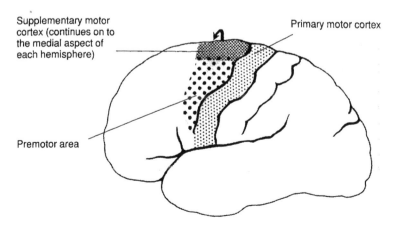

Figure 10.4 The motor cortex.

inflexibility of thought; thinking is very literal and complex analogies and metaphors are not understood. Social customs and conventions may be lost, producing inappropriate or embarrassing behaviour such as neglect of toilet and eating. Emotional reactions may be wildly exaggerated, such as crying for the most trivial reasons or laughing at inappropriate incidents.

The cerebellum and basal ganglia

Motor systems are also regulated by two regions that do not project directly onto motor neurons. These are the basal ganglia and cerebellum. Their role in movement control is not fully understood. The cerebellum projects to the cortex via the thalamus but also acts on descending pathways. It may act as an error detector that corrects for discrepancies between movements as they occur and the commands coming from the cortex, but it is likely to have other functions as well. The basal ganglia also act on the cortex via the thalamus and on the brainstem. They must act in planning and execution of movements but how they do so remains obscure. The basal ganglia participate in complex loop systems which link the sensory areas of the brain with the motor areas. Both these systems are loops that connect together different cortical regions. It is easier to describe the functions of these systems in terms of what goes wrong if they are affected by disease or brain injury rather than to describe what they do. Damage or disease of the basal ganglia results in unwanted abnormal movement known as **dyskinesia**, where there is either an excess or poverty of movement. The dance-like movements associated with Huntingdon's chorea are an example of the former, while an example of the latter is the rigidity seen in Parkinson's disease. One common result of cerebellar disease is **dysarthria**.

The cerebellum

The first major loop system connecting the posterior association cortex and the motor cortex involves the **cerebellum** (Figure 10.5). The cerebellum is an ipsilateral structure and the consequence of this is that all pathways originating from parts of the CNS in which representation of the body is on the contralateral side must therefore cross once more before entering the cerebellum.

The cerebellum consists of two hemispheres joined in the midline by the **vermis** (Figure 10.5). The inferior part of the vermis, together with a small part of each hemisphere – the flocculus, constitutes the **flocculo-nodular lobe**, which is phylogenetically the oldest part of the cerebellum. Though the gross anatomy of the cerebellum is complex and there are many terms used to describe the various subdivisions of each lobe, the

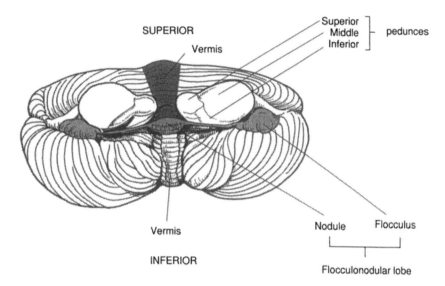

Figure 10.5 The cerebellum. The flocculonodular lobe (archicerebellum) is shaded dark grey and the vermis (paleocerebellum) is shaded light grey.

crucial divisions of the cerebellum are functional ones based on connectivity and these divisions are largely oriented in the mediolateral axis and without clear anatomical landmarks always separating them. The flocculonodular lobe forms the **vestibulocerebellum** or **archicerebellum**. The midline vermis together with the adjacent paramedian parts of the cerebellar hemispheres is the **spinocerebellum** or **paleocerebellum** and the lateral parts of each hemisphere comprise the **neocerebellum**. This may seem very complicated but each area controls different aspects of motor function.

The **vestibulocerebellum** is mainly concerned with balance. Information from the vestibular apparatus in the inner ear via vestibular nuclei in the medulla and from reticular nuclei in the brainstem reaches the ipsilateral half of the flocculonodular lobe. Efferent axons pass from the cerebellum back to the vestibular and reticular nuclei and many cross to the contralateral side as they do so. This part of the cerebellum influences motor neuron activity by influencing the ventromedial descending pathways, vestibulospinal and reticulospinal tracts (see above).

The **spinocerebellum** principally receives information from muscle and joint receptors via spinocerebellar tracts and influences muscle tone, hence posture. Efferent information passes to the contralateral red nucleus in the midbrain and this part of the cerebellum exerts its influence on motor activity through the rubrospinal tracts. Connections also pass to those parts of the motor cortex concerned with the control of distal muscles. Thus, this part of the cerebellum exerts its effects through dorsolateral descending pathways.

The **cerebrocerebellum** is the part of the cerebellum handling information received from the loop systems linking the sensory and motor parts of the cerebral hemispheres, described above. Axons of neurons within the posterior association cortices pass via the internal capsule to the pons where they synapse in **pontine nuclei**. The pontine nuclei send axons to the cerebellum after decussating. The cerebellum then sends efferent axons to the **ventral lateral** group of thalamic nuclei which, in turn, project back to the motor cortex. Efferent axons from the cerebellum also pass to the red nucleus in the midbrain where they connect with descending pathways from the motor cortex to the brainstem and spinal cord. The projections through the thalamus complete the **ponto-cerebello-cortical** loop. They can thus influence motor neuron activity through direct corticospinal and rubrospinal pathways. The neocerebellum is the part of the cerebellum that evolved most recently and deals with the most sophisticated aspects of motor activity and muscular coordination by ensuring that the rate, range, force and speed of muscular movement is appropriate to the task.

Cerebellar damage generally has widespread effects because of its widespread output and influence on several other motor pathways. Sometimes, circumscribed lesions such as tumours can produce specific symptoms. In such cases, the effect is seen on the same side as the damage and produces uncoordination of arm and leg movements resulting in an unsteady gait. This is usually accompanied by an **intention tremor**, a tremor of the hand and arm which increases in amplitude as movements are attempted and the intended target such as a cup or pen is approached. Bilateral cerebellar damage produces **errors in the rate, range, force and direction of movement** producing separation of complex movements into their components, overreaching of targets and intention tremor. Cerebellar dysfunction produces symptoms not unlike alcohol intoxication, with rolling gait and slurred speech being the most obvious manifestations of the errors of compound movement. This is known as **cerebellar ataxia** and may be due to a wide variety of causes such as hypothyroidism, alcoholic intoxication, CVA affecting the cerebellar blood supply, cerebellar degenerative diseases or multiple sclerosis.

Although the most obvious signs of cerebellar damage involve gait, other muscle groups are not immune and cerebellar ataxia has profound effects on eye movement and speech as well. Eye movements are uncoordinated and the patient exhibits **nystagmus**, a rapid oscillation of the eyeball. Nystagmus usually has a slow phase as the eye turns away from the visual target and a rapid phase as it turns back again. Nystagmus is described in terms of the direction of the rapid phase so if the eye moves rapidly to the left, this is a left nystagmus. **Dysarthria** is a disturbance to speech articulation in the absence of obvious muscular or peripheral nervous dysfunction and is one of the signs of cerebellar dysfunction. Articulation is often explosive with rapid utterances being followed by prolonged breaks. Syllables are often slurred or may be separated according to which phase of explosive speech the client is in.

The overall effect of cerebellar lesions is that the rate of errors made during movement increases. These observations, together with knowledge of cerebellar connections, suggest that the cerebellum compares the difference between the intention when executing a movement and the movement which actually occurs. It does this by comparing internal signals from the cortex with feedback signals coming from the muscles themselves and from the periphery. When an error is detected, the cerebellum computes an appropriate correction. In addition, the cerebellum is also believed to have a role in the learning of complex voluntary motor tasks and may also have a cognitive function.

The basal ganglia

The basal ganglia are located deep within the white matter of the cerebral hemispheres. They consist of a number of separate nuclei whose functions are to receive inputs, act as the source of outputs or act to connect together the various components of the basal ganglia. The input nuclei consist of the **caudate nucleus** and a nucleus called the **putamen**. The intrinsic nuclei that link the input nuclei to the output nuclei are a part of the globus pallidus called the **internal segment**, a part of the substantia nigra called the **pars reticulata** and the **subthalamus**. The output nuclei are the remainder of the globus pallidus, called the **external segment** and the remainder of the substantia nigra, the **pars compacta**. The overall pattern of connectivity within the basal ganglia is that cortical axons from widespread areas of cortex are routed through the basal ganglia and via its output nuclei are directed via the thalamus back to the frontal lobe of the cerebral hemispheres. Activity in these extrinsic cortical loops is modified by activity in intrinsic loops of which the most important are the striatonigral loop passing through the substantia nigra and the subthalamic loop passing through the subthalamus. There are four major cortical loops, the sensori-motor loop, the oculomotor loop, the association loop and the limbic loop.

The sensorimotor loop will be illustrated as an example of one of these loops. In the sensorimotor loop axons from primary sensory and motor cortices and the premotor area project through the **internal capsule** to the parts of the basal ganglia known as the putamen and caudate nucleus. These project to the globus pallidus internal segment and substantia nigra pars reticulata which projects in turn to the **ventrolateral** nuclei in the thalamus. Axons from the thalamus project to the supplementary motor area (Figure 10.6). It is important to realize that the output from the basal ganglia to the thalamus is inhibitory so that the effect of activating this circuit is to increase this inhibitory effect upon the thalamus. Two subsidiary reciprocal tracts arise from the major loops. Activity in the major loops is modified by the striatonigral and subthalamic loops. The striatonigral loop that passes from the putamen and caudate nucleus to the **substantia nigra** in the midbrain and back again activates the putamen and has the effect of decreasing the inhibitory effect of the basal ganglia. The subthalamic loop that passes from the globus pallidus to the **subthalamic nucleus** is also reciprocal and has the effect of increasing the inhibitory effect of the basal ganglia upon the thalamus.

As with so much of the brain, it is easiest to appreciate what these loops do by examining their malfunction. Damage to the basal ganglia or substantia nigra produce a group of symptoms known collectively as

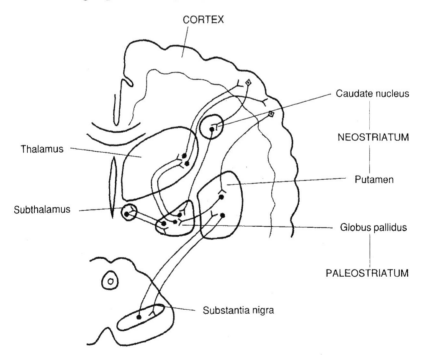

Figure 10.6 The loop systems connecting the cortex through the basal ganglia.

dyskinaesias (abnormal involuntary movement). The general effect on communication is dysarthria and impairment of non-verbal gesture and expression. Diseases of the basal ganglia can be characterized as either producing poverty of movement or excess of movement.

Parkinson's disease, resulting from inadequate amounts of the monoaminergic transmitter dopamine in the substantia nigra, is characterized by uncontrolled tremors, impairment of movement, slowness of movement and muscular rigidity and is an example of a disorder showing poverty of movement. The tremor often starts in the hand, especially the thumb and index finger, and is increased by stress but temporarily reduced by holding an object. It is the slowness and general impairment of movement that is often the most disabling aspect of Parkinson's disease. These signs can affect any muscles and often the muscles of facial expression are affected so that expression becomes fixed and mask-like with lack of expression of emotion. Coupled with lack of gesture generally, non-verbal aspects of communication are seriously impaired. Gait becomes shuffling and hurried. Muscular rigidity causes an uneven jerky resistance when a limb is moved passively. Speech is affected in the majority of clients with Parkinson's disease and worsens as the disease progresses. Characteristically, the voice becomes monotonous and reduced in volume. Rigidity of the respiratory muscles makes it difficult to alter force of expiration and therefore loudness cannot be varied. Sentences tend to fade away as the client runs out of breath. The vocal cords become rigid, producing dysphonia, which is characterized by low pitch and tremulous voice. The voice also becomes hypernasal, as palatal elevation and closure becomes more difficult (see Chapter 19). Dysarthria affects all the muscles involved in articulation but speech usually only becomes indistinct in the later stages of the disease. In the earlier stages, difficulty in initiating movement affects speech: the client is slow to respond but then there is often an acceleration of speech with repetition and words getting faster and faster until they slur and trail away. The cause of all these signs is the degeneration of the neurons in the substantia nigra that form the striatonigral loop which results in an increase in inhibitory activity from the basal ganglia and a reduction in movement.

Lesions of other parts of the basal ganglia can produce a variety of signs and symptoms. Dyskinaesia may be dance-like (**chorea**), or exhibit slow writhing movements (**athetosis**) or violent flailing movements. The latter are characteristic of **hemiballismus**, which is caused by vascular occlusion in the subthalamic nuclei. Chorea and athetosis cause jerkiness of speech which is sometimes explosive due to sudden involuntary movements of the respiratory, laryngeal and perioral muscles. In severe cases, speech is virtually unintelligible. Here, excess of movement is the abiding characteristic resulting from a reduction in inhibitory activity from the basal ganglia that releases the thalamus from inhibition.

A summary of motor function

The control of voluntary muscular activity is extremely complex. Nerve tracts from several sources project to the lower motor neurons in the spinal cord which then convey impulses to the muscle and cause them to contract.

Neurons from various areas of the cerebral cortex pass in loops through deeper areas of the cerebral hemispheres before returning to the motor cortex. One system forms a cortico-striato-cortical loop and passes through the basal ganglia. This loop appears to form an inhibitory system suppressing unwanted random movement. A second loop system is the cortico-ponto-cerebello-cortical system passing from the cortex through the pons to the cerebellum and back to the cortex. This system has a role in controlling the rate, range and force of movement (Figure 10.7).

No less than five pathways project to the lower motor neurons. The direct corticospinal pathways travel without intermediate synapses

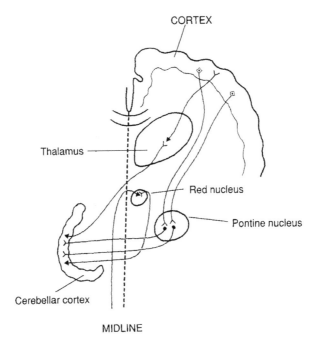

Figure 10.7 The loop system connecting the cortex through the cerebellum.

directly to the appropriate level of the spinal cord and control fine movement of the extremities. Other nerves leave the motor cortex but synapse at intermediate nuclei before reaching the lower motor neurons to form indirect corticospinal pathways. The corticorubrospinal tracts, with connections in the red nucleus of the midbrain and the corticoreticulospinal tracts, and with synapses in the reticular nuclei of the brainstem, form these indirect pathways. These pathways may play a part in coordination of complex movements requiring little dexterity. Most of the nerves in these pathways cross to the opposite side somewhere en route from the cortex to spinal cord; thus the right hemisphere controls movement of the left side of the body.

Visual information and positional information (balance) are paramount for coordinated muscular movement. Tectospinal pathways carry visual information from the tectal region of the midbrain to the lower motor neurons and vestibulospinal pathways convey information about head position and angular movement to the spinal cord. Finally, lower motor neurons receive information about the degree of stretch and contraction in the muscle they control from afferent fibres originating in the muscles or their tendons.

When motor pathways cross, the majority do so at the level of the lower medulla oblongata. Most of the cranial nerve motor nuclei lie above this level and receive a mixture of nerves originating from the ipsilateral and contralateral cortex. The effects of interruption of these corticonuclear pathways are not as serious as interruption of corticospinal pathways. There is generally some remaining input to the cranial lower motor neurons, as lesions tend to be unilateral and therefore only interrupt pathways in one side of the CNS.

CHAPTER 11

The cranial nerves

The peripheral nerves distributed throughout the head and neck, and in some cases beyond, are the **cranial nerves**. Twelve pairs of cranial nerves are distinguished and are given a numerical designation according to the order in which they arise from the brain; the most anterior nerves have the lowest number (Figure 11.1). Strictly speaking, the first and second cranial nerves are not peripheral nerves but are an integral part of the forebrain, connecting it to special sensory receptors, the olfactory epithelium in the nose and the retinae of the eyes respectively. Following head injuries, strokes and other trauma, the function of the cranial nerves and the integrity of their reflexes are examined to determine the extent of damage. A knowledge of the distribution and function of the cranial nerves is therefore essential to clinical practice but also serves as a basis for much of the anatomy of the head and neck and its function in speech.

The olfactory nerves

The first pair of nerves are the **olfactory nerves**. The specialized olfactory mucosa for reception of smell is found in the most superior part of the nasal cavity (see Chapter 19). The axons of neurosensory cells forming the mucosa pass through the bone separating the nasal cavities from the frontal lobe of the brain to synapse in the olfactory bulb, the peripheral dilated portion of the olfactory nerve (Figure 11.1). From the olfactory bulb, each olfactory nerve forms a prominent flat nerve on the base of the frontal lobe of each hemisphere and terminates in the olfactory cortex. The sense of smell is of relatively little importance in man compared with most other species. Clinically, loss of smell may pass almost unnoticed except that food tends to taste blander, an experience also found when the nose is blocked because of a heavy cold. The function of the olfactory nerves is tested by administering smelling salts or other strong smelling substances under the nostrils.

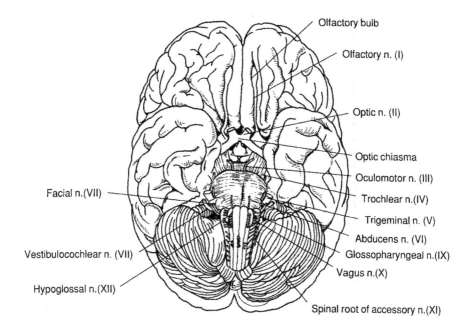

Figure 11.1 The exit of the cranial nerves from the inferior surface of the brain.

The optic nerves

Each optic nerve passes from the retina and exits the posterior medial part of the eyeball to pass through the **optic canal** into the middle cranial fossa (Figure 11.2). The two nerves are partially joined at the **optic chiasma** and diverge again to form the **optic tracts** which pass to the visual cortex in the occipital lobe. Damage to the retina or optic nerve results in blindness in the affected eye. Once the optic nerves have reached the optic chiasma, the effects of damage at these levels is much more complex due to the elaborate segregation of nerves from different parts of the retina within the optic tracts and visual cortex.

Visual pathways

The stimulation of visual pathways is an excellent example of the phenomenon of **disinhibition**, a sort of 'double-negative' way in which much of the central nervous system may operate. Put simply, many CNS pathways may not be positively stimulated to conduct impulses but may be held in a state of inhibition until the inhibition is released. Release of inhibition (disinhibition) allows nerve conduction to occur. The retina of

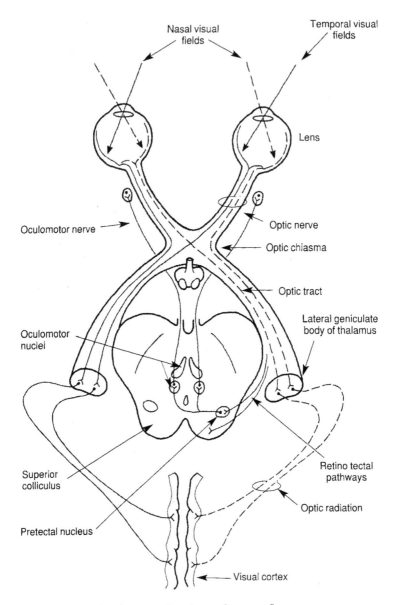

Figure 11.2 The visual pathways and pathways for eye reflexes.

the eye has visual receptors in the form of cells named **rods** and **cones** which release an inhibitory substance preventing transmission in the nerves in the deeper layers of the retina. When light enters the eye, the pigments in the rods and cones are converted into a material which prevents the release of the inhibitory transmitter, thus allowing the nerve fibres to propagate an impulse.

Due to the convex curvature of the cornea and the biconcave lens the visual image is inverted; the variable lens allows it to be focused (Figure 11.2). Thus objects on the ceiling form an image on the lower part of the retina and objects seen out of the lateral corner of the eye will project to the medial part of the retina. The fields of vision are divided into a **temporal** and **nasal** field for each eye (Figure 11.2) and lie laterally and medially respectively. Again, their representation on the retina is inverted.

The nerves leaving the retina from each eye form the two **optic nerves** which pass through the optic canal in the posterior part of the orbit to enter the cranial cavity. Just inside the cavity, the two nerves converge to form the **optic chiasma**. They then diverge posterior to the chiasma. Within the optic chiasma, nerve axons from the medial or nasal half of the retina (corresponding to the temporal fields of vision) cross to the opposite side at the chiasma (Figure 11.2). The axons from the lateral or temporal half of the retina receiving the nasal visual fields, do not cross. The optic nerves continue back to a nucleus in the thalamus, the **lateral geniculate body**, where they synapse. The continuation of the visual pathways from the lateral geniculate body constitute the **optic radiation**, a tract of nerve fibres passing through the posterior part of the internal capsule to reach the **visual cortex** situated along the upper and lower lips of the **calcarine sulcus** on the medial surface of the occipital lobe of the hemispheres. Point to point representation of the retina is retained throughout the visual pathways but partially changes sides at the optic chiasma.

Some axons from the optic tract leave the nerve after the optic chiasma, bypassing the lateral geniculate body to reach the area of the midbrain in and above the superior colliculi, known as the **tectum** (see Figure 8.7). These **retinotectal** pathways are involved in the **pupillary light reflex** and the **accommodation reflex**. Tectospinal pathways involved in motor function also originate in the tectum (see Chapter 10).

Before considering the remaining ten cranial nerves, it is worth diverting to discuss some general points about the organization of the central connections of the cranial nerves. Their sensory nerves and motor nerves terminate on or originate from **cranial nerve nuclei** in the brainstem. Some cranial nerves also have autonomic components and these nerves also have their own nuclei in the brainstem. You will recall that the dorsal half of the grey matter of the spinal cord is sensory and the anterior half is motor, with the autonomic components originating from the lateral horns between the dorsal and ventral horns. A similar relationship is preserved in the brainstem but because of the intrusion of the fourth ventricle causing an expansion of its roof, the brainstem is splayed out so that sensory nuclei lie laterally and motor nuclei medially with autonomic nuclei in between. It is relatively straightforward to anticipate the arrangement of the central connections of the cranial nerves by applying a few simple rules (which in some cases are, needless to say, broken).

- Each cranial nerve has one nucleus for each function so if it is a mixed sensory and motor nerve, it will have a sensory nucleus and a motor nucleus on each side. The sensory nuclei of cranial nerves are, however, associated with a single function so that all axons carrying a particular sensory modality converge on to the same nucleus irrespective of their nerve of origin; all axons carrying taste, which enter with two different nerves, terminate in the same nucleus. In contrast, motor axons in one motor nerve only originate from one motor nucleus.
- The nuclei lie at the same level as the nerve enters or leaves the brainstem so if a nerve is attached to the lower part of the pons, its nuclei will also be in the lower part of the pons.
- Sensory nuclei lie laterally, motor nuclei medially and autonomic nuclei in between, so the sensory nuclei of a mixed nerve would lie under the lateral surface of the brainstem and their motor nuclei near the midline.

The oculomotor, trochlear and abducens nerves

These three pairs of nerves innervate the **extraocular muscles** which move the eyeballs within the orbital cavities and thus control eye movement and the muscle which raises the upper eyelid and opens the eye. The oculomotor nerves also contain autonomic nerves which control the **pupils** and the **lenses**.

The **oculomotor (third) cranial nerves** arise from two pairs of nuclei in the midbrain, one pair for the motor nerves and the other pair for the autonomic nerves. The nerves emerge from the anterior surface of the midbrain (Figure 11.1) and enter the orbit through the **superior orbital fissures** in the posterior wall of the orbit. They supply the superior, inferior and medial rectus muscles which turn the eyeball up, down and medially respectively, the inferior oblique muscle which turns the eye upwards and outwards and the elevator muscle of the upper eyelid (Figure 11.3). The parasympathetic components of the oculomotor nerve control the **ciliary muscles** which alter the thickness of the lens and hence the focusing of the eye and the pupillary constrictor muscles which narrow the diameter of the pupil and control the amount of light falling on the retina. As the amount of light falling on the eye increases, the pupils contract; conversely, moving into the dark will stimulate pupillary dilation. The afferent pathway of the **pupillary light reflex** is the optic nerve and the efferent pathway is the oculomotor nerve (Figure 11.2). The reflex is **consensual**, that is, it occurs in both eyes, because the optic tracts send axons from both eyes to the oculomotor autonomic nuclei in both sides of the midbrain. A similar reflex of pupillary constriction, accompanied by eye convergence and thickening of the lens, make up the **accommodation reflex** when visually fixing on a near object.

The **trochlear nerves**, the fourth cranial nerves, are slender nerves which originate from the trochlear nuclei in the midbrain and exit from its posterior surface. They pass in the free edge of the tentorium cerebelli (see Figure 8.5) and enter the orbit by the same route as the oculomotor nerve to supply the superior oblique muscles which turn the eyeball downwards and outwards (Figure 11.3).

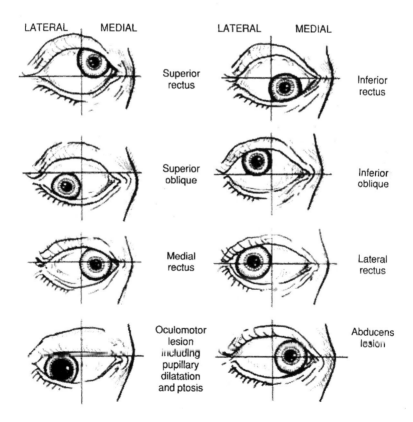

Figure 11.3 Normal eye movements (upper three panels) and the result of damage to the oculomotor and abducens nerves (lower panel).

The **abducens nerves** (the sixth nerves) originate from motor nuclei in the lower pons and exit from its anterior surface at its junction with the medulla oblongata (Figure 11.1). They run upwards along the cranial base to pass through the cavernous sinuses and **superior orbital fissures** into the orbit. They supply the lateral rectus muscles which turn the eyeballs laterally – or abduct them – hence the name of the nerves (Figure 11.3).

Clinical anatomy of the nerves supplying the orbital muscles

The three pairs of cranial nerves innervating the extraocular muscles may be affected by fractures involving the orbit or raised intracranial pressure or by localized stroke or tumours in the brainstem. The sixth nerves are particularly vulnerable when intracranial pressure is raised as they have a long course in contact with bone and are therefore easily compressed against it. Comparatively rarely, the cranial base may be fractured and this too can damage the abducens nerve. The first presenting symptom of damage to any of these three nerves is **diplopia (double vision)**. The integrity of the nerves may be tested by a combination of testing of reflexes, examination of the eye position of the client and **following tests** whereby the client is asked to follow an object moved in various directions across the visual field.

Damage to the abducens nerve causes a **medial strabismus** or squint with diplopia (double vision) because the eye cannot be turned laterally and the opposing muscles will eventually exert an unopposed medial pull (Figure 11.3). Damage to the oculomotor nerve causes an inferolateral strabismus for similar reasons that the medial pull on the eye is lost, pupillary dilatation because the autonomic supply to the constrictors is lost and drooping of the upper eyelid – **ptosis** (Figure 11.3). These are relatively easy to detect on inspection of the patient or with a following test. Loss of pupillary parasympathetic innervation may be ascertained by shining a pen torch into each eye in turn to stimulate the **pupillary light reflex**. Damage to the trochlear nerve rarely occurs in isolation and in such cases is quite difficult to detect. The superior oblique muscle turns the eye downwards and laterally. If the trochlear nerve is injured, diplopia is maximal when the patient looks in this direction; this may cause difficulty in walking downstairs because the subject cannot see the edge of the stairs clearly.

The trigeminal nerves

Functionally, the **trigeminal nerves** are straightforward: they are the sensory nerves to much of the skin of the face and scalp and to the deep structures of the face and they are the motor supply to the muscles of mastication and some other muscles. Anatomically, however, their course and distribution are complex (see Chapters 18 and 19).

The larger sensory components of trigeminal nerves enter the pons to terminate in the **trigeminal sensory nuclear complex** (TSNC) which extends from the midbrain cranially into the cervical spinal cord caudally. The sensory nucleus is so large because, in order to maintain spatial discrimination in the highly important sensory areas subserved by the trigeminal nerve such as the lips and tongue, one-to-one synapses between the trigeminal primary sensory neurons and the thalamic projection neurons in the nuclear complex are required. The requisite number of nerve cell bodies will simply not fit into the pons, hence the expansion of the nucleus into the midbrain and spinal cord. The TSNC comprises three nuclei: the main sensory nucleus in the pons; the spinal nucleus in the medulla and upper cervical spinal cord; and the mesencephalic nucleus in the midbrain. Each nucleus is associated with separate sensory functions. The main nucleus receives axons mediating discriminative touch, the spinal nucleus is the terminal site of axons carrying pain and temperature information and the mesencephalic nucleus deals with proprioception (see Chapter 9). The smaller motor root originates from the **trigeminal motor nucleus** in the pons and leaves at the same point as the sensory root enters. In common with spinal sensory nerves, cranial sensory nerves have their cell bodies in sensory ganglia external to the CNS. Each trigeminal nerve has a single **trigeminal ganglion** on the sensory root lateral to the pons. Peripheral to the ganglion, each trigeminal nerve has three major divisions designated the **ophthalmic**, **maxillary** and **mandibular** divisions (*trigemina* means 'triplets', hence the name). The motor root bypasses the ganglion to join the mandibular division, the only division which has a motor component.

The easiest way to remember the anatomy of the trigeminal nerve is to consider an important clinical point – the cutaneous distribution of the three divisions of the nerve (Figure 11.4). The upper, **ophthalmic**, division supplies the skin of the forehead as far back as the vertex of the skull and down as far as the upper eyelid, with a small extension to the tip of the nose. The **maxillary division** innervates the skin from the lower eyelids to the upper lips, excluding the bridge of the nose. The **mandibular division** innervates the skin of the lower lips and the lower jaw extending back in front of the ear as far as the temple. The deep structures underlying these three cutaneous areas are innervated by the same division of the nerve. Thus the ophthalmic division innervates the orbit and some of the air sinuses and part of the nasal cavity, the maxillary division innervates the nasal cavity, maxillary sinuses, palate, upper teeth and nasopharynx, while the mandibular division innervates the lower teeth, tongue and floor of the mouth.

Each **ophthalmic division** passes through the superior orbital fissure into the orbit where it branches to supply those structures and areas mentioned above. The **maxillary division** leaves the skull and almost immediately divides into numerous branches. Except for the terminal branches innervating the skin, the maxillary division is enclosed within the bones of the middle third of the face. The branches are named after the structures they innervate: the palatine nerves innervate the palatal mucosa for example. Each **mandibular division** emerges from the skull deep to the mandible, and divides into a small anterior motor division and a much larger sensory posterior division. The motor divisions supply motor nerves to the muscles of mastication and some other muscles in the floor of the mouth. The sensory divisions supply the lower teeth and skin of the chin and lower lip, the floor of the mouth and the anterior part of the tongue, the skin of the ear and temporal region. Some named branches of the trigeminal nerve will be considered in more detail in Chapters 18 and 19.

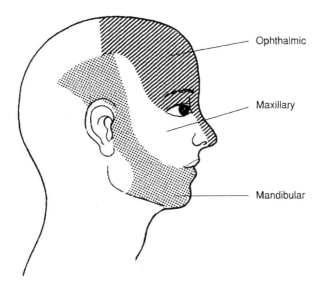

Figure 11.4 The cutaneous sensory distribution of the divisions of the trigeminal nerve.

Clinical anatomy of the trigeminal nerves

Individual branches of the nerve may be involved in facial injuries resulting in sensory loss in the affected areas of skin and oral mucosa. One branch which is not infrequently damaged is the **lingual branch** supplying the tongue; it passes close to the mandible at the level of the third molar (wisdom) tooth and may be damaged by surgical removal of that tooth resulting in anaesthesia of one side of the anterior part of the tongue (see Chapter 19). Sensory loss from the lips results in difficulty locating their position and articulation of speech tends to be affected. Anyone who has had a local anaesthetic for dental treatment with accompanying numbness of the lip will have experienced this effect temporarily. Damage to the motor components of the trigeminal nerve are comparatively rare but produce paresis of the muscles of mastication; the jaw will deviate to one side because of unopposed action of the unaffected contralateral muscles.

The facial nerves

The seventh cranial nerves, the facial nerves, have a large motor component supplying the subcutaneous muscles of the face, the **muscles of facial expression** which produce facial expression and lip movements (see Chapter 18). In addition, the facial nerves have parasympathetic components controlling secretion from salivary, nasal and lacrimal glands and also contain sensory nerves which carry taste sensation from the anterior part of the tongue.

The facial nerves therefore originate from three pairs of nuclei in the brainstem, one pair for each of the main functions they subserve. The motor nerves originate in the **motor nuclei of the facial nerve**, the parasympathetic nerves arise from **salivatory nuclei** and sensory nerves terminate in the **tractus solitarius**. The facial nerves leave the brainstem at the angle between the pons and cerebellum and enter the **internal auditory meatus** in the petrous temporal bone in company with the eighth cranial nerve. The seventh nerve passes around the middle ear cavity where parasympathetic efferent nerves leave the main nerve to take a complex course to the lacrimal glands. At a point where the motor nerves turn backwards to form a knee-like bend (the genu), where **geniculate ganglion** containing the cell bodies of the taste afferent nerves is found. Distal to the ganglion, the remaining parasympathetic nerves and the sensory components form a separate branch called the **chorda tympani**. This branch crosses the tympanic membrane and joins the mandibular division of the trigeminal nerve, travelling with it to supply the taste buds of the anterior two-thirds of the tongue and adjacent salivary glands in the floor of the mouth. A small branch also supplies the stapedius muscle which damps down vibrations in the ossicles of the middle ear (see Chapter 22). After the middle ear, the nerve consists entirely of motor axons. They emerge from the stylomastoid foramen on the inferior surface of the skull and pass on to the face to innervate the muscles of facial expression (Figure 11.5). The peripheral distribution of these branches is clinically important and is described more fully in Chapters 18 and 19.

Central connections of the facial nerves

The **nucleus tractus solitarius** is quite extensive but only its cranial part is concerned with taste reception. Taste sensation is ultimately received bilaterally in the lower primary somatosensory cortex. The lower part of the nucleus tractus solitarius receives visceral afferent inputs from various internal organs and the specialized baroreceptors and chemoreceptors monitoring blood pressure and chemistry (see the section on the glossopharyngeal and vagus nerves below).

The **motor nucleus** of the seventh nerve is peculiar in that the descending inputs to those parts of the nucleus supplying the muscles of the lower face are crossed, whereas the inputs to the upper face are both crossed and uncrossed. A unilateral lesion of corticonuclear pathways will

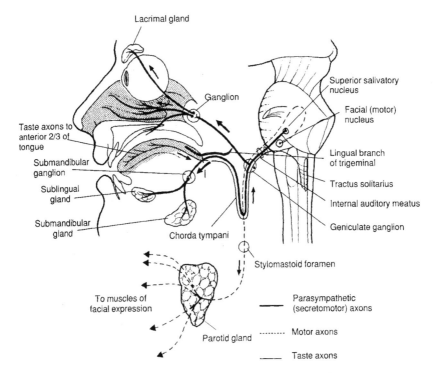

Figure 11.5 The nuclei and distribution of the facial nerve.

cause **contralateral** paralysis of the facial muscles below the eye. As yet unexplained on neuroanatomical grounds is the retention of involuntary responses of paralysed facial muscles to mood and emotion. One possible clue is the flat mask-like expression found in Parkinson's disease; the emotional control of the facial motor nucleus may pass through the cortico-striato-nigro-cortical loops described in Chapter 10.

Clinical anatomy of the facial nerve

Because of its elaborate course through narrow bony canals en route from brain to face, the facial nerve is on the one hand well protected from external injury, but on the other hand is susceptible to compression. Damage to the peripheral nerves produce facial hemiparalysis but the likely level of the lesion (and possible causes) can be determined using anatomical knowledge. If the lesion is distal to the middle ear, only motor activities are lost whereas taste, salivation and lacrimation will also be affected if the lesion is proximal to or in the middle ear. Taste deficiencies may be noticed as an unpleasant metallic taste in the mouth but are usually not discernible. Absence of lacrimation can result in soreness and ulceration of the cornea. Lack of innervation to the stapedius muscle results in **hyperacusis**: everything, even quiet conversation, seems abnormally loud. The facial nerve may be compressed in the internal auditory meatus by an **acoustic neuroma**, a benign neoplasm of the eighth cranial nerve. As well as loss of function due to damage to the facial nerve, ringing in the ears, deficiencies in comprehension and the inability to sustain hearing of pure tones indicate the presence of a neuroma before other signs are detected since hearing and balance are only markedly affected in the late stages.

The most common presentation of facial paralysis is **Bell's Palsy**. Onset of complete hemifacial paralysis is sudden and apparently without cause but is thought to be due to infections in the facial canal compressing the nerve. The infections may be subclinical or may be potentially serious conditions such as meningitis. Damage to the peripheral components of the facial nerve on the face through traumatic injury, surgery or parotid tumours are the other common causes of facial paralysis: these are described in Chapter 18.

The vestibulocochlear nerves

The vestibulocochlear nerves (also called the **auditory** or **acoustic** nerves) supply the inner ear which contains the **cochlea**, the sensory organ for hearing, and the **vestibular apparatus** containing sensory receptors for balance and motion. Each nerve passes from the inner ear through the internal auditory meatus alongside the facial nerve to enter the brainstem at the junction of the pons and medulla. Each nerve terminates in a complex of nuclei, **the cochlear nuclei** from which the auditory pathways originate and the vestibular nuclei from which various tracts concerned with balance begin.

Auditory pathways are anatomically very complex (Figure 23.1) but functionally are relatively straightforward. From the cochlear nuclei, nerves ascend through the superior olivary nuclei to the **inferior colliculi**. Projections are bilateral and may cross and recross at several levels. From the **inferior colliculi** axons pass to the **medial geniculate nucleus** of the thalamus and then to the **transverse temporal gyri** of the temporal lobe forming the **auditory cortex**. Because of the complexity of the pathway and its multiple decussations, lesions of the auditory pathways cause very little disability. Most deafness is associated with damage to the cochlea and cochlear nerve, the ear ossicles or tympanic membrane (see Chapter 22).

Direction and distances of sounds are determined by intensity or time differences between the stimulus in the two ears and are analysed in the **superior olivary complex**. However, to interpret the information meaningfully, it must reach the auditory cortex which is arranged tonotopically, that is areas of the cochlea responding to specific tones project to discrete areas of the cortex so that responses to particular tones are segregated from others. The auditory pathways are described in more detail in Chapter 23.

The glossopharyngeal and vagus nerves

Although both these pairs of nerves are technically mixed motor and sensory nerves, the glossopharyngeal nerves are essentially sensory to areas where the muscles are supplied by the vagus nerves. In this respect and in several others, the ninth and tenth cranial nerves have much in common.

The **glossopharyngeal nerves** contain somatosensory afferent and taste nerves from the posterior part of the tongue and pharynx. They also carry viscerosensory afferent nerves from the carotid sinus and bodies and also distribute parasympathetic secretomotor nerves to the parotid salivary glands. They have a very minor motor component to one pair of muscles. The **vagus nerves** innervate the muscles of the soft palate, the pharynx and the larynx and are also sensory to the larynx. In addition, they have a huge parasympathetic output to the thoracic and abdominal viscera and correspondingly extensive viscerosensory afferent components.

Despite the apparent complexity of function and distribution, the anatomy of both nerves is relatively straightforward as their central nuclear components are shared and they also make use of nuclei associated with other cranial nerves. The somatic afferent components of both nerves terminate in the trigeminal sensory nuclear complex and taste afferents end in the **nucleus tractus solitarius** with those from the facial nerve. Visceral afferent neurons end in the inferior part of the nucleus tractus solitarius. Parasympathetic components of the glossopharyngeal nerves to salivary glands originate in the **salivatory nuclei** along with those of the seventh nerve. Parasympathetic nerves of the vagus originate from two specific nuclei of the vagus nerve, the **dorsal nucleus** and the **nucleus ambiguus** (Figure 11.6). The nucleus ambiguus is also the origin of somatomotor nerves of the vagus. Both nerves leave the medulla oblongata posterior to the olives as a series of fine nerve rootlets (Figure 11.1). Each set combines into the two major nerve trunks and both exit the skull through the **jugular foramen**.

The glossopharyngeal nerves pass forward of either side of the pharynx, innervating its mucosa through the **pharyngeal plexus** of nerves as they do so, to enter the posterior third of the tongue where they supply

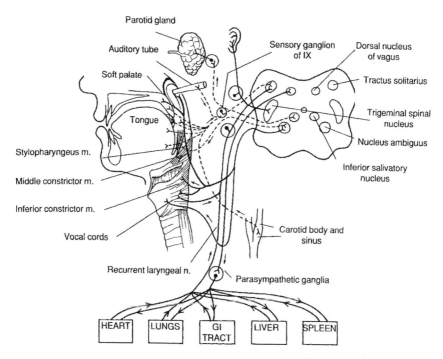

Figure 11.6 The nuclei and distribution of the glossopharyngeal (broken lines) and vagus nerves (solid lines).

the mucosa (Figure 11.6). Smaller branches to the parotid salivary glands and carotid sinuses and bodies are given off en route.

The **pharyngeal branches** of the vagus nerves arise very high in the neck and form the motor component of the pharyngeal plexus which supplies motor nerves to the muscles of the soft palate and pharynx. The **superior laryngeal nerves** innervate the mucosa of the larynx above the vocal folds. The vagus nerves then travel the length of the neck before the last somatic branches, the **recurrent laryngeal nerves**, leave the main nerve in the thorax. These branches, as their name suggests, double back up in the neck to supply the muscles of the larynx and its mucosa below the vocal cords. Their course and functions are described in Chapter 16. The thoracic and abdominal vagus nerves are entirely visceral, supplying the parasympathetic innervation of the thoracic and abdominal viscera through a series of plexuses and carrying visceral afferent nerves from these areas (see Figures 11.6 and 12.2).

Central connections of the glossopharyngeal and vagus nerves

The visceral afferents carried in both nerves are important in reflex control of cardiovascular, respiratory and gastrointestinal function through the autonomic efferent system. Irrespective of origin, these nerves terminate in the inferior part of the **nucleus tractus solitarius** (Figure 11.6). Efferent axons from this nucleus pass through various areas of the reticular system, midbrain and hypothalamus to the dorsal and ambiguus nuclei of the vagus nerve and intermediolateral columns of the spinal cord.

The motor nuclei of the vagus are the **dorsal nucleus** and **nucleus ambiguus** (Figure 11.6). The nucleus ambiguus is preponderantly the motor nucleus but parasympathetic nerves to the heart and oesophagus also originate there. The majority of parasympathetic nerves, however, originate in the dorsal nucleus of the vagus. The nucleus ambiguus, as well as receiving descending inputs from corticonuclear tracts, has important reflex inputs from sensory nerves in the respiratory and gastrointestinal tracts which form reflexes for protective actions such as gagging, vomiting and coughing and coordinate complex activities such as swallowing (see Chapter 21).

Clinical anatomy of the glossopharyngeal and vagus nerves

The glossopharyngeal nerves are rarely damaged in their peripheral course, but may be susceptible during tonsillectomy. Certain branches of the vagus, particularly the **recurrent laryngeal nerves**, are vulnerable; damage results in laryngeal paralysis (see Chapter 16). Central damage to the nuclei of these two cranial nerves is usually due to CVA affecting the brainstem. The nucleus ambiguus is frequently involved along with the trigeminal spinal nucleus when the blood supply of the lateral medulla is interrupted. This is often due to occlusion of the posterior inferior cerebellar arteries and produces a characteristic group of symptoms known as the **lateral medullary syndrome (Wallenberg syndrome)**. The trigeminal sensory nuclei and the nucleus ambiguus of the vagus are lost and the sensory pathways conveying temperature and pain sensations from the trunk and limbs are also affected. This produces ipsilateral loss of pain and temperature sensation on the face and contralateral loss of the same modalities on the body. Paralysis of palatal, pharyngeal and laryngeal muscles occurs ipsilateral to the lesion with attendant difficulties in swallowing (**dysphagia**) and speech (**dysphonia** and **dysarthria**). The consequences of lateral medullary syndrome are discussed more fully in Chapter 21.

The accessory nerves

The **accessory nerves** are not strictly cranial nerves in terms of mature anatomy. Developmentally, however, the motor neurons which constitute the spinal accessory nerve arise in the lower brainstem but migrate into the upper cervical spinal cord. The spinal accessory nerves retrace this migration route as they supply the sternocleidomastoid and trapezius muscles of the neck (see Chapter 16). Damage to the peripheral nerve produces flaccid paralysis of the two muscles. The integrity of the accessory nerves is tested by asking the client to shrug their shoulders against resistance, such as the investigator's hand on their shoulder. When the nerve is damaged this action cannot be performed on the injured side. It is important when testing for suspected motor nerve injury that the muscles are tested against resistance because the client may be able to use weaker muscles supplied by another nerve to produce the movement or, if the injury is long-standing, may have produced trick movements to overcome the deficiency.

The hypoglossal nerves

The twelfth cranial nerves are somatic motor nerves to the muscles of the tongue. The motor neurons lie in the **hypoglossal nuclei** at the caudal end of the medulla oblongata and the nerves leave as rootlets between the olives and pyramids. The nerves exit the skull and pass across the upper anterior neck into the floor of the mouth and then the tongue to supply its musculature.

Flaccid paralysis of the ipsilateral side of the tongue occurs if one peripheral nerve is damaged. When the tongue is protruded it will deviate to the injured side.

Stroke affecting the brainstem

Occlusion of the small **medullary** and **pontine** branches usually affects the direct corticospinal pathways, resulting in contralateral muscle weakness. In the medulla, the major sensory pathways from the dorsal column nuclei to the thalamus may be affected with impairment of proprioception and discriminative touch on the contralateral side. As many of the cranial nerves originate in the pons and medulla, various other effects may be seen depending upon which cranial nerve nuclei are affected.

CHAPTER 12

The autonomic nervous system

The autonomic nervous system (ANS), the other functional division of the peripheral nervous system, maintains **homeostasis** in the viscera and internal environment of the body. This is achieved by regulation of motility and secretion of the cardiovascular, respiratory and digestive systems and control of body temperature by various regulatory mechanisms.

There are two efferent components of the ANS, known as the **sympathetic** and **parasympathetic** systems, which may be distinguished on anatomical and pharmacological grounds. In most cases they also have distinct but interactive physiological functions. The activities of the two systems are sometimes antagonistic but are more often synergistic: their actions are cooperative. Much of the activity of the ANS is determined by reflex action in the lower levels of the brain, spinal cord and peripheral ganglia but higher levels can also influence autonomic output, especially in response to emotion.

Peripheral autonomic efferent nerves

Autonomic efferent axons originate from neurons in the **intermediolateral cell columns**, or more simply the lateral horns, of the spinal cord (see Figure 6.6) or from certain cranial nerve nuclei in the brainstem. The lateral horns lie laterally between the dorsal and ventral horns and the efferent axons exit the spinal cord with somatic motorneurons in the ventral root of spinal nerves. Between the CNS and the target organ, autonomic information does not reach its target directly but is carried by two or more neurons designated as **preganglionic** and **postganglionic** neurons respectively with an intervening synapse (Figure 12.1). The cell bodies of the postganglionic axons form **autonomic ganglia** and it is within these ganglia that the preganglionic neurons synapse with the postganglionic neurons.

187

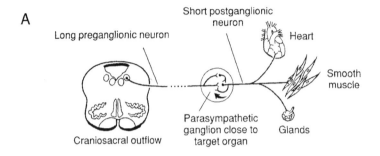

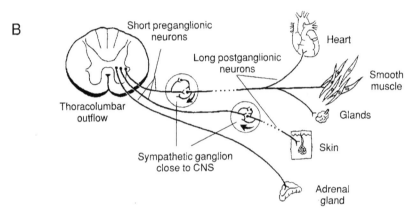

Figure 12.1 The general arrangement of (A) the parasympathetic and (B) the parasympathetic nervous systems.

Parasympathetic nerves

Autonomic efferent axons are not universally distributed with somatic peripheral nerve roots. **Parasympathetic** efferent components leave the CNS in four of the cranial nerves and the sacral spinal nerves and are thus referred to as the **craniosacral outflow** (Figure 12.2). The large intervening gap is covered by the widespread distribution of the vagus nerves. The relatively long autonomic preganglionic components run with the corresponding somatic nerves to the vicinity of their target organs. At this point, they diverge from the parent nerves to synapse in ganglia in or near the target organs. Short **postganglionic** axons then ramify throughout the target organs (Figure 12.1). In common with neuromuscular junctions, **acetylcholine** is the neurotransmitter at both the ganglionic and some target synapses. The **oculomotor**, **facial** and **glossopharyngeal** cranial nerves carry parasympathetic axons to the eyes and glandular tissues in the head and neck (see Chapter 11). The **vagus nerves** constitute the parasympathetic supply to the thoracic and abdominal viscera and the sacral parasympathetic nerves innervate the lower gastrointestinal and urinogenital tracts.

Sympathetic nerves

The **sympathetic** efferent components leave the CNS with all the thoracic and first three lumbar spinal nerves, exiting with the motor roots of the somatic nerves, hence the alternative term of **thoracolumbar outflow** (Figure 12.2). Shortly after the nerves pass through the intervertebral foramina, the preganglionic sympathetic neurons leave the spinal nerves to enter sympathetic ganglia lying adjacent to the vertebral column. The myelinated preganglionic axons form thin bundles, the **white rami communicantes**, between the spinal nerve and the ganglion. After

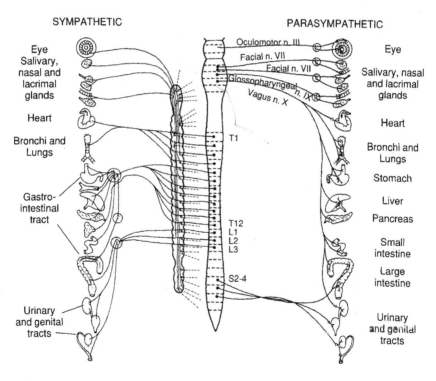

Figure 12.2 The distribution of the autonomic nervous system. For clarity, the distribution of the sympathetic system is shown on the left and the parasympathetic system on the right.

synapsing in the ganglia, relatively long unmyelinated postganglionic axons follow one of three routes (Figure 12.1). They may rejoin the spinal nerve via thin **grey rami communicantes** or, more commonly, run in the connective tissue surrounding arteries to distant organs and tissues supplied by the same arteries; these nerves also supply the arteries themselves. Thirdly, they may form independent visceral nerves to reach specific targets. Preganglionic nerves may run up or down to adjacent sympathetic ganglia before synapsing, their postganglionic axons taking one of the first two exit routes. These vertically disposed axons connect the sympathetic ganglia forming the **sympathetic chains** (Figure 12.2) which lie on the lateral aspects of the vertebral bodies on each side. The sympathetic chain continues beyond the thoracolumbar region into the neck as the **cervical sympathetic chain** and into the pelvic cavity as the pelvic sympathetic chain.

In the neck, the cervical chain has three prominent **cervical ganglia**. The postganglionic axons from these ganglia mainly travel along the carotid arteries to be distributed throughout the head and neck but some nerves enter the cervical spinal nerves to supply the skin of the neck. Other postganglionic nerves from the cervical sympathetic ganglia, together with neurons from the upper thoracic ganglia, innervate the thoracic viscera, especially the heart. In common with the parasympathetic nervous system, **acetylcholine** is the transmitter in sympathetic ganglia between pre- and postganglionic axons but the transmitter used between postganglionic axons and target organs is **noradrenalin**.

In both parasympathetic and sympathetic ganglia there are more postganglionic axons than preganglionic axons or other input axons, thus information at the ganglion is divergent.

The functions of the autonomic nervous system

The parasympathetic system acts to renew energy sources in the body by promotion of digestive activity and general lowering of metabolism, and hence energy utilization, in other systems. As some parasympathetic nerves stimulate secretion in various parts of the gastrointestinal tract, this system is sometimes referred to as the **secretomotor** system. The sympathetic system generates activities which are homeostatic in the short term but also happen to consume energy or provide energy sources locally. Sympathetic stimulation will increase heart rate, cardiac output and respiratory rate, and directs blood to muscle at the expense of cutaneous and gastrointestinal systems. The sympathetic nervous system is also involved in maintenance of body temperature by such devices as reduction or alteration of blood flow through specific areas, sweating, hair erection and muscle activity. The activities of the two systems on different organs and tissues are summarized in Table 6.2

For most of the time, the ANS acts locally to produce a homeostatic effect on a particular organ or system. These effects are mediated through reflexes either between visceral afferent nerves passing through autonomic ganglia or between afferents and autonomic efferents in the spinal cord. Special receptors for blood pressure (**baroreceptors**) and blood chemistry (**chemoreceptors**) located in the major vessels act through the cardiac and respiratory centres in the brainstem and diencephalon. The afferent nerves from these receptors terminate in a nucleus called the **tractus solitarius**, then pass to the reticular formation where their activities are coordinated and thence to the autonomic nuclei of the vagus nerves and the lateral horns in the thoracic and upper lumbar spinal cord. For example, running upstairs may incur an oxygen debt because of muscular exertion. This is balanced by sympathetic action which stimulates bronchodilatation thus increasing respiratory volume and oxygen flow to the lungs and cardiac output so that the oxygen may be distributed more quickly. The high metabolism necessary for exertion increases body temperature. Local sympathetic activity causes dilatation of blood vessels in the skin and sweating to carry away excess heat by evaporation of sweat and cooling at the surface.

The sympathetic part of the ANS can act in toto during stress or emergency to produce the '**flight or fight**' reaction. All possible effects of the sympathetic system are brought into play in preparation for the dramatic action anticipated, producing the well-known pre-examination or pre-interview symptoms of pallor, sweating, a 'thumping' heart, breathlessness and 'butterflies' in the stomach.

Higher control of the autonomic nervous system

The principal areas influencing activity of the ANS are the **hypothalamus**, the **limbic system** and the **prefrontal association cortex**, all of which are extensively interconnected. The limbic system is involved in cognitive functions such as memory, attention, detection of familiarity, behavioural inhibition and basic emotional responses such as fear and rage and is regarded as one of the oldest parts of the cortex phylogenetically. The prefrontal cortex exerts a more subtle influence generally referred to as 'mood'. These higher mental processes may affect autonomic function, sometimes by stimulation but often by inhibition of basic instincts.

The **limbic system** (Figure 12.3) is the marginal area of cortex roughly surrounding the diencephalon. It comprises the **cingulate gyrus** and its forward continuation, the subcallosal gyrus, the **parahippocampal gyrus** on the medial side of the temporal lobe, the **hippocampus** in the temporal lobe itself, the **amygdala** on the anterior end of the parahippocampal gyrus, the **hypothalamus** and the anterior thalamic nucleus. These are connected by well defined pathways which often form discrete structures and link the limbic structures in complex loops. The major output pathway from the limbic system is the hypothalamus.

Direct influences on the **hypothalamus** arise from ascending visceral afferent nerves and also from neurons within the hypothalamus itself which can detect changes in blood chemistry such as osmolarity and glucose levels as well as others. Most of the output from the hypothalamus reaches the parasympathetic nuclei of those cranial nerves with a parasympathetic component and the lateral horns of the spinal cord in the thoracic and upper lumbar segments through the reticular formation in the brainstem. The hypothalamus, through its control of the pituitary gland, has a profound influence on the activity of the endocrine system (see Chapter 7). Through the ANS and the endocrine system, the limbic system is able to influence many aspects of emotional behaviour, especially through modulation of visceral responses. The interconnections of the different structures comprising the limbic system and connections with the hypothalamus and most areas of the association cortex are extremely complex. Lesions in the limbic system, especially the hippocampus, have serious deleterious effects on short-term memory. Lesions in the amygdala reduce emotional excitability.

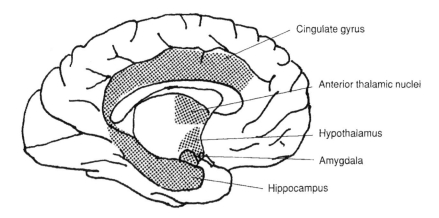

Figure 12.3 The limbic system.

CHAPTER 13

Language processing in the brain

The essential question to be asked about the role of the brain in language is whether there are specific cortical areas responsible for language? If so, are **aphasias** – disorders of language – the manifestations of disturbances of specific areas governing language comprehension and production or are they merely manifestations of more general disturbances of cognitive function already described in Chapters 9 and 10? The answers are that there are specific cortical areas involved in language comprehension and use and that disorders of language (**aphasia**) are due to specific dysfunction of these areas. Disorders of speech – **dysarthria** and **dysphonia** – are fairly clear-cut; they are usually consequent on damage to those parts of the brain concerned with control of motor activity which may be general, affecting muscular activity as a whole, or specific damage to areas controlling the muscles of the larynx and muscle groups involved in articulation such as the muscles of facial expression, mastication, soft palate and pharynx.

Historical perspective

Surprisingly, language areas in the brain were some of the first components to which a specific function could be attributed. We owe this knowledge to the careful clinical and post-mortem observations of Broca who, about a hundred and fifty years ago, studied a patient nicknamed 'Tan Tan' in the asylum where he was the doctor. Tan Tan acquired his nickname because these were the only words, apart from a few expletives, that he ever uttered. Nevertheless, his comprehension was perfectly good and he could understand instructions and respond to them to the extent that he was used as a ward orderly to look after the other patients. When Tan Tan died, Broca examined his brain post mortem and found that there was a large defect in the lower left frontal cortex anterior to what we now know to be the motor cortex governing movements in the head and neck.

He confirmed his observations on a further eight patients with similar language disorders and finally pronounced a landmark finding: 'Nous parlons avec l'hémisphère gauche' ('We speak with the left hemisphere'). This was the first time that localization of a particular function in the cerebral cortex was documented, and led to exploration of other regions in experimental animals to discover areas which served a particular function; it also laid the foundations for ideas of cerebral dominance in the cortex (see Chapter 9). It was quickly confirmed that Broca's findings were not isolated when the primary motor cortex and its somatotopic arrangement were discovered a few years later. Only a decade after Broca's discovery of a language area dealing with language production, Wernicke observed several patients with a different defect. These patients were unable to comprehend speech, but could initiate fluent speech. Post-mortem investigations demonstrated lesions in the left hemisphere around the posterior part of the lateral fissure at the junction of the parietal, temporal and occipital lobes.

The two areas in which defects were found to affect language subsequently became known as Broca's and Wernicke's areas. The defects consequent upon damage to these areas became known as **Broca's aphasia** and **Wernicke's aphasia**. **Broca's area** (Figure 13.1) comprises the **frontal operculum** just anterior to the lower part of the motor cortex and the **pars triangularis** anterior to the frontal operculum. **Wernicke's area** is much more difficult to define as there are no obvious boundaries delineated by conveniently placed gyri but it is usually taken to encompass an area on the superior margin of the temporal lobe posterior to the primary auditory cortex extending around the posterior margin of the lateral fissure. To avoid difficulties in defining specific brain areas, the term 'perisylvian language core' has been used to fudge the issue. ('Sylvian fissure' is the old name for the lateral fissure.) The core area extends from the auditory association cortex posterior to the primary auditory cortex through the angular gyrus and then anteriorly to the supramarginal gyrus in the parietal lobe just above the lateral fissure. As we will see below, these definitions have been modified in recent years.

On the basis of his own observations and those of Broca, Wernicke formulated a theory of language which predicted various manifestations of aphasia which had not at that time been observed clinically. Essentially, he claimed that interconnections between sites carrying out basic functions were the basis of more complex cognitive and intellectual functions of the brain and formulated a model for language processing which has stood the test of time, albeit with many modifications and refinements. He proposed that the auditory and visual perceptions of language are formed in the primary auditory and visual cortices. These are then integrated in

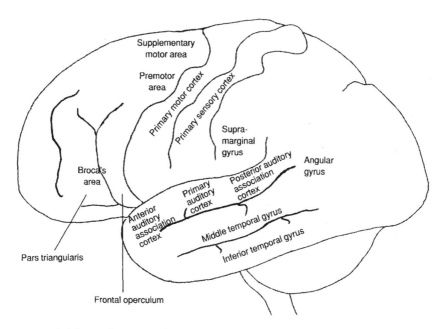

Figure 13.1 Cortical areas involved in language processing.

the adjacent association cortices and then passed to Wernicke's area where they are understood as language and associated with specific meanings. In language production, the encoded language is then passed from Wernicke's area to Broca's area by the **arcuate fasciculus**, a tract of white matter running from the temporal lobe posterior to the lateral fissure and forwards to the frontal lobe connecting Wernicke's and Broca's areas. In Broca's area, language concepts are transformed into a motor signal for either speech or written language which is then enacted by the motor cortex. Using this model, Wernicke predicted the existence of **conduction aphasia** when the two language areas are intact but the connecting arcuate fasciculus is damaged. As they were studied more critically, other manifestations of aphasia became apparent which did not fit into Wernicke's model of language. Lichtheim refined the model to include areas which dealt with cognitive aspects of language although he had no idea where these might be located in the brain. Various other models were put forward based on cognitive models of language which did not relate language deficiencies to specific areas of the brain.

The localization of language comprehension and production in the two proposed language areas was confirmed in the 1950s when it became possible to record electrophysiological responses from brain areas in patients undergoing surgery on the exposed brain under local anaesthetic. Using such methods, Penfield demonstrated that Broca's and Wernicke's areas did appear to act as discrete language areas as predicted. The Lichtheim–Wernicke model was revisited and revived in the early 1960s by Geschwind who argued that aphasic disorders that produced a given set of signs and symptoms could be described most easily by relating them to damaged areas of brain or the axonal tracts which connect them. This is known as the **Wernicke–Lichtheim–Geschwind model**.

One of the problems associated with post-mortem examination of brain tissue is that damage is rarely limited to the cortex alone, but also affects adjacent structures particularly '**fibres of passage**', nerve tracts passing through or adjacent to the damaged area. Furthermore, damage is rarely restricted to functionally or anatomically discrete parts of the brain. To complicate matters still further, clients with aphasia often show more than one cognitive deficit and these may be masked by compensatory strategies evolved by the client. There is then a certain amount of conflict as to whether the effects observed by Broca and Wernicke and predicted by the Wernicke model were due to the primary lesion in the cortex or were more complex entities involving fibres of passage. Many people claim that the proposed model is far too simple to account for the cognitive defects observed.

Recent studies using non-invasive methods, especially PET scanning and fMRI (described in Chapter 8), have confirmed aspects of the Wernicke–Lichtheim–Geschwind model but have also thrown up various observations which have led to further refinements:

- It is now known that signals generated in Broca's area do not pass directly to the adjacent motor cortex controlling the muscles used for phonation and articulation but pass through the supplementary motor and premotor area which are involved in the initiation of complex movement (see Chapter 10).
- Non-invasive studies of language dysfunction have also shown that adjacent structures as well as the specific cortical rim are involved to some extent in language processing and have highlighted several areas of the brain not historically associated with language which are used in language processing. Clinical and experimental observations on aphasic clients indicate that several subcortical structures, including the thalamus and basal ganglia, are also important for language processing.
- Functional studies have also confirmed that some concepts of parallel processing, alternative pathways for dealing with aspects of language, first proposed by cognitive psychologists also operate during language processing.

- They have also shown that several areas of the brain may be activated simultaneously for a particular aspect of language processing. This is known as **functional integration** and differs from the older models of sequential activation.
- Finally, functional imaging studies have shown that large areas formerly treated as one functional entity can be subdivided into different functional areas.

Although great strides have been made in functional neuroimaging in the last few years, it is still in its infancy in some respects. Most functional studies involve single word processing as opposed to sentence processing. Nevertheless, they have clarified our understanding of language processing but more remains to be discovered as technical advances increase the resolution of these techniques and these methods are applied to more complex studies of language processing.

One problem arising from Broca's initial claim that 'we speak with the left hemisphere' is what functions, if any, do the corresponding areas in the right hemispheres have. The answer is that they do have a function in language processing concerned with the **prosody** of language, the intonation and emphasis used to convey mood and subtle meaning. Defects of the right hemisphere language areas are sometimes referred to as **aprosodias**. A client with a right-side Wernicke's defect could not pick up change of tone for emphasis or sarcasm, for example, and one with a right-side Broca's defect would not be able to express emotion by speech tone or emphasis although the delineation of function in specific areas of the right cortex is not as clear-cut as in the dominant left hemisphere.

Language processing

The effective use of language requires the integration of sensory input systems and motor output systems with memory of aspects of language. We need to recall the sounds (**phonology**), spelling (**orthography**) and meaning (**semantics**) of words and semantic and grammatical rules of the language being heard or spoken. Of course, hearing is not the only sensory input; reading, the other major input, requires vision, and blind people use tactile sensory processing to read Braille. Motor output, likewise, is not restricted to speech but involves writing or signing as well as associated facial gestures and body language. Motor output, in whichever form, may occur as a response to a stimulus (written or spoken words) or can be generated internally in response to thought processes. It is therefore no great surprise that several areas of the brain are involved in language processing. The trick is deciding which areas are language-specific or are functionally integrated during language processing.

Visual or auditory input is received at the primary visual and auditory cortices respectively and is further processed in the adjacent secondary association cortices. It is now realized that making distinctions between methods of input (hearing, vision) and output (speaking and writing) are not too helpful in determining the role of different brain areas except in terms of the primary and secondary areas of reception (auditory or visual cortex) or transmission (head and neck or hand areas for speech and writing). It seems that selective areas of the brain deal with specific aspects of linguistic processing irrespective of the input or output.

There appear to be certain areas within the monomodal (secondary) **auditory association cortex** which respond to verbal input, whether written or spoken, and help to distinguish speech from background environmental sounds or writing from other visual symbols. The left association cortex anterior to the primary auditory cortex is a secondary area of auditory processing but is only activated by speech sounds and other human sounds such as coughing. It seems to be the area which distinguishes speech from background environmental sounds and connects directly with the frontal association cortex through the arcuate fasciculus. The left association cortex immediately posterior to the primary auditory cortex, which may be considered as a part of the original Wernicke's area, has no direct connection with the primary auditory cortex but is activated during semantic activities and retrieval of words from memory. Interestingly, the corresponding area of the anterior auditory association cortex on the right is activated by strong dynamic pitch variation (prosody and music) which correlates with the different functions of the two hemispheres in language processing.

These are not the only areas of the temporal cortex involved in language processing. In fact, virtually all of the **temporal cortex** is involved. The cortex of the **middle temporal gyrus** is activated during semantic processing and there is some evidence that the cortex in this area is arranged in a 'semantotopic' fashion. Different areas appear to be activated by different word groups such as nouns or verbs; nouns also appear to be arranged in different groups such as names, tools, parts of the body and so on. The **posterior inferior temporal gyrus** anterior to the cerebellum is concerned with visual recognition of words and pictures and thus appears to connect the semantic areas with the visual areas. The **anterior inferior temporal area** is involved in semantic decision-making (e.g. alive vs. dead, animal vs. vegetable) and may also be involved in analysis of phonemic content of words. Lesions in this area manifest as losses of semantic knowledge.

Because it is difficult to know where the classical Wernicke's area stops, it is hard to ascribe adjacent areas as part of Wernicke's area or separate entities. The **angular gyrus**, the cortex above and below the upward extension of the middle temporal sulcus, is activated in more complex semantic tasks such as sentence reading and lesions in this area cause severe comprehension deficits characteristic of Wernicke's aphasia (see below). The **supramarginal gyrus**, usually considered as part of the perisylvian language core, does not seem to be involved directly in language processing but is involved in tone discrimination, which can play a part in phonological processing.

Semantic knowledge and application is also necessary for language output and there are areas in the frontal lobe in and around Broca's area which are activated and therefore functionally integrated with the temporal areas during semantic tasks. For simple repetition, the pars triangularis of Broca's area is activated but not the frontal operculum. Semantic tasks involve the frontal operculum and extensive areas of the inferior and middle frontal gyri. The frontal operculum is also involved in planning of articulatory movements but another area is also crucial for this activity. This is the **anterior insula**. The insula is a deep lobe of the cerebral cortex hidden from view beneath the frontal, parietal and temporal lobes of the brain. It can only be seen if the lateral fissure is opened out. The insula connects with the adjacent lobes and the anterior insula is connected with the inferior part of the frontal lobe which contains the head area of the motor cortex and Broca's area anterior to it (Figure 8.8).

Other areas of the brain are also involved in language processing but their exact function is not entirely clear. To try to gain some appreciation of the role of the classical language areas of Broca and Wernicke, the newly discovered areas of the frontal and temporal lobes and other structures in language processing, we need to return to studies of aphasia.

Aphasia

The functions of various brain areas involved in language processing and the clinical consequences of brain lesions are best appreciated by examining the effects on language of the various clinically recognized types of aphasia together with other presenting signs and symptoms which give clues about other structures involved. These summaries are derived from the results of careful clinical observation with associated high resolution imaging techniques to verify location and extent of brain lesions.

Wernicke's aphasia

Wernicke's aphasia is classically associated with lesions in Wernicke's area in the **left posterior superior temporal lobe** (the auditory association cortex dealing with semantic tasks of word recognition described above) and the area around the posterior margin of the **lateral fissure**. The most obvious language defect is deficiency of comprehension. Depending on how extensive the lesion is, both visual and auditory language comprehension may be affected. Language output is well articulated and is delivered at the normal rate and rhythm, although it may be excessive, with the client using far more words than are necessary to convey the idea and the content may be almost meaningless. They often use the wrong word or place words in the wrong order (**paraphasia**). Wernicke's aphasics also tend to add additional syllables to words, especially nouns, or make up new words (**neologisms**). Repetition is also severely impaired. Generally, there are no other neurological signs, although there are severe reading (**dyslexia**) and writing difficulties (**dysgraphia**). It now appears that Wernicke's aphasia is also caused by damage to the middle temporal gyrus and the deep white matter interconnecting the different areas of the temporal lobe.

Conduction aphasia

Conduction aphasia is classically associated with lesions affecting the arcuate fasciculus connecting Wernicke's and Broca's areas while leaving the two language areas unaffected. The **arcuate fasciculus** passes through the white matter of the temporal lobe around the back of the lateral fissure, in the white matter deep to the superior marginal gyrus, the lower parts of the somatosensory and somatomotor cortices to Broca's area. It has rather rashly been assumed that the arcuate fasciculus was a one-way system from temporal to frontal lobe but it is now clearly established that it is a reciprocal pathway and carries information in the reverse direction as well. It may therefore be involved in a wide variety of lesions. Lesions may be located in the supramarginal gyrus of the left parietal lobe, the posterior superior aspects of the left temporal lobe, the insula or anywhere in the white matter underlying these areas. There is no evidence that conduction aphasia is caused by a damage to the arcuate fasciculus in isolation, but there is clearly functional disconnection between the frontal, parietal and temporal lobes.

Clients are usually less fluent than those with Wernicke's aphasia but are paraphasic, using inappropriate words or producing the wrong sounds. Significantly, they are unable to repeat or to name objects and cannot read aloud accurately. They usually exhibit severe **dysgraphia**, omitting, substituting or reversing letters. Clients with conduction aphasia often have some degree of impairment of voluntary movement. There may also be a right hemisensory defect and apraxia of the face and limbs. This is consistent with the lesion extending into areas of the parietal association cortex not specifically concerned with language function (see Chapter 9).

Anomic aphasia

Anomic aphasia is specific in that the only obvious deficiency is in finding and using correct words. Lesions may be present in the posterior part of the **inferior temporal gyrus** but many are not localized to a particular brain region. This indicates, not surprisingly, that widely distributed parts of the memory cortex are involved in word usage. One difficulty with classifying anomic aphasia is that clients with most other types of aphasia have word-finding difficulties and even non-aphasic clients with left or right hemisphere lesions have some deficits in this respect.

Transcortical sensory aphasia

Transcortical aphasias do not affect the classical language areas. Instead, the connections between the language areas and the association cortex are damaged. Transcortical sensory aphasia is usually due to lesions in the **tertiary association cortex** around the junction of the parietal, temporal and occipital lobes but it may also arise as a result of lesions in the inferior parts of the left temporal lobe and left thalamus through which some of the connections are probably routed. A characteristic of transcortical aphasias is that repetition of spoken language is fluent, indicating that Wernicke's and Broca's areas are still functionally connected by the arcuate fasciculus. Transcortical sensory aphasia can vary from a severe fluent aphasia with defective comprehension with intact repetition to a more subtle loss of memory of word meaning. It is probably a deficit in semantic aspects of language while syntactic abilities are preserved.

Transcortical motor aphasia

The second type of transcortical aphasia is due to disconnection of Broca's area from the supplementary motor cortex and other areas of the frontal association cortex, usually because of lesions in the frontal lobe anterior to Broca's area, although Broca's area itself may be involved. Such lesions produce a nonfluent aphasia in which the client will attempt conversation but produces only odd words or syllables. However, repetition is preserved. Writing may be affected. Clients with transcortical motor aphasia often exhibit right-sided hemiparesis consistent with connections to adjacent motor areas being involved.

Subcortical aphasia

Transcortical aphasias indicate that successful comprehension and production of language requires much more of the cerebral cortex than the classical language areas and their surrounding association cortex and their immediate connection through the arcuate fasciculus. It is now recognized that various subcortical structures are also involved as damage can produce aphasia, distinguished as subcortical aphasia.

Damage to the **left caudate nucleus** or **putamen** produces a fluent aphasia with extensive use of neologisms. For reasons which are not understood, the aphasia is sometimes only transient although there are case reports of persistent subcortical aphasia. Irrespective of the duration of aphasic symptoms, other aspects of dysfunction of the striate cortex – **dyskinesia** – persist and there is usually some degree of **dysarthria**.

Lesions in the **thalamus** produce effects similar to the transcortical aphasias with paraphasia, poor comprehension but intact repetition. The effects on language are again transient and the client will often make a full recovery. It is difficult to explain both the thalamic involvement and the recovery. Presumably, pathways connecting the language areas with other cortical areas project to and from the thalamus but this does not explain why the effects are only transient.

Broca's aphasia

Broca's aphasia results from damage to much more extensive areas than Broca's area itself. Lesions confined to Broca's area result in apraxia of speech (see below) but not Broca's aphasia. Lesions producing Broca's aphasia extend from Broca's area into adjacent areas of the left frontal association cortex or the premotor area or are limited to these areas. Recent analysis of brain images from Broca's aphasics indicate that the anterior insula is almost inevitably involved. Broca's aphasia varies from almost complete mutism at worst to slow speech constructed from the simplest elements at best. Essentially, Broca's aphasics use only key words, eliminating adjectives, adverbs and articles and using nouns in the singular and verbs in the infinite form. They find it extremely difficult or even impossible to link phonemes into words and words into sentences. Repetition is seriously impaired and writing is usually affected as well. Unlike Wernicke's aphasics, clients with Broca's aphasia are usually acutely aware of the errors they make. In addition to the direct effects on language, clients usually have right hemiparesis and right homonymous hemianopsia (loss of vision from the right eye) because of involvement of the adjacent motor areas and internal capsule.

Global aphasia

Global aphasia results from extensive lesions of the left hemisphere affecting Broca's area, Wernicke's area and the arcuate fasciculus and adjacent structures. Needless to say, all aspects of language are affected: they cannot speak or comprehend, read, write, name or repeat. Because of the extent of the lesions and their effects on other structures, these clients usually have complete right hemiplegia, right hemisensory defects and right homonymous hemianopsia. It is often due to damage to the left middle cerebral artery which supplies most of the lateral aspect of the left hemisphere (see Chapter 8). Some other aphasias manifest as global aphasia initially but resolve into one of the other types as resolution of blood clots occur. Neurons in the brain are not in direct contact with blood under normal circumstances. Blood has deleterious effects when it contacts neurons because it contains many high molecular weight proteins in the plasma and haemoglobin in red cells which disrupt the osmotic balance of any neurons they contact. When the clot resolves, these effects may be reversed so the chronic damage is much less than acute damage.

Aprosodias

Although it has been claimed that language areas in the right hemisphere mirror those in the left hemisphere, this is not widely accepted. Essentially, right hemispheric defects lead to **aprosodia**, the inability to use appropriate tone, rhythm and emphasis to express emotion or subtle nuances or to interpret correctly their use by others, thereby 'missing the point'. Aprosodias consequent upon right parietal lesions are usually accompanied by sensory neglect and dressing apraxia (see Chapter 9)

Cerebral dominance and language function

Ever since Broca's pronouncement that 'we speak with the left hemisphere', the majority of clinical and experimental evidence indicates that language function resides in the left hemisphere. However, functional studies using the **Wada test** have shown that this is not always the case. This test is conducted by injecting sodium amytal unilaterally into the common carotid artery. Despite the presence of the Circle of Willis (see Chapter 8), normal blood flow is unilateral so that, for example, blood from the left internal carotid artery will only enter the left anterior and middle cerebral arteries and will not cross to the right side or flow posteriorly into the areas supplied by the posterior cerebral arteries. The middle cerebral arteries supply the lateral aspects of the frontal and parietal cortex and the superior aspects of the temporal cortex and therefore the language areas and much of the association cortex involved in processing of language. The branches of the internal carotid arteries also supply most of the primary motor and sensory cortices and the auditory cortex too. The effect of injection of sodium amytal is immediate and dramatic: brain function is depressed in the areas that the drug reaches. Sodium amytal is, however, rapidly degraded so that function rapidly returns to normal. The client will lose control of both limbs on the opposite side to the injection and also experience a contralateral sensory loss. Language ability is examined by a battery of tests which include being asked to count, to name objects shown as pictures and to answer questions. Sodium amytal usually has a more profound effect on language on one side than the other. In one series of tests, language was represented in the left hemisphere in over 95 per cent of right-handed people but also in 70 per cent of left-handed people. A few subjects had bilateral representation of language, but even then, there were subtle differences in the function of each hemisphere: naming was stronger on one side whereas correct selection of word order was stronger on the other.

An interesting insight into this issue is provided by various studies of the deaf or users of sign languages. Sign languages vary in complexity from simple pictographic/iconic representations (e.g. cupped hands for 'drink') or spelling out of words by hand gesture corresponding to letter shape to complex languages such as British and American Sign Language. In these languages, use is made of hand, arm and facial gesture to produce emphasis and inflection and their semantic and grammatical rules differ from the rules of spoken language. If it is accepted that the right hemisphere deals with visuospatial phenomena and the left hemisphere with abstract functions including language, which hemisphere is dominant when using sign language? If the left hemisphere is the site of a lesion in deaf people, they become aphasic for sign language with the same manifestations of defects in comprehension, fluency or repetition as are observed in people using spoken language. This indicates that the left hemisphere is dominant for sign language as well as spoken language. Deaf clients with right-side lesions show little difficulty with use or interpretation of sign language since prosody is usually seriously impaired in profoundly deaf people anyway. In one isolated case of a fluent signer, the Wada Test produced parallel defects in interpretation and production of spoken and signed language when sodium amytal was injected into the left internal carotid artery, showing left cerebral dominance for a language which is predominantly visuospatial in execution but nevertheless abstract in structure.

Dyslexia and dysgraphia

One aspect of language disorders that is apparent from the considerations of aphasia above is that visual input (reading) and manual output (writing) of language are sometimes affected in some types of aphasias and are unaffected in others. This demonstrates that all aspects of language are not processed in the same areas of the brain and that distinctions can be made between processing of spoken and written input and output.

Dyslexia may be **developmental**, manifesting as reading difficulties as these skills are acquired in early school years, or **acquired** as a consequence of brain lesions. There are no obvious lesions in the brains of developmental dyslexics although there are reports of subtle brain abnormalities. In acquired dyslexia, quite small circumscribed lesions in the brain in the tertiary association cortex at the junction of the temporal, parietal and occipital lobe can produce dyslexia or agraphia without interfering with other aspects of speech and language. Essentially, clients cannot associate letters as symbols of sound with the sound itself. They can neither recognize written words nor spell.

Pure word blindness (alexia without agraphia) is due to lesions in the **visual association cortex** and the adjacent posterior part of the **corpus callosum** where visual information is passed between the two hemispheres. Information received by the right visual cortex cannot be passed to the left language areas. Such clients can associate meaning with words spelt out to them and can spell correctly.

Damage to the anterior **corpus callosum** interferes with writing, especially in left-handed people, as the left language areas cannot be accessed by the right motor cortex which controls the left hand. They also cannot name objects placed in the left hand as the right somatosensory cortex cannot pass the information to the left hemisphere.

Other language defects due to cortical damage

Two specific conditions affecting control of oral structures are recognized which are not manifestations of dysarthria or aphasia or other forms of dyspraxia. They are poorly understood. **Oral apraxia** is the impairment of non-speech volitional movements of structures involved in speech, usually the tongue. For example, a client with oral apraxia may not be able to stick their tongue out on command. **Apraxia of speech** is impairment of speech articulatory movements specifically in the absence of paresis or sensory impairment. A client thus affected may be able to lick biscuit crumbs from their lips but not place their tongue correctly for, say, alveolodental phonemes. The two conditions often coexist but apraxia of speech may present alone. It is uncertain whether they are different conditions or are a continuum of signs and symptoms with more severe conditions affecting gross oral movements as well as specific speech movements. Both oral apraxia and apraxia of speech are due to lesions in the language dominant (usually left) hemisphere and are *independent* of other manifestations of apraxia because the lesion is usually in the left frontal cortex as opposed to the parietal cortex (see Chapter 9). However, similar signs and symptoms have been reported in some clients with lesions in the left parietal cortex. Apraxia of speech thus seems to be a deficiency in formulation of complex movement rather than a defect in spatial guidance seen in other forms of dyspraxia. Apraxia of speech has now been associated with lesions confined to Broca's area.

CHAPTER 14

The structure of the respiratory system

The respiratory system comprises the **respiratory tract** conveying air to and from the lungs, the **lungs** themselves, their surrounding **pleural membranes**, the **thoracic wall**, formed by the thoracic vertebrae, ribs, sternum and intervening muscles, and the **diaphragm**. All these structures are involved in ventilatory movements to move air into and out of the lungs. The respiratory tract is divided in terms of function into a **conducting zone** consisting of reinforced tubes of decreasing diameter which lead into the **respiratory zone** in the lung alveoli where gaseous exchange between the lungs and the blood take place. Oxygen diffuses from the inspired air into the blood and carbon dioxide diffuses in the opposite direction to be expired. In clinical terms, the conducting zone is divided into the **upper respiratory tract** comprising the nose and mouth, pharynx and larynx and the **lower respiratory tract** comprising the trachea and bronchial tree. The upper respiratory tract, although essential for ventilation, plays a more significant role in articulation of speech and is more fully described in Chapter 19.

Ventilatory movements are designed to maintain adequate oxygenation levels in the lungs and to ensure removal of waste gases, in particular CO_2. This in turn ensures adequate oxygenation of and clearance of CO_2 from the blood by **external respiration**, the exchange of gases between the lungs and blood. By efficient gaseous exchange at this level, the requisite levels of oxygen and clearance of CO_2 will be sufficient to maintain the tissues by **internal respiration**, the exchange of gases between blood and the tissues. Bodily demands for oxygen vary according to the functions being performed at any one time, and changes in ventilation rate and volume are the key to ensuring that oxygen demand is met. CO_2 must be removed from the blood otherwise the blood pH will fall to the detriment of the bodily tissues; increases in blood CO_2 levels also stimulate changes in ventilation. In fact, the levels of blood CO_2 are more significant in determining the respiratory rate than is the oxygen demand.

Ventilation is controlled automatically by respiratory centres in the brainstem. However, the automatic control of respiration can be overridden and bypassed by higher centres in the brain and respiration can become voluntary if, for example, you are requested to take a deep breath. During vocal activities such as speech or singing, the respiratory centres are overridden and respiration moves into the realms of a learned motor skill and is not purely voluntary. Because we rarely think about our breathing during speech, it is often considered as being a trivial part of the speech and language chain when it is in fact all important. The coordination of respiratory activity during speech is extremely complex and probably compares with other compound aspects of speech and language such as linguistic encoding and decoding.

The upper respiratory tract

The conducting zone of the respiratory tract (see Figure 5.1) is more than mere gas piping. **Cleaning, humidification** and **warming** of the inspired air are important functions of the conducting zone. Humidification and cleaning take place in virtually the whole extent of the respiratory tract but the upper respiratory tract is particularly involved in warming inspired air. These functions are carried out by respiratory mucosa lining the whole of the conducting zone of the respiratory tract. **Respiratory mucosa** consists of respiratory epithelium (see Chapter 2) supported by very vascular connective tissue containing numerous mucous and serous glands. Respiratory epithelium is ciliated and contains numerous goblet cells which secrete mucus over the entire epithelial surface. Mucous glands in the connective tissue supporting the epithelium add to the volume of mucus secreted by the goblet cells. Large particles are removed by the nasal hairs in the entrance to the nose. Small particles and various noxious gases are trapped by or dissolved in the mucus which is continually swept backwards from the nasal cavities or upwards from regions below the laryngeal inlet towards the pharynx from where it is swallowed or expectorated. The mucous and serous secretions also humidify the inspired air. The respiratory mucosa in the nasal cavities in particular has a very rich vascular network, and heat exchange between blood and inhaled air warms the air (see Figure 5.2). Bony projections from each lateral wall of the nasal cavity enlarge their surface area to increase efficiency of heating and humidifying inhaled air. The paranasal air sinuses, four paired air-filled cavities in the bones adjacent to the nasal cavity, are lined with respiratory mucosa continuous with that of the nose. They provide a reservoir of mucus which is outside the direct air stream and is therefore less susceptible to dehydration in extremes of temperature and humidity.

The sinuses also amplify basic vocalization and act as resonance chambers (see Chapter 19); resonance is noticeably reduced in upper respiratory tract infections.

In areas of the respiratory tract subject to abrasion and friction, stratified squamous epithelium replaces respiratory epithelium; this is found where the gastrointestinal and respiratory tracts share a common pathway in the pharynx and where it is subject to vibrational stress at the vocal cords in the larynx. A small area in the roof of the nasal cavities contains olfactory epithelium specialized for detection of smell.

Returning to the basic function of movement of air into and out of the lungs, the conducting zone must remain open irrespective of the changes in air pressure within it. Patency is maintained by cartilage in the walls of the respiratory tract augmented by bone in the nose. The cartilage forms incomplete rings with posterior deficiencies in the larynx and trachea and consists of irregular plates or complete rings in the bronchial tree. As the respiratory tract passes through areas where much movement occurs, some degree of flexibility and extensibility is essential. These requirements are met by a combination of the physical properties of cartilage together with connective tissue which has a relatively high content of elastic fibres. Elastic fibres form an important component of both respiratory and conducting portions of the respiratory system and are most numerous in the smaller diameter tubes; the energy which inflates the lungs is also used to a large extent to deflate them by means of their passive elastic recoil.

The pharynx

The pharynx (see Figure 21.2) is a muscular tube extending from the level of the base of the skull to the oesophagus in the neck and is shared by the respiratory and gastrointestinal tracts. It is divided into three regions. The nasopharynx lies behind the nasal cavities and above the soft palate and has an entirely respiratory function. Collections of lymphoid tissue, the pharyngeal tonsils or adenoids, lie on its posterior wall. The nasopharynx communicates with the middle ear cavity via the auditory tube. This tube keeps the air pressure on both sides of the tympanic membrane equal under varying atmospheric conditions. The tubes are normally closed but swallowing opens them. For example, the discomfort in the ears encountered when ascending or descending in an aeroplane is relieved by swallowing. The auditory tubes provide a natural passage for the spread of infection between the nasopharynx and the middle ear.

The **oropharynx** lies behind the oral cavity and extends from the soft palate as far as the tip of the epiglottis above the laryngeal inlet below. It contains the **palatine tonsils** which lie between the palatoglossal and palatopharyngeal arches. When the soft palate is raised, the nasopharynx is closed off from the oropharynx. The **laryngopharynx** extends from the tip of the epiglottis to the oesophageal entrance. The nasopharynx is lined with respiratory epithelium but stratified squamous epithelium lines the oropharynx and laryngopharynx because food as well as air passes through these areas. The pharynx is described more fully in Chapter 21.

The larynx

The larynx opens into the laryngopharynx above and is continuous with the trachea below. The larynx is supported by a cartilaginous skeleton which differs from that in other parts of the respiratory tract, in that the cartilages are joined by synovial joints and are moved by voluntary muscles so that the configuration of the larynx can be altered for voice production. Its primary role is, however, the protection of the lower respiratory system: during swallowing the vocal folds are reflexly closed to prevent anything inadvertently entering the larynx from progressing into the lower respiratory tract. Its mucosal lining is covered by respiratory epithelium except over the vocal folds where it is covered by stratified squamous epithelium. The larynx and its role in phonation is described in detail in Chapters 16 and 17.

Clinical and applied anatomy of the upper respiratory tract

Infection of and allergic reactions in the upper respiratory system are common. Irrespective of the aetiology, the tissues become inflamed: **rhinitis** is inflammation of the nasal cavities; **sinusitis** is inflammation of the paranasal sinuses. Because of their role in the conditioning of inspired air, the nasal cavities have a well-developed blood supply. During inflammation, the blood vessels dilate and produce an exudate which is rich in antibodies and host defence cells to remove the offending organisms. The exudate forms a watery discharge which, if excessive, may drain anteriorly through the nostrils or posteriorly into the pharynx. During infections, bacterial toxins may temporarily damage the cilia, reducing the efficiency of the removal of nasal secretions to the pharynx, thus blocking the nose. Infected secretions generally contain pus and become thickened and change colour and texture. Because the nasal cavities communicate with the air sinuses and middle ear via the auditory tube in the nasopharynx, infection can spread quickly to these sites. Nasopharyngeal infection can cause temporary partial deafness by producing swelling which blocks the auditory tube. In children, the auditory tube is short and middle ear infections are common following an upper respiratory tract infection. Excess mucus produced by the inflamed mucosa can also track posteriorly into the pharynx and the larynx, not only spreading the infection but also causing congestion in these areas; excess mucus in the larynx can interfere with vocal fold function and hence phonation (see Chapter 16). The increased vascularity produced by inflammation or allergy greatly distends the nasal mucosa and may narrow the opening of the paranasal sinuses, impairing drainage. Rhinitis leads to mouth breathing because of congestion of the nasal cavities. **Nasal polyps**, areas of oedematous mucosa which bulge into the nasal cavity are often associated with chronic allergic rhinitis and cause severe nasal obstruction. They can be surgically removed relatively quickly and simply under local or general anaesthesia but do, however, tend to recur. Malignant disease of the lining epithelium of the respiratory system is relatively common and can affect the nasal cavities, pharynx or larynx, once again leading to obstruction of the affected part of the respiratory tract.

The lower respiratory tract

The trachea and bronchi

The **trachea** forms the airway between the larynx and the lungs and is about 10 cm long and between 1.5–2 cm in diameter (Figure 14.1). It lies mainly in the midline and terminates by dividing into **left** and **right main bronchi** deep to the sternum. The patency of the trachea is maintained by incomplete C-shaped rings of cartilage which are deficient posteriorly. During swallowing, the deficiency allows for expansion of the oesophagus which lies posterior to the trachea. The cervical part of the trachea is subcutaneous and the cartilaginous tracheal rings may be palpated in the lower part of the midline of the neck.

The bronchial tree

The right and left main bronchi supply the corresponding lungs. They divide almost immediately on entering the lungs into three lobar bronchi on the right side and two in the left lung and each supplies a separate lobe of each lung (see below). The **lobar bronchi** divide repeatedly into successively smaller diameter tubes. The smallest are **terminal bronchioles**, which terminate by dividing into two or more **respiratory bronchioles**, connecting the conducting and respiratory parts of the respiratory tract. The division of the bronchial tree into distinct components is largely artificial: there is a gradual merging with subtle alterations of structure between them.

Generally the structure of the larger bronchi is similar to that of the trachea, but the shape of the cartilages is more irregular. Their walls

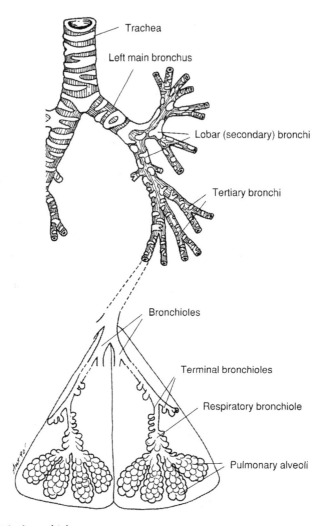

Figure 14.1 The bronchial tree.

contain substantial amounts of smooth muscle and mucous and serous glands discharging into the lumen. When the bronchi reach a diameter of 1 mm or less, they are called bronchioles. **Bronchioles** lack cartilage and glands in their walls. Instead, their walls consist largely of smooth muscle under autonomic control. Sympathetic stimulation produces relaxation of the smooth muscle, increasing the diameter of the bronchioles and thus permitting an increased flow of air into the lungs whereas parasympathetic stimulation produces the opposite effect by inducing contraction of this muscle and reducing bronchiolar diameter. As the diameter of the bronchioles decreases further, goblet cells in the respiratory epithelium also become rarer as even a relatively small amount of mucus would block these very small diameter tubes. The greater part of the walls of respiratory bronchioles are smooth muscle and elastic fibres. As respiratory bronchioles enter the sac-like alveoli, there is a transition from respiratory to simple squamous epithelium.

Clinical and applied anatomy of the trachea and bronchi

As mentioned above, malignant disease of the lining epithelium of the respiratory system is common. Carcinoma of the bronchus accounts for more than 30 000 deaths each year in England and Wales and cigarette smoking is a predisposing factor. Carcinomas invade and damage adjacent normal tissues and their related nerves and blood vessels. Bronchial obstruction can occur which usually results in infection of the bronchial tree distal to the lesion (**pneumonia**). Malignant cells may enter the lymphatic and vascular systems to produce metastases at distant sites. Symptoms usually involve coughing, often producing blood stained-mucus (haemoptysis) and difficulty in breathing (**dyspnoea**). The tissues of the lung are not innervated by sensory nerves and pain is usually absent unless the pleura or thoracic skeleton become involved. Wide surgical resection of the lesion is the treatment of choice although radiotherapy and chemotherapy are also used separately or in conjunction with surgery. Malignant disease in other parts of the respiratory system usually produces haemorrhage and obstruction. **Bronchoscopy** can also be used to examine the greater part of the conducting portion of the respiratory system and to obtain biopsies of potentially diseased areas.

Bronchitis is inflammation of the lining of the lower respiratory tract and may be acute or chronic. The bronchial glands hypertrophy and the number of goblet cells increase resulting in excess mucus production. Acute bronchitis is often a complication of common colds or influenza, and children, the elderly and debilitated people are often susceptible. The main symptoms are wheeziness and difficulty in breathing (dyspnoea). Acute bronchitis can be treated with antibiotics to remove the source of infection and bronchodilators to help overcome the obstruction to air movement caused by the excess mucus. Many geriatric clients will have some degree of respiratory compromise and cannot sustain exhalation, important for maintenance of vocalization and for achieving loudness. As a result their speech tends to be weak and expressionless (see Chapter 15). Chronic bronchitis is usually due to long-term exposure to atmospheric and industrial pollutants such as car exhaust fumes or coal dust or cigarette smoke. It is characterized by dyspnoea and an early morning cough producing thick infected sputum. Another condition in which there is excess mucus production is **cystic fibrosis**, a genetic condition in which excess mucus is produced in several areas of the body including the respiratory tract. As mucus builds up then, dyspnoea follows. An increasingly common non-infectious condition affecting the diameter of the lower tract is **asthma**, an allergic condition in which the allergen produces spasm of the smooth muscle causing acute bronchoconstriction. The client will often 'fight for breath' and attempt to use the accessory muscles of respiration (see below), although this has no effect until the bronchospasm is relieved by bronchodilators which asthmatics should carry with them at all times if prescribed.

Spirometry is a technique for measuring respiratory volumes and rates. The client breathes into a tube connected to flow valves and a computer. A useful measure of the effect of chronic obstructive conditions is using a spirometer to measure **forced expiratory volume per second (FEV$_1$)**. The client takes a deep inspiration then breathes out forcibly and the spirometer measures flow rate and volume. Because of the raised airway resistance, flow rate is low compared with normal subjects and the volume of air breathed out (forced vital capacity) is lower for the same respiratory effort. Measurement of respiratory rates and volumes is more fully described in Chapter 15.

Clients who are chronically ill with respiratory disease, who are depressed or fatigued or in some discomfort often breathe shallowly. This affects loudness, intonation and stress during speech, as well as their ability to sustain long sentences or even speak for anything other than short periods. These effects are discussed more fully in Chapter 15.

The lungs

The lungs are contained within the thoracic cavity along with the heart and great vessels entering and leaving the heart. The thoracic cavity extends from the root of the neck above to the diaphragm below and is enclosed by the thoracic cage. The left **lung** is slightly smaller than the **right lung** because of the presence of the heart. The right lung is divided into **upper**, **middle** and **lower** lobes by an upper **horizontal** and a lower **oblique fissure**. The **left lung** comprises only **upper** and **lower** lobes separated by a single **oblique fissure** (Figure 14.2). The **root (hilum)** of the lung is where the main bronchi enter their respective lung accompanied by blood vessels. If the lungs are removed from the body, they collapse around the bronchi. If, on the other hand, you have the opportunity to examine lungs which have been removed from an embalmed cadaver, they remain inflated and their shape conforms to the thoracic cavity and the heart intervening between right and left lungs. Each lung has a blunt **apex**,

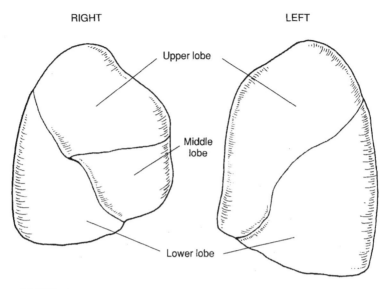

Figure 14.2 The lungs.

which extends upwards into the root of the neck for about 2–5 cm above the medial third of the clavicle. The outer costal surface is in contact with the thoracic wall and often has faint grooves where the ribs leave an impression. The inferior surface of each lung is concave where it rests on the diaphragm and the medial surface is also concave where it is indented by the heart.

The pulmonary arteries carrying deoxygenated blood from the right ventricle enter the lung at the hilum and follow the course of the bronchial tree as it divides. The arteries decrease in diameter until they end in a rich capillary network around the alveolar sacs of the lung where gaseous exchange takes place. The capillaries then join to form veins which also tend to follow the bronchial tree, getting larger as they do so, to exit the lungs at the hilum as the pulmonary veins which return oxygenated blood to the right atrium of the heart.

The respiratory zone

The **respiratory zone** is where gaseous exchange between the lungs and cardiovascular system takes place through very thin-walled alveolar sacs lined with simple squamous cells although other cell types are also present (see below). The openings of the alveoli into the alveolar duct are surrounded by a network of smooth muscle which acts as a sphincter for groups of **alveolar sacs** and can therefore regulate the amount of air entering the alveoli. The squamous cells are supported by a few delicate collagen and elastic fibres and a complex capillary network. Elastic fibres permit expansion during inspiration and assist in the passive contraction of the alveoli during expiration.

The **alveoli** themselves are small sac-like spaces. Their walls comprise very thin, simple squamous epithelial cells lining the alveoli (Figure 14.3) lying on a basal lamina which separates them from a thin layer of cytoplasm of the endothelial cells lining the small capillaries. The regions of gaseous exchange thus comprise only three components: the alveolar epithelial cytoplasm, the capillary endothelial cytoplasm, and a basal lamina sandwiched between the two. The total width of the air–blood exchange region is between 0.2 and 0.6 μm. It has been estimated that the human alveolar lining contains about 300 million alveoli with a total surface area of about 80 square metres.

Gaseous exchange occurs through squamous **alveolar (Type I) cells**, the major cell type lining the alveolar surface. They are also involved in the

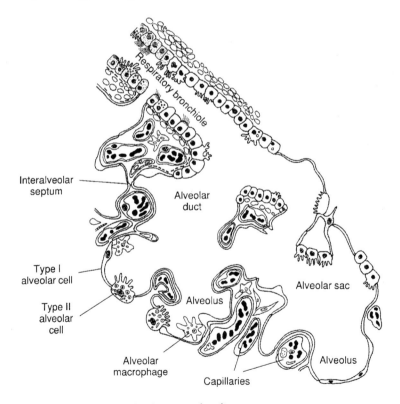

Figure 14.3 The structure of pulmonary alveoli.

turnover of surfactant (see below) and the removal of small particles from the alveolar surface. Type I cells are held firmly together by desmosomes and tight junctions to prevent leakage of tissue fluid into the alveoli. **Surfactant (Type II)** cells interspersed between Type I cells are secretory cells which synthesize **pulmonary surfactant**, a material which spreads over the alveolar surface and has several functions. **Alveolar macrophages** phagocytose foreign material like bacteria, carbon and dust particles and then migrate into the alveolar lumen. Once in the lumen, macrophages cannot pass back between the lining epithelial cells. They move up the bronchial tree to be eventually swallowed or migrate along lymphatic vessels on to the lung surface, keeping the undigested material they contain away from the area where it could damage the delicate alveolar lining. Environmental pollution results in the inhalation of particulate matter which cannot be broken down and remains within the macrophages. For this reason, the lungs of coal miners or inhabitants of polluted urban regions are discoloured because of the presence of numerous alveolar macrophages laden with carbon within and on the surface of the lung.

Pulmonary surfactant is an oily secretion consisting of protein in an aqueous phase covered by a single layer of phospholipid secreted by Type II cells. It undergoes constant turnover and is removed by Type I cells. Surfactant reduces the surface tension of the squamous epithelial cells and thus enables them to assume the smallest possible diameter. By reducing the surface tension, less work is needed during inspiration to inflate the alveoli. Although the surface tension is reduced by surfactant, the surface tension forces account for about two-thirds of the elastic recoil in the lungs during expiration. Surfactant also facilitates the transport of gases between air and fluid phases, and it contains a bactericide which kills any bacteria which manage to reach the respiratory portion of the pulmonary tree.

The thoracic wall

The thoracic cavity is continuous above with the neck. Below, the thorax is separated from the abdominal cavity by the musculotendinous **diaphragm**. The thoracic cavity is surrounded by the thoracic wall which is covered externally by skin and by muscles which attach the upper limb and shoulder girdle and the neck to the trunk. The thoracic wall is formed by the **thoracic vertebrae** in the posterior midline; they articulate with each other and with the ribs. The twelve pairs of **ribs** arch forwards and downwards forming the posterior, lateral and part of the anterior walls of the thoracic cage. Anteriorly the ribs terminate in the **costal cartilages**.

The ribs articulate either directly or indirectly through their costal cartilages with the **sternum** which completes the anterior thoracic wall in the
midline. The **intercostal spaces** between the ribs contain the intercostal
muscles, blood vessels and nerves.

The vertebrae

There are 33 vertebrae: seven cervical vertebrae, twelve thoracic vertebrae,
five lumbar vertebrae, five fused vertebrae which form the sacrum
posterior to the pelvis and four vestigial coccygeal vertebrae. Each vertebra
is separated from its neighbour by an intervertebral disc which is made of
fibrocartilage with a soft centre of gelatinous material.

Each vertebra consists of a **body** with projections which meet posteriorly to enclose the spinal cord in the **vertebral canal**. Two **transverse
processes** project laterally and a **spinous process** projects posteriorly
from the bone surrounding the vertebral canal. These processes are
attachments for the muscles of the vertebral column. There are also
superior and **inferior facets** which form the articulations between
adjacent vertebrae. The spinal nerves exit to innervate peripheral structures through the **intervertebral foramina** formed each side between
two adjacent vertebrae.

The **thoracic vertebrae** (Figure 14.4) have facets on their bodies for
articulation with the ribs. Each adjacent vertebra contributes half the
articular surface and each rib therefore articulates with two vertebrae, its
corresponding vertebra and the vertebra above, and the intervening intervertebral disc. Each rib also articulates with a facet on the transverse

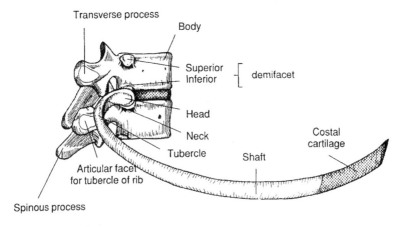

Figure 14.4 Articulation between thoracic vertebrae and ribs.

process of its corresponding vertebra. There are exceptions to this general scheme: the lowest two ribs do not have articulations with the transverse processes and the first ribs only articulate with the first thoracic vertebra.

The ribs

Each rib is markedly curved when viewed from above and also shows a downward curve when viewed laterally. Each rib has a **head** where it articulates with the vertebrae and a narrow **neck** separating the head from the **tubercle** which articulates with the transverse process of the vertebra (Figure 14.4). The **shaft** forms the major part of each rib and its distal end is extended by the **costal cartilage**. The upper six pairs of ribs articulate through their costal cartilages directly with the sternum, a blade-like bone lying in the midline of the thorax. The cartilages of the next four pairs of ribs articulate, through the cartilage of the one above, indirectly with the sternum. The lowest two pairs of ribs are free, having no anterior articulation.

Intercostal muscles

The **intercostal spaces** lie between adjacent ribs. Each space contains intercostal muscles and the intercostal neurovascular bundles. The intercostal spaces are covered in many places by muscles associated with the shoulder girdle or anterior abdominal wall which may be used to assist in forced ventilation.

There are three layers of **intercostal muscles** but only two are functionally significant (Figure 14.5). The fibres of the **external intercostal muscles** pass downwards and forwards from the inferior border of the rib above to the superior border of the rib below. Each muscle is continuous from the tubercle of the rib posteriorly to the costochondral junction anteriorly. Between this junction and the sternum, muscle is replaced by fibrous tissue. The **internal intercostal muscles** lie deep to the external intercostal muscles. Their fibres lie at right angles to the external intercostals and are directed downwards and backwards from the inferior border of the rib above to the superior border of the rib below. Each muscle extends from the sternum and costal cartilages anteriorly to the angles of the rib posteriorly where muscle is replaced by fibrous tissue occupying the interval between the angle and tubercle of the ribs.

The intercostal muscles draw adjacent ribs closer together. If the first rib is fixed by the action of other muscles attached to it superiorly, then the intercostal muscles will raise the second to twelfth ribs towards the first rib. However, if the twelfth rib is fixed by abdominal muscles, the first to eleventh ribs will be pulled down towards the twelfth rib. However, because

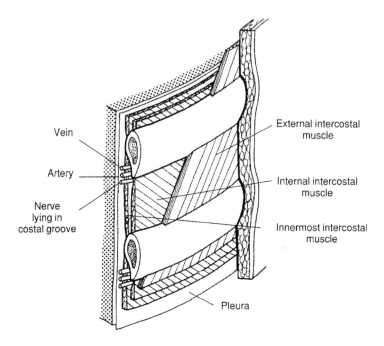

Figure 14.5 The intercostal muscles.

the ribs have an anterior attachment to the sternum and a posterior attachment to the thoracic vertebrae, they cannot concertina together. Instead the ribs pivot on both attachments so that they swing outwards, thus widening the thoracic cavity; this movement is most noticeable in the lower ribs. The upper ribs also swing upwards carrying the sternum forward, thus increasing the anteroposterior diameter of the thoracic wall.

The **intercostal nerves** are the first eleven thoracic spinal nerves emerging from the corresponding intervertebral foramina into the intercostal space between the parietal pleura and the internal intercostal muscle. They then run in the costal groove on the underside of the corresponding rib. Cutaneous branches pierce the intercostal muscles and are sensory to the skin on the thoracic wall and muscular branches supply the intercostal muscles; sensory branches also innervate the parietal pleura. The lower intercostal nerves also innervate the muscles of the anterior abdominal wall.

The diaphragm

The thoracic and abdominal cavities are separated by the **diaphragm**, a dome-shaped musculotendinous sheet which is pierced by structures passing between the two cavities (Figure 14.6). The peripheral area is muscular whereas the central area is tendinous; the **central tendon** is trefoil shaped and is partially fused with the fibrous pericardium above. The dome is convex superiorly, rising to the level of the fifth rib in the midline. The muscular periphery of the diaphragm is attached to the lower posterior surface of the sternum, the inner surfaces of the lower six costal cartilages and to the first three lumbar vertebral bodies by two muscular slips, the left and right crus (crura). The two crura cross each other as they blend with the central tendon, extending around the oesophageal opening (see below). Lateral to the crura, the diaphragm is attached to thickened bands of fascia covering the abdominal surfaces of the muscles of the posterior abdominal wall.

The diaphragm contains three major openings. Posteriorly the descending aorta passes through the aortic opening between the crura to enter the abdomen. Muscle fibres derived from the crura encircle the oesophageal opening through which the oesophagus and vagus nerves pass; the muscles act as a sphincter to prevent reflux of the stomach contents into the oesophagus. The inferior vena cava passes through an opening within the central tendon which is non-contractile. Venous return from the lower limbs and abdomen is thus not restricted by diaphragmatic contraction.

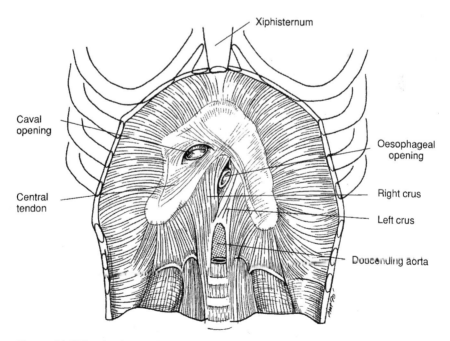

Figure 14.6 The diaphragm from below.

The diaphragm is innervated by the paired **phrenic nerves**. These nerves are derived from the third, fourth and fifth cervical spinal nerves and pass down the neck and the entire length of the thorax to reach the diaphragm. On the face of it, this may seem a very strange arrangement but is explained by the embryological development of the diaphragm. The diaphragmatic muscle develops from muscle from these cervical segments during the formation of the embryo and is displaced downwards as the heart develops and enlarges. The phrenic nerves are dragged down with the diaphragm as it is displaced, hence their long course.

The pleura

We now have almost all the components necessary for ventilation, a respiratory tract, the lungs with their alveoli for gaseous exchange and the components of the thoracic wall to alter its size. There is, however, one other component which is essential for ventilation. The lungs are not in direct contact with the thoracic wall but are surrounded by two layers of pleural membranes (Figure 14.7). The **parietal pleura** line the inside of the thoracic wall, the thoracic surface of the diaphragm and the lateral aspect of the pericardium surrounding the heart. The visceral layer intimately covers the outer surface of each lung, extending into the

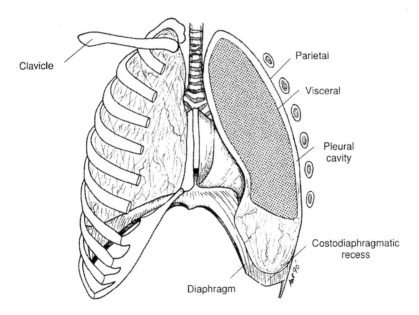

Figure 14.7 The pleura from the front.

fissures. The two layers become continuous with each other at the roots of the lungs where there is a loose fold which can accommodate increases in volume during inspiration. Elsewhere, the parietal and visceral layers are separated from each other by a very narrow potential space, the **pleural cavity**, which is completely filled by a thin film of **pleural fluid**. This fluid, an exudate from blood plasma, is a lubricant between the two layers enabling them to slide smoothly over each other. It has a high surface tension which firmly adheres the parietal and visceral pleura to each other and prevents them from being pulled apart. In quiet ventilation, the parietal pleurae lining the lower ribs and the diaphragm are apposed below the lower border of the lung and the lungs do not intervene. This region is known as the **costodiaphragmatic recess.** During deep inspiration, the inferior margins of the lungs expand and extend into the recess.

You may question why the lungs are not simply attached directly to the thoracic walls so that they could be moved directly by movements of the ribcage. Essentially, the thoracic cavity is of a very complex shape, and as the thoracic wall and diaphragm move, the dimensions of the thoracic cavity change in a non-linear fashion. The lungs fill more efficiently if they can expand to comply with the shape of the cavity irrespective of how much or little it expands. This is achieved by allowing the visceral pleura attached to the lungs to slide across the parietal pleura attached to the thoracic wall. The reduction in friction produced by the lubricant action of pleural fluid also lessens the effort required to expand the lungs.

CHAPTER **15**

The mechanisms of respiration

Respiration is the movement of air into and out of the respiratory system caused by alteration of the volume of, and hence pressure within, the thoracic cavity. Gases in the inhaled air are then exchanged between air and blood in the lung alveoli. As the thoracic wall moves, the parietal pleura will move with it. The visceral pleura will conform to this movement because they are adherent to the parietal pleura through the pleural fluid. Because the lungs are attached to the visceral pleura, they will also expand. Thus, as thoracic volume increases, so does the volume of the lung and the pressure within them decreases. As pressure reduces, air is drawn into the respiratory zone of the lungs down the conducting zone of the respiratory tract. This is **inspiration**. The lungs themselves, as well as the larger elements of the conducting zone of the respiratory system, contain substantial amounts of elastic tissue. To make the lungs inflate during inspiration, it is necessary to exert muscular force to overcome their elastic recoil. Inflation of the alveolar sacs and smaller bronchioles stretches the elastic fibres in their walls. Likewise, muscular activity during inspiration alters the configuration of the chest wall and increases the elastic strain in the muscles, joints and cartilages comprising the chest wall. When the muscles which produce expansion of the thoracic cavity relax, the inherent elasticity of the thoracic walls and lungs makes them revert to their original dimensions with a subsequent reduction in volume and with a consequent increase in pressure in the thoracic cavity which forces air out. This is **passive elastic recoil**, an important mechanism in the expulsion of air from the lungs, or **expiration**.

At rest, there is a rhythmic flow of a small volume of air into and out of the lungs; this is **quiet respiration**. However, this volume can be increased in response to increased demand for oxygen during exertion or if there is a need to alter intrathoracic pressure to assist other bodily functions, such as during expulsion of faeces or during childbirth. Altering the thoracic volume beyond that used for quiet respiration is called **forced**

respiration and is also rhythmic. During **speech**, respiratory patterns are altered considerably; they are non-rhythmic and must be carefully and minutely regulated to maintain a constant outflow of air into the upper respiratory tract and to vary volume and tone.

Respiratory performance and volume changes

It goes without saying that breathing is a continuous process so it is difficult to imagine what might happen, short of death, if breathing was suspended. If breathing were arrested, the lungs have a natural tendency to collapse due to their elastic properties and the chest wall has a natural tendency to expand if respiration is suspended, again due to its elastic properties. Because the lungs are linked to the thoracic wall by the pleura, the two opposing forces will cancel out, therefore the lungs do not collapse and the thoracic wall does not expand. The equilibrium position is referred to as the **neutral** or **balanced position**; at equilibrium the volume of the respiratory tract is equal to the amount of air left in the respiratory tract at the end of a quiet expiration. This is the **resting expiratory level,** the point achieved naturally between inspiration and expiration when no muscular forces are operating.

To appreciate things in context, some physiological terms used to describe respiratory movements need to be defined (Figure 15.1). The **total lung capacity** (TLC), in reality the total capacity of the whole respiratory tract, is about 6–7 litres of air. Of this total, there is a **residual volume** (RV) of about 2 litres which remains in the airway even after a maximal expiratory effort. The air constituting the residual volume is important for maintaining oxygenation of the blood between breaths to avoid excess fluctuation in blood gas levels. This leaves a total of 4–5 litres which is the maximum amount of air which can be inspired: this is the **vital capacity** (VC). During quiet inspiration and expiration, the residual volume is not reached and there is usually about another 2 litres of **expiratory reserve volume** (ERV), the amount of air which could be exhaled with maximum expiratory effort. Expiratory reserve volume plus residual volume add up to 4 litres: this is the **resting expiratory level** in physiological terms and represents the balanced position in anatomical terms.

Tidal volume (TV) is the amount of air inspired or expired during a respiratory cycle and its value will depend upon the oxygen demand at the time. In quiet inspiration and expiration, the tidal volume is about 0.5 litres. In such circumstances a comparatively small amount of the total lung capacity is used. In extreme use, such as exercise or singing, then inspiratory volume approaches the **inspiratory capacity** of about 3 litres:

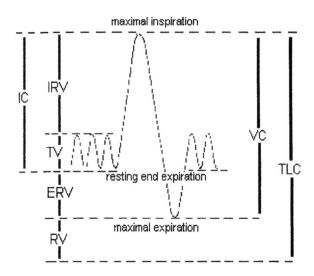

Figure 15.1 Respiratory volume relationships (see text for abbreviations).

equal to TLC – (ERV + RV). During exercise, the resting expiratory level will be exceeded and forced expiratory effort may bring the amount of air left in the respiratory tract down to the residual volume.

The average vital capacity is about 4.5 litres in young adult males and 3 litres in females. Vital capacity depends on body build and also decreases with age. Vital capacity and consequently other lung volumes increase in fit athletic individuals and are smaller in people who are relatively sedentary. Respiratory volumes also decrease when lying down. Vital capacity is reduced in any disease states affecting the lungs such as bronchitis, emphysema, tuberculosis, asthma or bronchial carcinoma. Diseases of the heart which cause pulmonary congestion also decrease vital capacity because there is an increase in fluid in the lungs.

When used clinically, two other measures are extremely useful. **Forced vital capacity** (FVC) is the volume of air exhaled during a forced expiratory manoeuvre. If the lungs are normal, then it should enable sufficient air to be exhaled to leave only the residual volume. A reduced forced vital capacity is indicative of **restrictive lung disease** such as pulmonary fibrosis. Forced expiratory volume (FEV_1) is the flow rate of air in the first second of a forced vital capacity manoeuvre and is reduced in **obstructive lung diseases** such as asthma and emphysema; the forced vital capacity is, however, unchanged. Chronic obstructive pulmonary disease (COPD), including chronic bronchitis, is in reality a combination of restrictive and obstructive lung disease and results in reduced FEV_1 and FVC.

Quiet respiration

During quiet respiration, breathing is rhythmic and the time taken to inspire and expire is approximately equal. The quiet respiratory rate is somewhere between 12 and 15 cycles per minute so a complete cycle of inspiration and expiration lasts about 4 or 5 seconds. This rate is faster in children and slower in old age. The amount of air taken into the lungs (tidal volume) with each breath is about 0.5 litres. There are minute variations in tidal volume and cycle time during steady state quiet respiration but these average out over several cycles.

As tidal volumes are small during quiet respiration, relatively little effort is needed to expand the lungs but it still requires energy expenditure. This is achieved by contraction of the **external intercostal muscles** which raise the rib cage, thus expanding the thoracic volume both anteroposteriorly and laterally. The vertical dimensions of the thoracic cavity are increased by contraction of the **diaphragm** which flattens from its dome-shaped resting position. Although the capacity of the thorax can be increased in all dimensions, the vertical dimension is the most significant: the movements of the diaphragm account for about 75 per cent of thoracic volume change during quiet respiration.

To raise the ribs, it is necessary to fix the first rib. This is achieved by muscles which extend upwards in the neck from the first rib. With the first rib firmly fixed, the intercostal muscles contract, which produces the overall effect of elevating all the ribs, making them lie more horizontally; the sternum to which they are attached moves outwards and upwards. The articulations of the ribs with the thoracic vertebrae posteriorly and the sternum via their costal cartilages anteriorly coupled with their downward and forward curvature have been likened to a bucket handle: by raising the ribs, they move upwards and outwards, thus increasing the transverse dimensions of the thorax. The diaphragm descends upon contraction, exerting pressure on the abdominal viscera, and this is accompanied by relaxation of the musculature of the abdominal wall, which can be seen to move in and out during respiratory movements. During inspiration, a point is reached when no further abdominal relaxation is possible. The abdominal viscera, in particular the superior surface of the liver, then act as a platform to support the diaphragm. Any further diaphragmatic contraction will result not in descent, but in lateral or anteroposterior expansion of the lower ribs. The bronchi and bronchioles elongate and dilate and this is accompanied by dilatation of pulmonary capillaries. The lubricating action of pleural fluid enables the pleural layers to slide across each other but its surface tension maintains them in intimate contact. The pressure in the pleural cavities falls to about −7 mmHg during inspiration. As the lungs expand, they descend into the costodiaphragmatic recess to occupy the potential space between the two apposed pleural layers at this site.

During inspiration, the ribs are displaced from their position at the resting expiratory level and the costal cartilages are distorted. When the desired tidal volume has been inspired, the inspiratory muscles relax. Due to the elastic strain built up in the thoracic wall, it will elastically recoil aided by the elastic recoil of the lungs themselves until the balanced position is reached and another inspiration starts the next respiratory cycle. An increase in muscular tone of the abdominal wall increases intra-abdominal pressure which pushes the relaxing diaphragm upwards. The lungs contract passively out of the costodiaphragmatic recess and the two layers of parietal pleura in this region come together.

Forced respiration

Forced respiration occurs when oxygen demand is high or tissues are producing excess CO_2. Respiratory rate and volume increase such that inspiration uses most of the vital capacity and expiration approaches the residual volume. During inspiration, the external intercostal muscles are used maximally if necessary and the internal intercostal muscles also assist in elevation of the ribs. The diaphragm is lowered considerably, thus expanding the thoracic cavity towards its maximum limits. The intercostal muscles and diaphragm are assisted by **accessory muscles**, muscles whose primary function is not respiration but which can be used for respi-ration when necessary. Those used during inspiration comprise two groups (Figure 15.2); both are attached to the thoracic wall but one group is attached to the arm and the other to the cervical vertebral column and base of the skull. The **pectoralis muscles** are the obvious examples of muscles inserting into the arm, and the arm must be stabilized for their efficient use so that their action is exerted on the thoracic cage and not on the arm. Arm stability is achieved by placing the hands on the hips or, *in extremis*, by grasping a fixed object such as a table, a response often observed in someone having a severe asthma attack. These muscles aid the intercostals in expansion of the rib cage. The accessory muscles attaching to the cervical spine and skull include the scalene and sternocleido-mastoid muscles. They elevate the upper ribs either directly or indirectly via action on the clavicle, enabling the intercostal muscles to elevate the lower ribs to a greater extent. The intrapleural pressure falls to about −30 mmHg in forced inspiration.

When the rib cage is expanded maximally, the elastic recoil generated is so high that when the intercostal and accessory muscles relax, the rib cage recoils with considerable force. However, muscular effort is also required

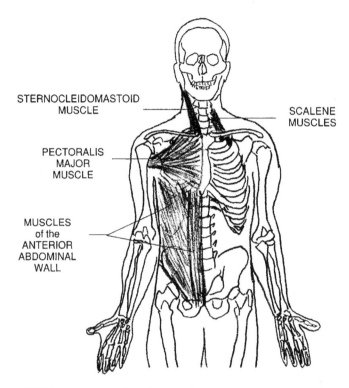

STERNOCLEIDOMASTOID
MUSCLE

SCALENE
MUSCLES

PECTORALIS
MAJOR
MUSCLE

MUSCLES
of the
ANTERIOR
ABDOMINAL
WALL

Figure 15.2 Accessory muscles of respiration.

during forced expiration when the lung capacity decreases to about halfway between the vital capacity and the expiratory reserve volume. At this point, the internal intercostal muscles contract to depress the rib cage and the **accessory muscles of expiration** are also used. The most important accessory muscles of expiration are the muscles of the **anterior abdominal wall** which attach the lower margins of the rib cage to the pelvic bones (Figure 15.2). Their effect is twofold: their direct pull lowers the ribcage and their contraction also increases the intra-abdominal pressure. Providing the muscles which form the pelvic floor are also in tone, the raised intra-abdominal pressure will force the diaphragm upwards, thus decreasing the vertical dimensions of the thorax. Although the respiratory rate increases during forced respiration, it is still rhythmic such that the inspiratory and expiratory parts of the cycle are equal. Air flow can be as high as 3 litres per second during forced respiration and higher flow can be maintained more effectively through mouth breathing as the resistance is less than in the nasal cavity.

Types of respiratory movements

Two types of normal respiratory movement exist. **Thoracic** respiration relies mainly on movements of the thoracic cage for breathing. On the other hand, **abdominal** respiration uses the descent of the diaphragm. In young children, the ribs are almost horizontal and consequently they have to rely on abdominal respiration until the course of the ribs becomes more oblique: this begins at about three years of age. Abdominal respiration is characterized by movements of the abdominal wall. Sexual differences exist in the type of respiration. In women, the thoracic type predominates and may be related to childbearing, preventing excessive pressure being exerted on the abdomen. In males, the abdominal form predominates.

In clients who are tense or nervous or who are trying to force their voice as a result of respiratory compromise consequent on an underlying disease process, the clavicles can often be observed to rise and the neck muscles to stand out. This is known as **clavicular breathing** and makes use of the upper thoracic muscles and accessory muscles of respiration in the neck at the expense of the diaphragm in particular. Clavicular breathing is inefficient as the volume increase produced by use of this type of breathing is small. Any client exhibiting this type of respiration should be given exercises to help them achieve normal thoracic or abdominal breathing.

Control of respiration

Respiration usually proceeds *automatically*, without any conscious thought: we rarely think about our breathing and it continues during sleep or even when unconscious. Respiratory movements and rates are automatically adjusted to meet oxygen demands or clearance of excess CO_2 and are phasic. Automatic control of respiration should not be confused with control of involuntary function by the autonomic nervous system. The respiratory muscles are under control of the somatic nervous system through the **intercostal** and **phrenic nerves**. Respiration can therefore be controlled. A simple example is holding your breath or taking a deep breath to command; a more complex example is the fine control of respiration during speech. Respiration also varies in response to emotional stimuli (see below).

Quiet and forced respiration is under the control of **respiratory centres** in the brainstem. Originally, it was believed that specific groups of neurons comprised the respiratory centres but respiratory neurons are scattered throughout the pons and medulla where they constitute the **reticular respiratory formation**. Despite their widespread distribution, neurons in certain areas have specific roles in the control of respiration.

Groups of neurons in the pons are also involved to some extent but their role is uncertain as respiration continues in a rhythmic fashion even if the brainstem is sectioned between the pons and medulla. **Medullary respiratory neurons** have an intrinsic rhythmicity: some control inspiration whereas others control expiration. In quiet respiration, inspiratory neurons respond to various stimuli and drive the contraction of inspiratory muscles while inhibiting expiratory muscles; as passive elastic recoil is the normal mechanism of quiet expiration, there is no need for the activation of the expiratory muscles.

Two factors comprise the main driving force of the inspiratory neurons, pulmonary stretch receptors and the partial pressure of CO_2 (pCO_2) in the blood (Figure 15.3). Pulmonary stretch receptors are scattered throughout the walls of the conducting zone of the lower respiratory tract, with 40 per cent in the trachea and bronchi outside the lungs, and 60 per cent in the intrapulmonary bronchial tree. Despite their name of stretch receptors, they actually respond to pressure differences across the bronchial walls rather than the actual stretch of the walls. As the pressure changes across the walls (transmural pressure) during inspiration, the stretch receptors are stimulated and inhibit the inspiratory neurons so that expiration by passive elastic recoil takes place. The pCO_2 in the blood is monitored by chemoreceptors in the carotid bodies at the bifurcation of

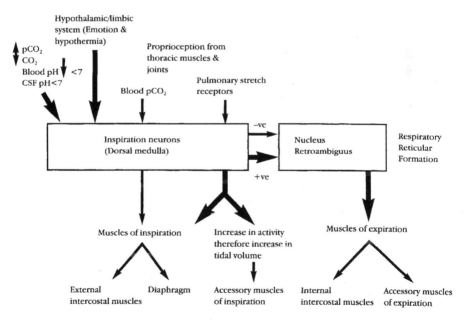

Figure 15.3 Neural control of respiration.

the common carotid arteries into the external and internal carotid arteries and in the aortic body in the aortic arch. The chemoreceptors also monitor pO_2 and blood pH.

Under normal circumstances, volume changes and hence transmural pressure changes are sufficient to control phasic respiration. However, when pCO_2 rises, pO_2 falls or blood pH falls and blood becomes acidic, chemoreceptors stimulate the inspiratory neurons in the medulla to increase tidal volume and respiratory rate by stimulation of the inspiratory muscles and accessory muscles of respiration. Unlike quiet respiration, stimulation of inspiratory neurons by blood chemistry changes also stimulates expiratory neurons which activate the muscles of expiration and the accessory muscles of expiration: this shortens the expiratory phase of respiration. Chemoreceptors are more sensitive to increases in pCO_2 than they are to a decrease in pO_2 but are stimulated maximally when both occur together. Increases in CO_2, amongst other factors, decrease blood pH and this also stimulates chemoreceptors. Another factor which drives inspiratory neurons is a fall in the pH of cerebrospinal fluid (CSF) which may alter independently of blood pH. The CSF pH is monitored by chemoreceptors on the ventrolateral surface of the medulla, and inspiratory neurons are stimulated if pH falls as the CSF becomes acidic.

Information from pulmonary stretch receptors and aortic chemoreceptors is conveyed to the reticular respiratory system by the vagus nerves and from the carotid body by the glossopharyngeal nerves; afferent axons from both nerves terminate in the **tractus solitarius** (Figure 15.3). The lower motor neurons to the primary and accessory muscles of respiration arise at various levels of the spinal cord and travel with the corresponding spinal nerves. The upper motor neuron inputs into the inspiratory muscles arise from neurons located dorsally in the medulla and control the activity in the phrenic nerves controlling the diaphragm and the neurons in the thoracic spinal segments controlling the external intercostals. A separate group of neurons (the **nucleus retroambiguus**) control the lower motor neurons in the thoracic spinal cord innervating the internal intercostal and abdominal muscles. The **nucleus ambiguus** is the main motor nucleus of the vagus nerve (see Chapter 11) and, amongst other things, controls the muscles of the larynx. The larynx must be open during respiration and is opened as far as possible during forced respiration. The respiratory reticular system coordinates the activity of these different groups of upper motor neurons supplying the muscles of respiration and other muscle groups involved in respiration so that muscular activity is coordinated with the desired rate and depth of respiration according to the demands of the body for oxygen or removal of CO_2.

The reticular respiratory formation also receives other important inputs (Figure 15.3). **Proprioceptors** in the joints of the thoracic wall and the intercostal muscles can affect respiratory rates if there are sudden changes in airway resistance, for example, when the vocal tract is stopped by valving in the larynx or at the velopharyngeal or articulatory levels, so that the muscles can accommodate to the change. The **hypothalamus** also has connections to the reticular respiratory formation and alters respiratory rates in response to hyperthermia (heat stroke) or fevers and in response to activity of the autonomic nervous system. If you are very nervous or frightened, your respiratory rate increases rapidly. The **limbic system** also has excitatory or inhibitory effects on the reticular respiratory formation in response to different emotions. Respiratory changes are marked, for example, during sexual activity or crying.

During speech, as described in the next section, the controls of respiration are largely overridden. However, the bodily demands for gaseous exchange at an effective rate take precedence over speech. Similarly, it is extremely difficult to override the inputs from the hypothalamus and limbic system so that smooth phonation and articulation become difficult when we are affected by extreme emotions or are rigid with fright.

Respiration during speech

To achieve phonation and articulation, a pressurized airstream is transformed into a series of pulses by constricting the airstream at the vocal folds in the larynx or at other places in the respiratory tract and oral cavity (the **vocal tract**). For each phoneme, a fundamental frequency of vibration is generated which passes through the vocal tract. During its passage, the fundamental frequency and certain multiples of this frequency are enhanced whereas other frequencies are damped. Which frequencies are transmitted or damped depends upon the length and shape of the vocal tract. Therefore to generate any phoneme, a pressurized airstream is necessary; the frequency of the sound is determined by the pressure and rate of airflow.

There are specific respiratory requirements during speech which must also be compatible with delivery of oxygen and removal of CO_2. Essentially, speech respiration is so different from normal respiration that the controls of normal respiration are voluntarily overridden. The first requirement for speech is that the **subglottal pressure** in the larynx, the difference between pressure beneath and above the vocal cords, is increased to and maintained at the appropriate level for the duration of the utterance. The increased pressure will generate vibration in the vocal folds or generate turbulent flow through the larynx or other constrictions in the vocal tract. In addition, the pressure is varied to regulate overall voice intensity (**loudness**), linguistic stress (**emphasis**) or the fundamental frequency (**pitch**). Speech is created during the expiratory phase, and muscular exertion as well as passive elastic recoil has to be used to maintain the subglottal pressure or vary its pressure. The respiratory cycle must also be coordinated so that appropriate divisions of speech into phonemes, syllables, words, phrases and sentences are conserved to maintain the linguistic sense.

Unlike quiet or forced respiration, respiration during speech is non-rhythmical. The inspiratory cycle increases in volume and is more rapid, taking about 0.6 seconds compared with about 2 seconds in quiet inspiration and the expiratory cycle is prolonged to conserve the speech divisions. Typically, inspiration lasts for about 10 per cent of each respiratory cycle and the expiratory component may last up to 30 seconds depending upon the linguistic context. The range of vital capacity used during speech differs from that used during quiet respiration. Although respiration for speech may be initiated from the balanced position at residual expiratory volume, expiration does not usually extend to the residual expiratory volume but stops short of this. Subsequent cycles are thus initiated at a lung volume above residual expiratory capacity. The tidal volume used during conversational speech is about 1.5 litres but for loud speech, such as presenting a lecture or other public speaking, it may be raised to 2.5 litres which is approaching inspiratory capacity. In quiet inspiration, diaphragmatic contraction accounts for a substantial proportion of the volume changes in the lungs but diaphragmatic movement is supplemented considerably by the external intercostal muscles during speech inspiration.

The pressure difference across the glottis or other parts of the vocal tract is the driving force for vocal fold vibration or turbulent flow in other areas. The pressure difference results from a combination of passive elastic recoil during expiration and active contraction of the muscles of the thoracic wall. The subglottal pressure determines the energy of vibratory motion in the vocal folds or other articulators and therefore the amplitude of vibration which determines the loudness. Although speech can be produced with a subglottal pressure as low as 3 cmH_2O, it is generally between 10 and 20 cmH_2O for conversational speech and can rise as high as 60 cmH_2O if you scream at the top of your voice. If the lungs are inflated maximally to reach total lung capacity (TLC), the force generated by elastic recoil is about 30 cmH_2O, greater than the subglottal pressure required for most speech activity (Figure 15.4). Below 60 per cent TLC the pressure generated by elastic recoil falls below the necessary subglottal pressure and reaches zero once the lungs deflate to about 40 per cent of TLC;

below this the pressure is negative. It follows therefore that above about 60 per cent TLC, elastic recoil will generate too strong a subglottal pressure. Tone is maintained in the external intercostal muscles to counteract elastic recoil and therefore maintain the desired subglottal pressure. Once the lungs have deflated to below 60 per cent vital capacity, active contraction of the expiratory muscles – the internal intercostals – is required to maintain sufficient subglottal pressure as lung volume

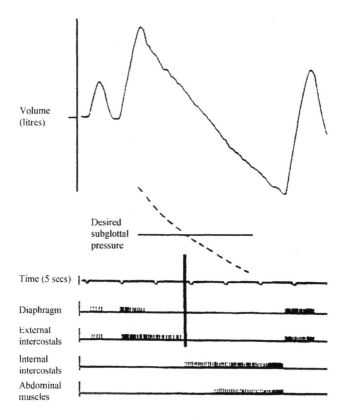

Figure 15.4 The relationship between subglottal pressure, elastic recoil and muscular activity during speech. (A) A spirometer trace of a normal respiratory cycle followed by a speech cycle. (B) The dotted line shows the pressure which would be generated at different phases of the speech cycle and the horizontal line indicates the desired subglottal pressure. Above the horizontal line, the pressure would be too high unless passive elastic recoil is counteracted by inspiratory muscle activity. Below the line, pressure would be too low and must be augmented by use of the expiratory muscles and accessory muscles. (C) The activity of different muscles at different phases of the cycle. (Drawn after Draper *et al.*, *J. Speech Hear. Res.*, 2, 16–27, 1959.)

decreases. Subtle changes in the activity of the external and internal inter-costal muscles irrespective of lung deflation produce variations in pressure and flow rate to produce the prosodic qualities of speech.

As well as subglottal pressure, the **flow rate** through the larynx and other cavities involved in articulation is also important. In quiet respiration, the flow rate is 0.3–0.5 litres per second (lps) at the glottis but, surprisingly, flow rate is less during speech, falling as low as 0.06 lps and only rising to about 0.4 lps at maximum rate. In conversational speech, flow rate is relatively constant at around 0.14 lps. The relationships between the two variables is complex and changes in both often occur out of phase. For example, to articulate /a/ subglottal pressure is high but flow rate is low whereas the converse is true during articulation of /h/ which requires an open glottis. Voiceless consonants require a high flow rate whereas voiced consonants require a low flow rate. Exact control of respiration is required to achieve the correct pressure and flow rate for a particular phoneme whilst maintaining the desired volume. If used correctly, a low flow rate will generate a quieter sound and high flow rates produce a louder sound. Untrained singers will increase the pressure rather than the flow rate to sing louder. Given a constant tension in the vocal folds, pitch rises as subglottal pressure increases, therefore vocal fold tension must be increased to maintain a constant pitch. Pressure and airflow changes are often very rapid and of considerable range. They vary according to where in the vocal tract phonatory and articular activity is taking place, the specific phoneme generated and its relationship to preceding and following phonemes and the rate, stress and pitch of speech to provide the necessary prosody. The pressure requirements for a given phoneme last somewhere between 75 and 150 milliseconds and pressure changes between phonemes for a given volume of speech are between 1 and 5 cmH_2O.

To achieve the rapid changes in pressure and airflow rates, respiration must be finely controlled. As a general principle, skilled motor events require both efferent motor signals to generate contraction and afferent feedback to modify the motor activity. However, many skilled movements are performed too rapidly for the conduction time required for afferent feedback and modification of motor activity. To overcome this limitation, we learn complex movements by repeated trial and error or have certain sequences of movement pre-programmed. You will be aware from any phonetic analysis you have encountered so far that a complex sequence of muscular activity must occur in a prescribed order to articulate any given phoneme. Instructions for each phoneme must fit into a larger programme to structure phonemes into syllables and words. The complexities required to formulate speech must be reflected in the motor activities required to produce audible speech beginning with the generation of pressure and flow rate during expiration. Above all, the respiratory movements during speech must fulfil the basic requirements for oxygen supply and CO_2 removal so there is often a compromise between the demands of speech and metabolic respiratory movements.

The control of speech respiration as well as other motor speech activities, irrespective of whether it is learned or pre-programmed, is achieved by a combination of auditory feedback (see Chapter 22) and proprioceptive information from the relevant muscles and joints. In the thorax, the intercostal muscles have many muscle spindles and the costovertebral joints have many proprioceptive nerve endings; each intercostal nerve comprises about 45 per cent sensory axons although a proportion of these innervate the skin of the chest wall. In comparison, the diaphragm has only a small number of muscle spindles and each phrenic nerve contains about only 10 per cent sensory axons. The control over the intercostal nerves is therefore much greater and more refined than the diaphragm. In addition, the diaphragm moves passively during expiration except when some tone is maintained at lung volumes approaching TLC to counteract passive elastic recoil. It is also worth bearing in mind that about 60 per cent of the lung surface is in contact with the chest wall compared with about 25 per cent in contact with the diaphragm, therefore much less rib movement is required to effect changes in pressure and flow rate than would be required of the diaphragm.

Cough reflexes

Coughing expels mucus or foreign bodies from the respiratory system. Irritation of the lining epithelium of the respiratory tract may instigate the cough reflex. A **non-productive cough** is due to minor irritation such as inflammation of the pharynx (pharyngitis), resulting in a cough which produces nothing but irritation for the patient. In many of the diseases of the respiratory system described in Chapter 14, excess purulent mucus may be produced which is removed from the bronchial tree by coughing (a **productive cough**). Infected mucus may affect the action of the cilia on the surface of the lining epithelium which may be unable to transport the mucus at a sufficiently rapid rate. A deep inspiration is taken which is followed by forceful adduction of the vocal folds. Intrathoracic pressure is increased by contraction of the muscles of the anterior abdominal wall and then the pressure is released suddenly by rapid abduction of the vocal folds. This high speed expired air stream forces the mucus up the bronchial tree, trachea and into the pharynx from where it is usually swallowed or into the mouth whence it can be expectorated.

A lesser degree of non-productive cough is **throat clearing** in which a slight cough is used to dislodge perceived irritants from the larynx. Although deep inspiration followed by forced expiration is not used to the same degree, the vocal folds are adducted and forcibly abducted by the increased pressure. When used excessively, this can traumatize the vocal folds leading to various pathologies described in Chapter 16.

It is not uncommon for food or drink to pass inadvertently into the larynx instead of the oesophagus during swallowing. The laryngeal mucosa, both above and below the vocal folds, is extremely sensitive to touch and an immediate adduction of the vocal cords occurs, followed by abdominal wall contraction, thus increasing intrathoracic pressure and then coughing. This may dislodge a foreign body sufficiently far up the pharynx to prevent its subsequent inhalation following the inspiration which precedes the next coughing phase, as coughing is repeated until the foreign body has been expelled.

Clinical considerations

It should be obvious from the foregoing description of respiration during speech, that it is a finely regulated process which, at a gross level, coordinates the expiratory phase with the linguistic context and, at a more minute level, regulates loudness, emphasis and pitch. If such regulation is lost, then speech will be disrupted to varying degrees.

Any conditions which affect the control of muscles, as described in Chapter 10, will also have adverse effects on speech. A good illustrative example is **Parkinson's disease**: the voice volume is reduced because of the inability to generate sufficient force during expiration or to maintain the expiratory cycle for the necessary duration. Prosody is virtually absent because of the lack of control over the intercostal muscles necessary to generate small changes in flow rates or pressure needed to vary loudness and pitch for emphasis. In Parkinson's disease, the absence of vocal prosody is compounded by the absence of some components of non-verbal communication: a mask-like facial expression is typical, and reduced control of upper limb muscles precludes hand gestures. A client with a **high spinal injury** affecting the lower cervical or upper thoracic region of the spinal cord will be paralysed below that level. This will affect most or all of the intercostal nerves and therefore the intercostal muscles but will not affect the diaphragm as the phrenic nerves arise from the upper parts of the cervical spinal cord and will thus be preserved. Because of the paralysis, the client's oxygen demands will be small and diaphragmatic breathing is adequate. However, control of breathing is difficult during speech because the diaphragm is poorly supplied with intrinsic proprioceptive muscular control systems such as stretch receptors, thus prosody and the ability to sustain utterances is poor. Any conditions affecting motor systems such as dyskinesias and other manifestations of upper and lower motor neuron damage will also have an effect on speech which you may be able to anticipate from the descriptions provided in Chapter 10.

Clavicular breathing has been mentioned above: this inefficient use of the respiratory muscles leads to phonation with reduced loudness and an expressionless voice because there is little use of intonation and stress.

One aspect of impaired respiratory performance that is often overlooked is general debility and fatigue. Illnesses causing general debility may affect the respiratory tract directly or be apparently unconnected with the respiratory system. Very often depression or stress are contributory factors to general fatigue or listlessness. Respiration requires energy expenditure and breathing for speech requires more energy than quiet respiration. Clients with any of the above conditions may only breathe sufficiently for barely audible communication. Volume is low and prosody may be virtually absent because of the additional effort required to vary pressure and flow rate for pitch and emphasis. A full case history must be taken to help distinguish whether the effects on speech are due to some primary cause or are secondary to general debility, depression or fatigue.

CHAPTER **16**

The structure and function of the larynx

Air passing to or from the lungs and food passing from the mouth to the stomach share a common pathway through the upper part of the pharynx. A variety of mechanisms have evolved to ensure that, where the respiratory and gastrointestinal tracts separate, food is directed into the oesophagus through to the stomach and air into the larynx and trachea through to the bronchial tree. The larynx is the lowest component of the upper respiratory tract and its primary vital function is as an important sphincter mechanism for lower airway protection. It also has the important non-vital function of phonation during speech.

The larynx is located anteriorly in the neck and is the lowest part of the upper respiratory tract above the trachea (see Figure 5.1). Vertically, the larynx is located at a level corresponding to between the third and sixth cervical vertebrae but its precise position varies with its function. The larynx is surrounded laterally and posteriorly by the laryngopharyngeal part of the pharynx and by the upper part of the oesophagus lower down. The larynx thus forms the anterior wall of the laryngopharynx and opens into it. The whole larynx is suspended from the hyoid bone by membranes and ligaments and the hyoid bone is in turn suspended from the skull.

In common with the rest of the respiratory tract, the larynx must remain open during respiration and not collapse when air pressure decreases. However, the lumen must also be periodically narrowed and opened during phonation and fully closed when it acts as a sphincter to protect the lower airway. A series of cartilages joined together by ligaments and membranes form the skeleton of the larynx and function to keep the lumen of the larynx patent. Unlike the rest of the respiratory tract, these cartilages articulate with each other by synovial joints. The laryngeal muscles are capable of moving the cartilages at these joints. The tube of the larynx is narrowed at two points by two pairs of mucous folds. The vestibular, or false, vocal folds lie superiorly; these folds are accentuated by a collection of mucous glands beneath the lining mucosa. The true vocal folds lie inferiorly and are composed of predominantly muscular and elastic tissue. The true vocal folds can be actively opened by muscular action to maintain airway patency or pulled together when the larynx is acting as an airway protector or during phonation.

The default position of vocal folds is open so that air can pass freely between the upper and lower respiratory tract during respiration. During swallowing, the vocal folds and vestibular folds are tightly closed and respiration is temporarily suspended, thus preventing food from being inadvertently taken into the larynx and the lower respiratory tract as it passes the laryngeal entrance en route from the pharynx to the oesophagus. If this mechanism should be defeated and foreign bodies do inadvertently enter the larynx, then the larynx can close and allow a build up of pressure between the vocal folds which is suddenly released in a cough to dislodge the foreign body. This is the cough reflex already described in Chapter 15.

During phonation the degree of closure of the vocal folds can be adjusted, thus changing the flow of air through the larynx. In addition, the length, tension and bulk of the vocal folds can be altered to vary the pitch and loudness of the voice.

The anatomy of the neck

For descriptive purposes, the neck is divided into **triangles** whose boundaries are determined by muscular and skeletal structures (see Figure 1.2). The **sternocleidomastoid muscles** form the boundaries between the **anterior** and **posterior** triangles and are attached to the mastoid processes superiorly and to the sternum and clavicle inferiorly. They run obliquely downwards and forwards across the lateral aspect of the neck and function to turn the head to the opposite side. The upper border of the **anterior triangle** is formed by the lower border of the mandible, its anterior border by the midline of the neck and its posterior boundary by the sternocleidomastoid muscle. The most important structure in each anterior triangle is the **carotid sheath** lying lateral to the larynx and trachea. The fibrous carotid sheath encloses the common and internal carotid arteries, internal jugular vein and vagus nerve. In the lower part of the neck, the sheath is covered by the sternocleidomastoid muscle but it emerges above the anterior border superiorly. The **carotid pulse** may be detected here. The posterior triangle contains nothing of importance to speech and language therapy. It lies behind the sternocleidomastoid muscle and in front of the trapezius muscle and the base of the triangle is formed by the clavicle (Figure 1.2).

The surface anatomy of the face and neck

It is important that those structures forming the larynx that are palpable in the body can be identified as such manipulations often form part of the clinical examination and treatment of clients. The easiest way to study surface anatomy is to use yourself or a partner as the subject to palpate the structures mentioned. Some of the laryngeal cartilages determine the surface anatomy of the anterior neck to a considerable degree. When the neck is extended by tilting the head back, several structures can be palpated by running a finger down the *midline* from the point of the chin to the suprasternal notch.

The lower border of the mandible is easily palpable for most of its length. Below the mandible, superficially fatty subcutaneous tissue and the submandibular gland smooth the skin contour as it passes from the lower border of the mandible down on to the neck (Figure 16.1). As the finger is moved back in the midline from beneath the chin across the muscles forming the floor of the mouth, the next solid structure encountered at the top of the neck is the hyoid bone. The **hyoid bone** is the only bone in the body which does not articulate with other bones. Instead, it is attached by muscles, ligaments and membranes to the mandible and skull above and the laryngeal skeleton below. There is a gap about the size of the finger tip below the hyoid bone before the **thyroid cartilage** is felt. A groove is present on its superior surface before the **laryngeal prominence** of the thyroid cartilage (the 'Adam's Apple') is met. Careful palpation at the lower level of the thyroid cartilage reveals a slight gap between it and the **cricoid cartilage**. Below the cricoid, the more flexible **tracheal rings** of cartilage may be felt until they disappear behind the sternum. Although the laryngeal skeleton is easily palpable in most subjects, it is separated from the skin and subcutaneous tissue by muscles.

The suprahyoid muscles

Two groups of muscles, the suprahyoid and infrahyoid muscles, attach the hyoid bone to the skull and sternum (Figure 16.2). The suprahyoid muscles comprise four pairs of muscles which are attached to the hyoid bone below but have widespread attachments to the skull above. The **geniohyoid muscles** pass from the internal surface of the mandible at the chin to the hyoid bone. The two **mylohyoid muscles** form the floor of the mouth and are attached to the mylohyoid lines on the internal surface of each side of the mandible. The two muscles meet each other anteriorly in the midline between the mandible and hyoid bone but their posterior

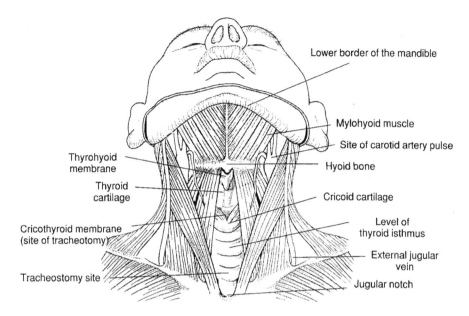

Figure 16.1 The surface features of the neck which can be palpated.

portions are attached along the length of the hyoid bone. The posterior border of each mylohyoid muscle is free. The **stylohyoid muscles,** as their name implies, attach to the styloid processes above and the hyoid bone below. The other muscles in this group, the **digastric muscles,** each have two distinct muscle bellies joined by a tendon. The anterior bellies attach to the digastric fossae of the mandible and the posterior bellies insert into grooves on the medial aspect of the mastoid processes. The two bellies are connected by a central tendon running through a fibrous sling which attaches them to the hyoid bone so that each muscle forms a shallow V with its apex at the hyoid bone.

The suprahyoid muscles have several actions during speech, swallowing and mastication but essentially they elevate the hyoid bone and, with it, the skeleton of the larynx. This is an important movement during swallowing (see Chapter 21) and is also used in speech. By using the hyoid as a fixed base, the muscles which attach to both the hyoid and the mandible, the anterior bellies of the digastrics, the geniohyoids and the mylohyoids, aid in depressing the lower jaw (see Chapter 18). A prerequisite for this action is fixation of the hyoid bone by another group of muscles, the infrahyoid muscles.

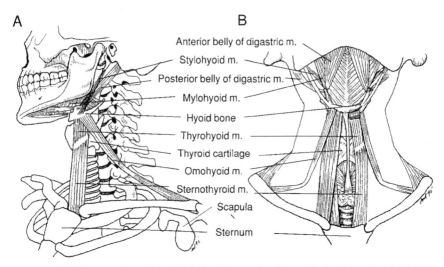

A B

Anterior belly of digastric m.
Stylohyoid m.
Posterior belly of digastric m.
Mylohyoid m.
Hyoid bone
Thyrohyoid m.
Thyroid cartilage
Omohyoid m.
Sternothyroid m.
Scapula
Sternum

Figure 16.2 The suprahyoid and infrahyoid muscles from (A) the lateral and (B) the anterior aspect.

The infrahyoid muscles

Four pairs of strap-like muscles make up this group. The **sternohyoid**, **thyrohyoid** and **omohyoid muscles** (Figure 16.2) are all attached to the hyoid bone above and to the sternum, thyroid cartilage and scapula respectively below. The **sternothyroid** muscles connect the thyroid cartilage and hyoid bone. This muscle group depresses the hyoid bone and the laryngeal skeleton after swallowing. They also counter the upward pull on the hyoid bone from the suprahyoid muscles enabling the suprahyoid muscles to act from a fixed hyoid bone to aid in opening the mouth. Their individual actions are poorly understood but the sternothyroid and thyrohyoid connect the thyroid cartilage with the sternum and hyoid respectively. These two muscles probably function to alter the position of or to stabilize the thyroid cartilage so that various muscles which move the laryngeal cartilages in relation to each other can operate to vary vocal pitch and loudness (see below).

The suprahyoid and infrahyoid muscles function in concert to adjust the overall position of the larynx. The geniohyoid and thyrohyoid muscles have the most significant effect upon elevation of the larynx and the other infrahyoid muscles on depressing the larynx. The overall position of the larynx alters the length of the resonating tube from the vocal folds to the lips, formed by the laryngeal vestibule, pharynx and the oral cavity thus changing fundamental frequency and resonance and is an important factor in varying the voice during speech.

The thyroid gland

The thyroid gland is another important structure in the neck whose functions have already been considered in Chapter 7. It consists of paired left and right pear-shaped lobes whose apices are directed upwards (Figure 16.3). They extend superiorly as far as the oblique line on the lateral surface of the thyroid cartilage and inferiorly to the level of the fourth or fifth tracheal rings. The lobes are connected by a narrow isthmus crossing the second, third and fourth tracheal rings. The lobes are covered anterolaterally by the infrahyoid muscles and the anterior borders of the sternocleidomastoid muscles. The lobes extend deeply around the sides of the larynx, trachea and the recurrent laryngeal nerves. Posterolaterally, the thyroid lobes are closely related to the carotid sheaths. The **posterior border** of each lobe contains superior and inferior **parathyroid glands**. The thyroid is surrounded by a connective tissue capsule which anchors it firmly to both the larynx and trachea.

Because of its endocrine function, the thyroid gland is a very vascular organ and the blood supply to the thyroid gland is derived from two sources. The **superior thyroid arteries** are branches of the external carotid arteries and descend to the upper pole of each lobe. The **inferior thyroid arteries** originate from the subclavian arteries and ascend behind the gland to the level of the cricoid cartilage to reach the posterior border

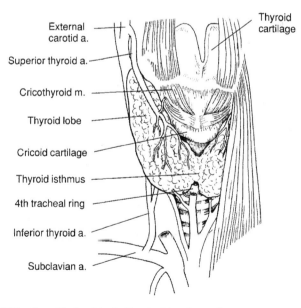

Figure 16.3 The thyroid gland including its blood supply.

of the gland. The recurrent laryngeal nerves are closely associated with these arteries, passing behind or in front of them. Damage to the recurrent laryngeal nerves as the inferior thyroid arteries are isolated during thyroid operations is one possible cause of laryngeal palsy (see below).

The laryngeal skeleton

Three paired and three unpaired cartilages make up the laryngeal skeleton (Figure 16.4). The three unpaired cartilages are the thyroid and cricoid cartilages and the epiglottis. The three paired cartilages are the arytenoids, and the smaller corniculate and cuneiform cartilages. The thyroid, cricoid and arytenoid cartilages are made of hyaline cartilage and the epiglottis, corniculate and cuneiform cartilages are made of elastic cartilage.

The laryngeal cartilages

The **thyroid cartilage** is formed of two flat plates, the **laminae**, which meet anteriorly at the thyroid angle to form the **laryngeal prominence** or Adam's apple. The anterior fusion is not complete and there is a V-shaped thyroid notch superiorly. An oblique line on each lamina is the site of attachment of several muscles, including the thyrohyoid and sternothyroid muscles. The superior and inferior cornua extend upwards and downwards respectively from the posterior edges of the lamina. The thyrohyoid ligament attaching the thyroid cartilage and hyoid bone is attached

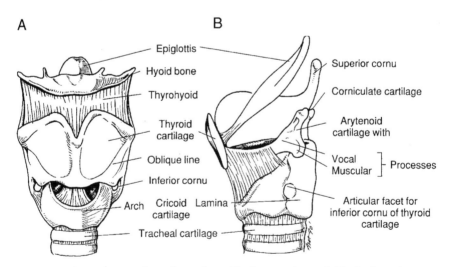

Figure 16.4 The laryngeal cartilages from (A) the anterior and (B) the lateral aspect with the left half of the thyroid cartilage removed.

to the superior horn. The tip of the inferior cornu forms a joint with cricoid cartilage.

The **cricoid cartilage** forms the only complete ring of cartilage in the respiratory system. It lies beneath the thyroid cartilage at the level of the sixth cervical vertebra. It is in the form of a signet ring with a narrow anterior arch, similar in size to the tracheal cartilages situated below it and a wide flat lamina posteriorly. A vertical midline ridge divides the posterior surface of the lamina into two shallow concave depressions, the site of attachment of the posterior cricoarytenoid muscles. Two small facets forming articulations for the arytenoid cartilages are located on either side of the superolateral surface of the lamina on the sloping shoulders of the lamina. Another pair of facets is located on the lateral surface of the cricoid cartilage at the junction between the lamina and the anterior arch. These facets articulate with the inferior cornua of the thyroid cartilage (Figure 16.4).

The small paired **arytenoid cartilages** lie on the superior surface of the lamina of the cricoid. They approximate in shape to a three-sided pyramid with a base, apex and three sloping surfaces. The base of the arytenoid cartilage is concave and forms a synovial joint with the lamina of the cricoid cartilage. The medial surfaces of the arytenoid cartilages face one another and are slightly convex towards the midline. The posterior surfaces are concave and end in a backward curving apex. The antero-lateral surfaces are concave; each has two depressions, the fovea triangularis above and an oblong depression lateral to the vocal process (see Figure 16.6). The base of each cartilage has two projections extending from it. The **vocal process** projects anteriorly from the anterior angle of the arytenoid cartilage and the vocal ligament is attached to it. The muscular process projects posterolaterally and is the site of attachment for various muscles of the larynx.

The **epiglottis** (see Figures 16.4 and 16.6) is a leaf-shaped elastic cartilage which is attached below by a narrow stalk of connective tissue to the internal surface of the thyroid angle just beneath the thyroid notch. The convex lingual surface of the epiglottis faces anteriorly and is separated from the tongue by the valleculae. The posterior surface is concave above but becomes convex below.

The **corniculate cartilages** are small elastic cartilages joined to the apices of the arytenoid cartilages. The **cuneiform cartilages** are small rod-like structures found in the aryepiglottic folds.

Joints of the larynx

There are two pairs of synovial joints between the laryngeal cartilages, the cricothyroid and cricoarytenoid joints. Movements at these two joints are responsible for all the opening and closing movements of the vocal folds and movements during adjustment of length, tension and thickness of the vocal folds during phonation.

The **cricothyroid joints** are formed between the inferior cornua of thyroid cartilage and the lateral facets on the cricoid cartilage. The joint is surrounded by a capsule strengthened by ligaments. The primary movement at the joint is one of rotation about an axis that passes between the two cricoid facets. There may also be some limited gliding in the sagittal plane when the ligaments are slack. The effect of rotation at this joint is to move the cricoid and thyroid cartilages in such a way that the laminae of the thyroid and arch of the cricoid cartilage are brought closer together as the cricoid lamina is moved away from the thyroid cartilage (Figure 16.5). As the vocal folds are attached anteriorly to the thyroid laminae and posteriorly to the arytenoid cartilages which are attached in turn to the cricoid lamina, the effect of moving these joints is to lengthen the vocal folds as the cricoid lamina rotates posteriorly. This may also increase tension in the vocal folds. It is unclear which of the two cartilages moves. The accepted wisdom is that the cricoid cartilage is the fixed component. In reality, there is no mechanism to fix the cricoid in place whereas the sternothyroid and thyroid muscles are capable of fixing the thyroid lamina: thus, it is likely that the cricoid cartilage moves to a greater extent.

The **cricoarytenoid joints** are also synovial joints surrounded by a capsule strengthened by ligaments. They are formed between convex facets on the sloping shoulders of the cricoid cartilage and corresponding concave facets of the bases of the arytenoid cartilages. The facets on the

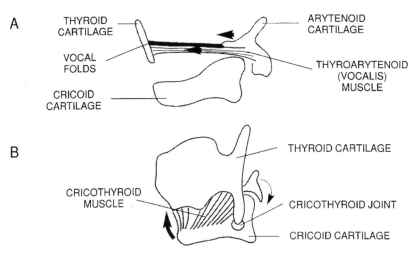

Figure 16.5 Movements at (A) the cricoarytenoid joint and (B) the cricothyroid joint.

cricoid cartilage are oval and convex and are directed downwards, laterally and anteriorly from behind. Movements at this joint are still not clearly understood but their effects are to open and close the vocal folds and alter their length and tension. There appear to be three main movements made at this joint (Figures 16.5 and 16.10). The most obvious movement is that of the arytenoid cartilages gliding along the long axis of the cricoid articular facet. If the cartilages glide upwards on the cricoid, then this brings the vocal processes together closing (adducting) the vocal folds; downward gliding has the opposite effect of opening or abducting the vocal folds. The other two movements which occur at these joints are a rotational movement through an axis approximately through the long axis of the arytenoid cartilage and a rocking of the arytenoids backwards and forwards on the cricoid lamina (Figure 16.5). There is considerable debate about how much these movements contribute to altering the position and physical state of the vocal folds. The rotational movement produces a movement of the vocal process upwards and outwards on lateral (or backwards) rotation abducting (separating) the vocal folds or inwards and downwards on medial (or forward) rotation abducting (bringing together) the vocal folds. The range of rotational movement is restricted by the shape of the joint surfaces and the processes of the arytenoid cartilages. Forward rocking movement of the arytenoid cartilages brings the vocal process forward and downwards, thus shortening the vocal folds whereas backward rocking lifts the vocal processes upwards and backwards, thus lengthening the vocal cords. It is likely that in most movements of the arytenoid cartilages on the cricoid at least two of these movements occur simultaneously.

Laryngeal membranes

The cartilages of the larynx are linked to surrounding structures by a series of extrinsic ligaments and membranes. They are also joined to each other by a series of intrinsic ligaments and membranes (Figure 16.6).

The **thyrohyoid membrane** joins the larynx to the hyoid bone. The membrane is attached to the superior border and cornua of the thyroid cartilage below and to the hyoid bone above. It is pierced by the superior laryngeal nerve and vessels. The **cricotracheal membrane** connects the lower border of the cricoid cartilage to the first tracheal ring.

The **intrinsic laryngeal membranes** essentially form one continuous sheet above and below, separated only by a small space between the true and false vocal folds (Figure 16.6C). The membrane below the true vocal folds is called the cricothyroid membrane and the membrane above the false vocal folds is called the quadrangular membrane.

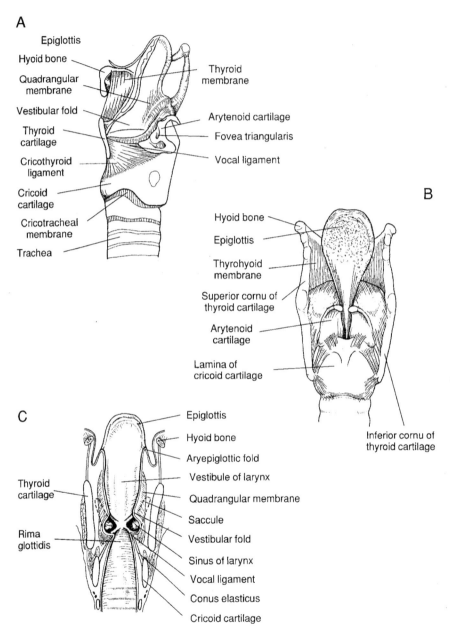

Figure 16.6 The laryngeal membranes from (A) the lateral aspect and (B) the posterior aspect. (C) shows the laryngeal membranes from the posterior aspect with the larynx cut coronally.

The **cricothyroid membrane** is attached between the cricoid, thyroid and arytenoid cartilages. It passes upwards from the arch and lamina of the cricoid cartilage to the inner surface of the thyroid cartilage to attach anteriorly to the deep aspect of the thyroid cartilage and posteriorly to the vocal process of the arytenoid cartilage. The anterior attachments on each side are fused to form the anterior commissure but the posterior attachments are separated if the arytenoid cartilages are abducted when the larynx is in the default setting of the vocal folds being opened to allow respiration. The upper free margins of the cricothyroid membrane thus form a narrow 'v' with the apex of the thyroid cartilage. The free margins are thickened to form the **vocal ligaments** and these form the basis of the **true vocal folds**. The internal part of the cricothyroid membrane is known as the **conus elasticus** because of its shape which narrows the profile of the lower larynx to a funnel or cone-shaped structure.

The anterior aspect of the **quadrangular membrane** is attached to the lateral side of the epiglottis and extends downwards to the deep side of the thyroid angle. The upper free border forms the **aryepiglottic folds** extending posteriorly from the sides of the epiglottis to the arytenoid and corniculate cartilages and are strengthened by the cuneiform cartilages. The lower border of the quadrangular membrane is attached anteriorly to the thyroid angle just above the attachment of the vocal ligaments and runs posteriorly to the fovea triangularis of each arytenoid cartilage. Between these two attachments, the free inferior border forms the framework of the **vestibular folds**.

The vocal folds and ligaments are attached to the vocal processes of the arytenoid cartilages but the vestibular folds are attached to the fovea triangularis which lies lateral to and above the vocal folds. These attachments ensure that there is space between the two sets of folds to allow for the vibration of the vocal folds and that the vestibular folds are situated more laterally than the vocal folds except near their anterior attachments to the thyroid cartilage. Both sets of folds are attached to the arytenoid cartilage and will therefore be moved when the arytenoid cartilages are moved. However, for virtually any movement of the arytenoid cartilages, the movement of the vocal folds will be accentuated because the displacement of the vocal processes, hence the vocal folds, is greater than the displacement of the body of the arytenoid to which the vestibular folds are attached. Simply, this means that the vocal folds will be, at most times, nearer the midline than the vestibular folds and that the vestibular folds will not be in the direct airstream.

The laryngeal inlet and cavity

The cartilages and membranes that form the skeletal framework of the larynx surround the laryngeal cavity which is continuous with the trachea below and opens into the anterior wall of the laryngopharynx above through the laryngeal inlet. The vestibular folds and vocal folds divide the laryngeal cavity into three parts, the supraglottic and infraglottic cavities separated by the laryngeal ventricle.

The **laryngeal inlet** faces upwards and backwards (Figure 16.7). Its margins are formed by the posterior surface of the epiglottis anteriorly, the aryepiglottic folds laterally and by the mucosa covering the two arytenoid cartilages and intervening muscles posteriorly.

The laryngeal cavity extends anteriorly and downwards to the lower border of the cricoid cartilage where it becomes continuous with the trachea. The upper part of the laryngeal cavity from the laryngeal inlet to the false vocal folds is known as the **supraglottic cavity** or laryngeal

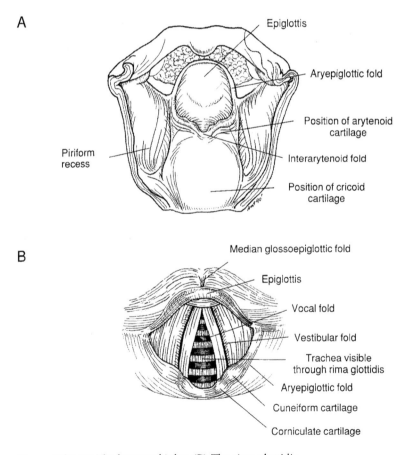

Figure 16.7 (A) The laryngeal inlet. (B) The rima glottidis.

vestibule. The supraglottic cavity is roughly triangular and narrows towards the false vocal folds. The **laryngeal ventricles** (or sinuses) lie on the lateral walls of the larynx between the vestibular folds and the true vocal folds. Each cavity, which is longer in males, provides a space that allows the true vocal folds to vibrate. From each ventricle, the blind-ended laryngeal saccules extend in an anterior direction between the ventricular folds and the thyroid cartilage. Many mucous glands are located within the walls of the saccules.

The lower part of the laryngeal cavity is known as the **infraglottic cavity** and extends from the true vocal folds to the inferior border of the cricoid cartilage. The infraglottic cavity is narrow and elliptical in cross section superiorly, and wider and more circular below. During phonation the walls of the infraglottic cavity are shaped like a nozzle and have exponentially curved surfaces. This particular shape may help to reduce the energy cost of phonation by accelerating the flow of air, ensuring lamina flow and minimizing turbulence as the expiratory air at high pressure is directed through the narrowed laryngeal cavity at the vocal folds (see Chapter 17).

The **true vocal folds** are located at the narrowest point of the laryngeal cavity. The horizontal space between the two vocal folds is known as the **rima glottidis** or the **glottis** (Figure 16.7B). The anterior three-quarters of the glottis is enclosed on either side by the vocal ligaments, the upper free margins of the cricothyroid membrane. This portion of the glottis is the **ligamentous glottis**. The posterior quarter of the glottis is bounded on either side by the vocal processes and medial surfaces of the arytenoid cartilages, forming the **cartilaginous glottis**. The overall length of the ligamentous glottis at rest is about 15 mm in males and 12 mm in females while the cartilaginous glottis is about 8 mm in males, 7 mm in females. The size and shape of the glottis can vary greatly as the result of movement of the arytenoid cartilages at the cricarytenoid joints.

The whole of the cavity of the larynx is lined with a mucous membrane that is continuous with that of the laryngopharynx superiorly and the trachea inferiorly. There are regional differences in both the mucous membrane and the underlying submucous tissue that reflect differences in function in the different regions. The structure of the true and false vocal folds are more complex reflecting their highly specialized functions.

Most of the supraglottic and infraglottic cavities, with the exception of the true vocal folds and a region of the supraglottic cavity close to the laryngeal inlet, are lined with a respiratory epithelium (see Chapter 2). The submucous tissue in these regions that separates the epithelial lining from the underlying tissues is lax and contains mixed serous and mucous glands.

The structure of the true and false vocal folds

The **vestibular folds** overlying the vestibular ligaments are thick and rounded and covered by respiratory mucous membrane (see Chapter 2). Sometimes the epithelium over the very edge of the vestibular folds is covered by a unique form of epithelium; the deep cells adjacent to the connective tissue are columnar like respiratory epithelium but they are covered by a few layers of squamous cells rather like stratified squamous epithelium (Figure 16.8). The folds themselves are very soft and flexible and the underlying connective tissue contains a large number of elastic fibres. There is an especially high concentration of mucous glands in the vestibular folds and particularly along the lower border of the quadrangular membrane. These glands form part of the bulge that constitutes the vestibular folds. Secretion from these glands together with those in the saccules are the major source of lubrication to the vocal folds during phonation.

The **true vocal folds** are covered with stratified squamous epithelium (see Chapter 2) in those parts of the vocal folds that come into contact

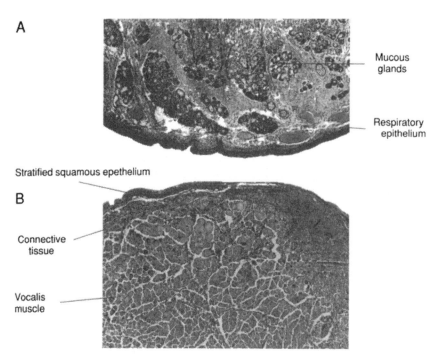

Figure 16.8 The microscopic structure of the vocal folds. (A) The vestibular folds. (B) The vocal folds.

with each other. This epithelium helps to protect the underlying tissues from the frictional stresses that arise as the vocal folds come into contact during phonation. Elsewhere, the mucous membrane covering the folds is lined with respiratory epithelium and the cilia help to remove the debris that collects on the vocal folds. There are no mucous glands within the vocal folds: instead the bulk of the vocal folds is formed by the thyroartenoid muscle. The connective tissue that supports the epithelium and separates it from the deeper lying muscle is arranged into three layers. The superficial layer directly under the epithelium is made up of loosely arranged elastic fibres. The intermediate layer is also composed of elastic fibres organized into dense bundles of fibres running parallel to the longitudinal axis of the vocal folds. The deep layer of connective tissue next to the muscle contains collagen fibres that are also organized in dense arrays oriented in an anteroposterior direction. Some of the deeper collagen fibres form the upper free border of the cricothyroid membrane and some form the covering of the thyroarytenoid muscle lying within the vocal folds. The connective tissue layers are about 2–3 mm thickness in total. The bulk of the vocal fold is made up of muscle, and this muscle layer is 7–8 mm thick. The muscle fibres are also oriented in an anteroposterior direction.

Different terminologies have been used to describe the soft tissues of the vocal folds. The above system describes five layers within the vocal folds. These have also been described as being grouped into three layers: the mucosa comprising the epithelium plus the superficial layer of connective tissue; the ligament that comprises the intermediate and deep layers of connective tissue; and the muscle. A third system uses the term 'body' to refer to the muscle and deep layer of connective tissue and the term 'cover' to refer to the remaining superficial layers.

Clinical and applied anatomy of the vestibular and vocal folds

Dysphonia is any disturbance in sound produced while voicing in the larynx and there are several possible causes. Dysphonia, usually with dysarthria, is often a consequence of damage to the nerve supply to the larynx; this may be due to neurological disease affecting motor pathways or other structures involved in motor control (see Chapter 10) or the nuclei of the nerves controlling the larynx (see Chapter 11). Dysphonia without dysarthria may be due to damage along the peripheral course of the nerves supplying the larynx (see 'Laryngeal nerve injuries' below). Dysphonia may also be caused by pathological changes to the vocal folds themselves. A prerequisite for the investigation of dysphonia is a clinical examination of the larynx carried out by laryngoscopy.

Laryngoscopy

Laryngoscopy is the examination of the larynx carried out by Ear, Nose and Throat (ENT) surgeons. Direct laryngoscopy involves the insertion of a long-handled dental mirror along the palate with the mirror facing downwards so that the larynx may be viewed through the oropharynx. This procedure is not very efficient. Extreme care must be taken to avoid stimulating the mucosa of the soft palate or posterior pharyngeal wall which will elicit a gag reflex when placing the mirror (see Chapter 21). The preferred method of examination of the larynx is **fibreoptic nasoendoscopy** in which a fibre optic tube with a lens on the end is passed through the nasal cavity and down into the oropharynx. The other end of the tube is connected to a viewing mechanism. It is possible to attach a second viewing lens to the laryngoscope which enables other observers to follow the examination including the client, if they are happy with the idea: this is particularly useful when clients need to change their vocal behaviour in such conditions as vocal nodules (see below). The picture of the larynx is now often transmitted directly to a television screen so that several observers can see the results simultaneously. After as full explanation of the procedure, the most patent of the right or left nasal cavity is anaesthetized with topical anaesthetic and the patient is given a lozenge containing local anaesthetic to suck. Generally, about ten minutes is allowed for the anaesthetic to take effect, then the tube is manipulated through the nasal cavity into the nasopharynx. Once in place, the viewing tip can be manipulated to produce the best view.

Figure 16.7B shows the general appearance of the normal larynx viewed by nasoendoscopy. The laryngeal inlet, formed by the epiglottis anteriorly and the aryepiglottic folds posteriorly, can be seen. Two bumps in each fold are observed close to the midline: the more lateral bump is the cuneiform cartilage and the more medial bump is the corniculate cartilage on the apex of the arytenoid cartilage. The vestibular folds are seen below the laryngeal entrance and, at a deeper level, the rima glottidis with the vocal folds on either side. Ridges made by the tracheal cartilages are visible through the open rima glottidis. It is usual to ask the client to phonate during the examination so that the movements of the vocal folds and their degree of closure can be observed. In experienced hands, laryngoscopical examination takes only a few minutes. Most clients, while not enjoying the experience, tolerate the procedure fairly well. A few have problems tolerating the laryngoscope in which case it is often difficult to observe long enough to see the folds and their actions clearly.

Pathology of the vocal folds

Many pathological conditions can be observed by laryngoscopy. A biopsy may be taken by using a modified endoscope with small scissors attached and is then sent for histopathological examination by microscopy to confirm the diagnosis.

One of the most common conditions producing dysphonia are **vocal nodes** (also known as 'singer's nodes' or 'screamer's nodes' – a heavy clue to their cause) and **vocal polyps**. There is considerable debate about the distinction, if any, between these two conditions. The consensus at present is that they are different manifestations of the same condition, and the term 'vocal nodule' is used in a generic way. Polyps are the early and nodes the later manifestation of the same condition.

Essentially, nodules arise due to vocal abuse or overuse of the voice, for which there may be many reasons. They appear a third of the way along the vocal folds from the anterior end (i.e. halfway along the ligamentous part of the vocal fold). This is the area of maximum contact and therefore the area which is most likely to be traumatized. Polyps appear as fleshy red or whitish lumps of variable size which may be symmetrical but are usually asymmetrical (one vocal fold only). They may be sessile, meaning that they are fixed to the vocal folds or may have a stalk. If they are stalked, polyps may disappear below the vocal folds and not be easy to detect. Nodes are symmetrical, firm, opaque, whitish lumps between 1 and 5 mm in antero-posterior dimension on the free edge of the vocal folds although the lumps may be of unequal size on each fold. Both lesions show changes in the epithelium and the subepithelial tissues. Polyps show oedematous changes often with haematomatous changes (intratissue bleeding), proliferation and degeneration of collagenous tissue and hyperkeratosis (thickening) of the epithelium. Nodes show oedematous changes and collagenous proliferation with epithelial hyperplasia. Their effect on phonation is the same, namely that the lump or lumps prevent the close apposition of the vocal folds during phonation. This in turn leads to air leakage around the lesion and difficulty in sustaining phonation. In addition, the mass of the vocal folds is increased and the vocal folds are stiffer. Hoarseness of the voice is the most common presenting symptom; the pitch may be lowered, pitch breaks may occur and there is vocal fatigue and lack of power in the voice. Treatment should always involve vocal re-education to minimize vocal abuse and prevent recurrence. In many clients, nodules will regress with appropriate voice therapy without additional medical intervention. In some cases, non-specific anti-inflammatory drugs (corticosteroids) which reduce oedema may be prescribed although the problems associated with corticosteroid therapy outlined in Chapter 7 should be borne in mind. The lesions may be surgically removed but this should always be followed by voice re-education, otherwise recurrence is very likely. Surgery results in scarring and voice quality will, inevitably, deteriorate with repeated operations.

Reinke's oedema is local oedema in the vocal folds, as opposed to generalized laryngeal oedema described below. Fluid accumulation in the vocal folds occurs in the superficial connective tissue, sometimes referred to as Reinke's space along the length of the vocal folds and is usually bilateral but asymmetrical. It may be a consequence of several conditions including laryngitis, premenstrual oedema, or fluid accumulation accompanying hypothyroidism: Reinke's oedema is often the presenting feature of hypothyroidism. Oedema due to any of these causes does not interfere with closure of the vocal folds. However, the oedema is pushed above the vocal folds and vibrates during expiration and phonation producing a characteristic hoarse voice. As the mass of the vocal folds is increased, pitch is lowered (see Chapter 17).

Cancer of the larynx is usually **squamous cell carcinoma** which occurs in stratified squamous epithelium and therefore appears on the vocal folds. Squamous cell carcinoma begins as dysplastic changes in the epithelial cells in which the cells look abnormal under the microscope. Nasoendoscopic examination may reveal a variety of appearances of the cancerous lesion. They are usually asymmetrical and can manifest as a circumscribed white patch, as extensive white lumps or as large ulcerative lesions. The white colouration is due to hyperkeratinization of the epithelium. If the lesion is restricted to the epithelium, it is known as **carcinoma in situ**. Removal of the carcinoma at this stage usually has an excellent prognosis. As the cancer grows, it invades the underlying tissues and may metastasize to distant sites (see Chapter 2). Prognosis worsens with local spread and is very poor once metastasis has taken place. Surgical excision of the lesion accompanied by chemotherapy or radiotherapy may be attempted for early cancer, but once the cancer has invaded other structures, it is usually necessary to carry out a **laryngectomy** in which part or all of the larynx is removed. A **tracheostomy**, a permanent opening in the airway, is performed. This is usually carried out at the level of the trachea which has cosmetic advantages because the tracheostomy may be hidden under clothing. There are a number of designs of valve which can be inserted at the tracheostomy. The valves enable air to enter and leave during respiration but they have a posterior extension that is attached to the oesophagus. By swallowing air and then regurgitating (belching) it through the oesophageal part of the valve, phonation may be achieved, albeit of reduced quality. However, not everyone can carry out the requisite manoeuvres successfully.

Laryngitis, inflammation of the larynx, is very common and can be caused by a bewildering array of agents, such as bacterial and viral upper respiratory tract infections, smoking, allergens, dusty or dry atmosphere, excessively prolonged speaking such as lecturing or talking loudly to overcome environmental noise. In many of these causes, the laryngitis is exacerbated by drying up of the mucus in the vestibular folds and saccules, either because of the underlying cause or simply because the glands have secreted all the mucus they can and require a period of inactivity to recover. The glands can also be inhibited by various drugs which have a sympatheticomimetic effect (see Chapters 12 and 19). The most obvious signs and symptoms are hoarseness and soreness. In acute laryngitis, the folds are red and there may be small dilated blood vessels on the surface. Chronic laryngitis often shows as epithelial hyperplasia in which case the folds are whitish in colour; it can lead to vocal abuse with the appearance of nodules. Because of the inflammatory condition, possibly with inadequate lubrication, vocal fold vibration is asymmetrical and the two folds are often out of phase with each other.

The submucous tissue separating the epithelial lining of the larynx from the underlying connective tissues is tightly bound to those tissues in the region of the vocal fold covered with stratified squamous epithelium but is lax elsewhere in the laryngeal cavity and this has important function consequences should **laryngeal oedema** occur. The major causes of generalized laryngeal oedema are allergic reactions to drugs or naturally occurring substances such as the toxins in bee stings or infection due to acute laryngitis. Various complex reactions occur, one consequence of which is that capillaries become more permeable and fluid from the blood accumulates in the connective tissues. This is especially so where the mucosa is loose. If fluid accumulates in the supraglottic cavity, it will naturally gravitate downwards until it is arrested where the epithelium is tightly bound down to the connective tissue of the vocal folds. As a result, fluid accumulation in the mucosa of the laryngeal vestibule and above distends the mucosa. If left untreated, fluid distension will eventually occlude the airway and is life-threatening. Injection of antihistamine drugs is usually successful in diminishing the oedema but occasionally a tracheotomy, an emergency opening into the respiratory tract performed through the cricothyroid membrane, is necessary to bypass the laryngeal obstruction.

Age changes in the vocal folds

The connective tissue in the vocal fold is relatively thick and uniform at birth and only differentiates into elastic and collagenous layers between the ages of six and twelve. Its adult structure is reached by the end of adolescence. One of the secondary sexual changes which occurs during puberty in males is that the thyroid cartilage enlarges, accounting for the greater size of the laryngeal prominence in adult males. This enlargement of the thyroid cartilage elongates the vocal folds; on average, adult male vocal folds are 5 mm longer than those of adult females and male voices are about one octave lower than female voices. During the pubertal growth spurt, males essentially have to learn to phonate with longer vocal folds. They may make errors leading to pitch breaks which are often embarrassing for the individual concerned. **Puberphonia** is the persistence of a high-pitched childlike voice beyond the age when voice changes should have occurred. If hormonal or other organic abnormalities have been ruled out as possible causes, puberphonia often has a psychological aetiology.

There are also changes to the structure of the vocal folds in old age but these can be very variable. In general, the superficial tissues become more oedematous and therefore thicken and elastic fibres degenerate. These changes are usually more obvious in males than females. The thyroary-tenoid muscles tend to atrophy with increasing age. There may be increase or decrease in pitch, and less control over volume, clarity and speed of phonation and articulation. When evaluating geriatric clients, it is important to distinguish between changes due to ageing and those due to disease states which increase in frequency with advancing age. For example, the laryngeal cartilages may exhibit some degree of ossification in older clients; this is not unique to the larynx as it also occurs in the costal cartilages and the xiphisternum too. Ossification may make movements of the laryngeal skeleton stiffer with some changes to voice. Arthritis, inflammation of joints, can affect any synovial joints in the body including those of the larynx. If the cricothyroid or cricoarytenoid joints are affected, voice characteristics will be altered. It is often difficult to distinguish joint ankylosis (fusion) from laryngeal palsy (see below), but arthritic changes are usually painful whereas palsies are not.

The laryngeal musculature

Functional movements of the larynx are brought about by the actions of the skeletal muscles that are attached to the laryngeal cartilages. The muscles attached to the larynx can be divided into two groups, the extrinsic muscles and the intrinsic muscles. The extrinsic muscles have one attachment to the larynx and the other attachment to another structure outside the larynx. The extrinsic muscles, the suprahyoid and infrahyoid muscles move the larynx as a whole during the production of speech and swallowing and have been described above.

The intrinsic muscles are attached at both ends to the laryngeal framework. These muscles are best understood in the context of laryngeal functions. As described above, the default setting of the larynx is open to maintain patency of the airway. It is then closed forcefully when it acts as a sphincter during protection of the lower airway but also during fixation of the thorax and abdomen to aid the functions of the muscles of the thoracic and abdominal muscles themselves. The larynx is closed less forcefully during phonation.

The larynx also has important functions in regulating ventilation, and to a lesser extent, circulation. The larynx, at the level of the vocal folds, represents the point of maximum constriction in the respiratory tract so that, in order to minimize the laryngeal contribution to the resistance to ventilation, the larynx needs to be open widely, especially during forced or vigorous ventilation. Closure of the larynx during expiration can raise intrathoracic pressure sufficient to impede venous return, hence the red face that accompanies exertion when lifting heavy objects.

The lifting of a heavy weight is often preceded by glottal closure. This action raises intrathoracic pressure and stabilizes the thorax and thus allows greater efficiency of action for the muscles of the arm that have one of their attachments to the thoracic cage. One of the frequent complaints of clients with laryngectomies is that they experience a loss of power when lifting. This is because they are no longer able to close their larynx in this way to increase the efficiency of action of the muscles of their arms. In a similar manner the larynx can be closed to aid the action of the abdominal muscles during functions such as defecation, urination or childbirth.

Intrinsic muscles of the larynx

Taking the functions of the larynx in turn, the muscles involved in maintaining an open larynx and producing forceful closure for its sphincteric functions will be described followed by those muscles involved in phonation. The sphincteric actions of the muscles are relatively simple but the actions of the muscles that occur during phonation are more complex. The sphincteric muscles are, however, also involved in phonation as any one functional movement or adjustment of the vocal folds during phonation may require the simultaneous contraction of several muscles. Thus it can be difficult to decide what the action of an individual muscle might be and there is often overlap in the functions of the intrinsic laryngeal muscles. The muscles of the larynx are an excellent example of the group action of muscles described in Chapter 3.

Muscles controlling the glottis and laryngeal inlet

The **posterior cricoarytenoid muscles** are the only muscles capable of opening, or abducting, the vocal folds (Figure 16.9). Each fan-shaped muscle is attached inferiorly to the posterior surface of the lamina cricoid cartilage up to the vertical midline ridge. Each muscle converges on to the muscular process of the arytenoid cartilage above. The superior fibres of the muscle are short and nearly horizontal while the inferior fibres are longer and nearly vertical. The main action of the muscle is to cause the vocal processes, to which the vocal ligaments are attached, to separate, thus opening the glottis (Figure 16.10A). This is brought about by the muscle acting to slide the arytenoid cartilages dorsolaterally. The posterior cricoarytenoid muscles are continuously active during respiration to keep the vocal folds apart and maintain the airway. The posterior cricoarytenoid muscles also have a subsidiary action of lengthening the vocal folds by tilting back the arytenoid cartilages if the positions of the thyroid and

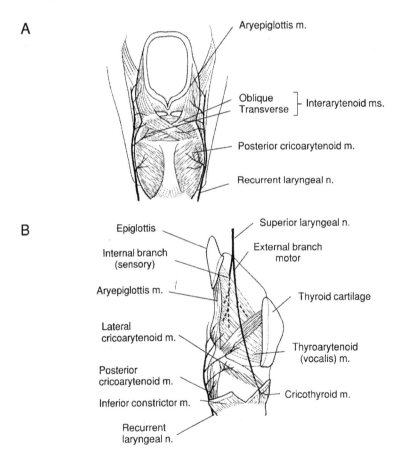

Figure 16.9 The laryngeal muscles and their innervation from (A) the posterior aspect and (B) the lateral aspect with the right half of the thyroid cartilage removed.

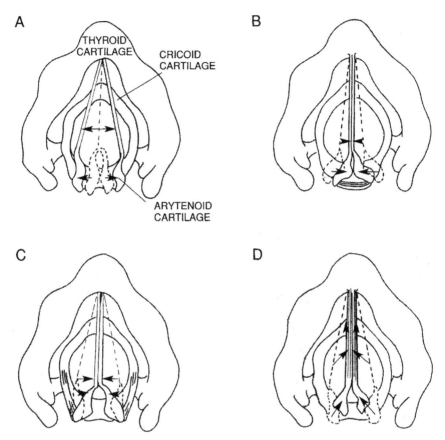

Figure 16.10 The actions of the intrinsic laryngeal muscles on the vocal folds. (A) The posterior cricoarytenoid muscles. (B) The interarytenoid muscles. (C) The lateral cricoarytenoid muscles. (D) The thyroarytenoid (vocalis) muscles. The starting position of the vocal folds and arytenoid cartilages is shown by dotted lines and the final position is shown by solid lines.

cricoid cartilages remain unchanged. The posterior cricoarytenoids are therefore used when using high register to counteract the forward pull of muscles shortening and tensing the vocal folds. These muscles are also active during the production of unvoiced sounds when the vocal folds are also separated.

Several muscles close, or adduct, the larynx. The **transverse interarytenoid muscle** is unpaired. It extends horizontally from the posterior surface and lateral border of the arytenoid cartilage on one side to that of its neighbour on the opposite side filling the concave posterior surfaces of the arytenoid cartilages and bridging the gap between cartilages at the back of the larynx. Its action is to bring the arytenoid cartilages together and thus close the glottis by adducting the vocal folds (Figure 16.10B). The **oblique interarytenoid muscles** are paired and lie superficial to the transverse interarytenoid muscles. The muscles are attached inferiorly to the lower, posterior aspect of the muscular process of each arytenoid cartilage. The fibres pass superiorly crossing each other in the midline to attach to the apex of the arytenoid cartilage on the opposite side. The action of these muscles is to draw the arytenoid cartilages together and thus to close the glottis by adducting the vocal folds with the transverse interarytenoid muscles above. The oblique interarytenoid muscles may be more effective than the transverse interarytenoids as adductors of the vocal folds because of their greater mechanical advantage. As the oblique interarytenoids draw in the arytenoid cartilages they will also adduct the vestibular folds, which only occurs during sphincteric actions of the larynx but not during phonation. Adduction of the arytenoid cartilages also produces a degree of narrowing of the laryngeal inlet. The oblique inter-arytenoid muscles extend beyond the apex of the arytenoid cartilage into the aryepiglottic fold as the aryepiglottic muscles (see below).

The **lateral cricoarytenoid muscles** are small paired muscles located in the lateral wall of the larynx outside the conus elasticus. They are attached inferiorly to the superior border of the lateral arch of the cricoid cartilage and ascend posteriorly to attach to the muscular process of the arytenoid cartilage. The main action of these muscles is to adduct the vocal folds (Figure 16.10C). The muscles pull the muscular processes of the arytenoid outwards and forwards. As the muscular processes rotate outwards, the vocal processes rotate inwards and backwards, thus adducting the vocal folds and closing the glottis. By bringing the tips of the vocal processes together the muscle closes the glottis along its ligamentous part. The lateral cricoarytenoid muscles also rock the arytenoid cartilages backwards and downwards on the cricoid, elevating the vocal process and moving it backwards, thus altering the length and tension in the vocal folds. Which action of these muscles predominates in a given situation is dependent upon the action of other muscles. It is likely that the transverse and oblique interarytenoids and lateral cricoarytenoids are all active when forceful closure of the larynx is required. These two muscles have little, if any, effect on the vibrational qualities of the vocal folds.

As well as closure of the glottis, the laryngeal entrance is also narrowed when the larynx is used as a sphincter. As well as the narrowing caused by approximation of the arytenoid cartilages as described above, there are two pairs of muscles whose specific function is to regulate the laryngeal opening. They are the aryepiglottic muscles and the thyroepiglottic muscles. The **aryepiglottic muscles** are the upward continuation of the oblique interarytenoid muscles and are located around the margin of the laryngeal inlet in the aryepiglottic folds. Below that, they are attached to the apices of the arytenoid cartilage and are attached to the lateral margin of the epiglottis above. The function of the muscle is to shorten the aryepiglottic folds and approximate them. These muscles are fairly weak and are trying to pull against the strong elastic effect of the epiglottis. They produce little, if any, movement of the epiglottis. Instead, their effect is to narrow the laryngeal inlet rather in the manner of the cord on a drawstring purse. The **thyroepiglottic muscles** consist of a few fibres attached to the deep surface of the thyroid lamina superior to the thyroarytenoid muscles. The fibres pass upward to attach to the aryepiglottic fold and the margin of the epiglottis and tend to widen the laryngeal inlet. These two muscles are very variable in extent and are never very prominent.

Muscles affecting the length, tension and mass of the vocal folds

During phonation for the production of vowels and voiced consonants, the vocal folds are adducted to some degree and must be under some degree of tension. In addition, the length, tension and mass per unit length (effective mass) of the vocal folds can be minutely adjusted to alter pitch and other variables of the voice during phonation. The relationships of these variables and their effects on speech are discussed in Chapter 17. The adductors of the glottis described above are therefore involved in phonation and the abductors, the posterior cricoarytenoids are used when unvoiced phonemes are being generated. Other muscles act specifically to lengthen or shorten the vocal folds.

The **cricothyroid muscles** lengthen the vocal folds. Each muscle has two bellies. The anterior belly is attached to the anterior part of the lower border and outer surface of the cricoid cartilage and ascends almost vertically to attach to the anterior half of the thyroid lamina. The posterior belly is attached to the cricoid arch more posterolaterally than the anterior belly and ascends but in a posterosuperior direction to attach to the inferior border of the posterior half of the thyroid lamina and to the inferior cornu (Figure 16.5B). Contraction of the anterior part of the muscle brings together the inferior border of the anterior end of the thyroid cartilage and the superior border of the anterior part of the cricoid arch by rotation at the cricothyroid joint. At the same time the posterior part of the muscle acts to pull forward the thyroid cartilage in relation to the cricoid cartilage. Both these actions result in an increase in the distance between the arytenoid and the thyroid cartilages, providing that the arytenoid cartilage is fixed in its position on the cricoid cartilage, and thus the vocal folds lengthen. As length is adjusted, there are also alterations in tension and the vocal folds are decreased in thickness.

The lengthening action of the cricothyroid muscles is opposed by the **thyroarytenoid muscles** whose main action is to shorten the vocal folds. Though some details of the anatomy of the thyroarytenoid muscle remain unclear it is generally agreed that there are two parts to each muscle. Its lateral part is attached anteriorly to the inferior half of the inner surface of the thyroid cartilage and runs parallel to the vocal fold to attach to the whole of the dorsolateral ridge of the arytenoid cartilage and the anterior aspect of its muscular process. Between these two attachments, some muscle fibres are attached to the outer surface of the lateral part of the cricothyroid membrane (the conus elasticus). The medial part of the muscle is attached anteriorly to the inner surface of the thyroid cartilage alongside the vocal ligament and posteriorly to the vocal process of the arytenoid cartilage. The medial portion of the muscle is usually called the **vocalis muscle**. There is no intermingling of the fibres of the two parts of the muscle but there is also no distinct fascial plane between them to make them separate muscles. The action of the medial part of the muscle is to move the arytenoid cartilage closer to the thyroid lamina and thus shorten and thicken the vocal folds (Figure 16.10D). The lateral part of the muscle moves the vocal processes medially as the result of its attachment of the muscular process of the arytenoid cartilage, thus adducting the vocal folds. The two parts of the muscle acting together, as well as shortening the vocal folds, help to approximate and straighten the vocal folds, thus helping to ensure an accurate fit of the vocal folds on both sides.

The cricothyroid and thyroarytenoid together act to regulate the length of the vocal folds but changes in vocal fold length do not necessarily presuppose changes in vocal fold tension. As described above, the action of the posterior and lateral cricoarytenoids also affects the length of the vocal folds. To put this in context, studies on isolated normal larynxes where individual muscles are electrically stimulated have shown the following effects on movements of the vocal folds:

- The only muscles capable of abduction are the posterior cricoarytenoids.
- The adductive effect of the lateral cricoarytenoid is greater than that of the thyroartenoid which is greater than the interarytenoids.
- The posterior cricoarytenoids can increase the length of the vocal folds by up to 20 per cent of their resting length; the lateral and posterior cricoarytenoids produce an increase of up to about 5 per cent of

resting length. The thyroarytenoids can shorten the vocal folds by up to 20 per cent of their resting length.

These findings presuppose that only one set of muscles is acting at any given time which in reality is unlikely except during laryngeal opening. It is likely that the adductors are used in concert to produce firm closure of the glottis and in variable degrees to produce varying degrees of glottal closure during phonation. It is also probable that the cricoarytenoids are responsible for the gross setting of vocal fold length and other muscles which affect vocal fold length are used to fine tune the setting. This is important when it is considered that as soon as the length, tension and mass of the vocal folds are set prior to phonation, these settings are promptly disturbed as the vocal folds are set into vibration. To prevent sudden changes in pitch, for example, the vocal folds can be minutely adjusted to compensate by using auditory feedback to monitor the voice and feedback mechanisms within the muscles and joints of the larynx.

Laryngeal innervation

The larynx is innervated by the superior and recurrent laryngeal branches of the **vagus nerves**.

The **superior laryngeal nerves** (Figure 16.9) branch from the vagus nerves high in the neck. Each superior laryngeal nerve then passes deep to the internal and external carotid arteries before descending to the larynx along the lateral aspect of the pharynx. At about the level of the hyoid bone, each superior laryngeal nerve divides into internal laryngeal and external laryngeal branches.

The **internal laryngeal nerves** enter the larynx by piercing the thyrohyoid membrane. As each nerve pierces the membrane it divides into an upper and a lower branch. The upper branch supplies the valleculae, anterior and posterior surfaces of the epiglottis and the mucosa of the supraglottic cavity as far inferiorly as the level of the vocal folds. The lower branch descends in the medial wall of the piriform fossa, which it supplies along with the aryepiglottic folds, to end by anatomozing with branches of the recurrent laryngeal nerves. The superior laryngeal carries sensory information from the laryngeal mucosa, proprioceptors within the intrinsic muscles of the larynx and mechanoreceptors in the capsules of the laryngeal joints. Finally it innervates low threshold mechanoreceptors in the wall of the laryngeal cavity that respond to changes in air pressure. Some reports indicate that it may also contribute to the nerve supply of the transverse interarytenoid muscle. The sensory innervation of the supraglottal cavity is important in initiating the protective cough reflex should a foreign body defeat the sphincteric mechanism and enter the larynx. The proprioceptors and joint receptors are important for the control and adjustment of movements of the larynx particularly during phonation. Clients with a supraglottal laryngectomy, in which the larynx from the vestibular folds above has been surgically removed together with the superior laryngeal nerves, can phonate at the pitch they intend to use but show pitch fluctuations because of loss of proprioception carried in the superior laryngeal nerves. The low threshold mechanoreceptors are believed to be important in the control of the larynx during ventilation. The superior laryngeal nerves also contain autonomic nerves that cause vasoconstriction of the laryngeal vessels and secretion for the laryngeal mucous glands.

The **external laryngeal nerves** descend external to the thyroid cartilage closely related throughout their course to the superior thyroid arteries. The nerves lie on the inferior constrictor muscle which they pierce inferiorly before curving around the inferior thyroid cornua to supply the cricothyroid muscles.

The **recurrent laryngeal nerves** (Figure 16.11) branch from the vagus nerve in the thorax; their branching and the initial part of their course differs on the left and right because of the asymmetry of the great blood vessels in the thorax. The **right recurrent laryngeal nerve** branches from the right vagus nerve anterior to the right subclavian artery. It curves under the artery just making contact with the apex of the right lung before ascending obliquely to the trachea. The **left recurrent laryngeal nerve** branches from the left vagus nerve as the latter crosses the arch of the aorta. It curves below the aorta passing up between the upper part of the left lung and the heart to leave the thorax on the side of the trachea. Both left and right nerves ascend to the larynx in the groove between the oesophagus and trachea. As the nerves approach the larynx they are crossed by the inferior thyroid arteries as they run from the subclavian arteries to the thyroid gland. The relationship between the recurrent laryngeal nerve and the inferior thyroid artery is variable with the nerve passing either posteriorly or anteriorly to the artery or even passing between arterial branches as they enter the thyroid gland. The recurrent laryngeal nerves then ascend to the lower border of the inferior constrictor muscle to enter the larynx by curving behind the cricothyroid joint and inferior cornu of the thyroid cartilage. The recurrent laryngeal nerves innervate all the intrinsic muscles of the larynx with the exception of the cricothyroid muscles. The muscles are innervated by the ipsilateral recurrent laryngeal nerve with the exception of the transverse interarytenoid muscle that crosses the midline and is bilaterally innervated. The recurrent laryngeal nerves are also sensory to the mucosa of the laryngeal cavity and proprioceptive to joint receptors beneath the level of the vocal folds although the recurrent laryngeal nerves only carry 30 per cent of the sensory nerves from the larynx; the superior laryngeal nerves have therefore a much more important role in sensory control of the larynx.

The arterial supply to the larynx is from the laryngeal branches of the superior thyroid arteries from the external carotid arteries and the inferior thyroid arteries, branches of the subclavian arteries. Superior and inferior laryngeal veins drain into the superior and inferior thyroid veins respectively.

Laryngeal nerve injuries

The four major nerve branches that supply the larynx are all susceptible to damage in certain circumstances. The resulting paralysis of any affected muscles is called **laryngeal nerve palsy**. The commonest laryngeal nerve injury is to the left recurrent laryngeal nerve and accounts for about 90 per

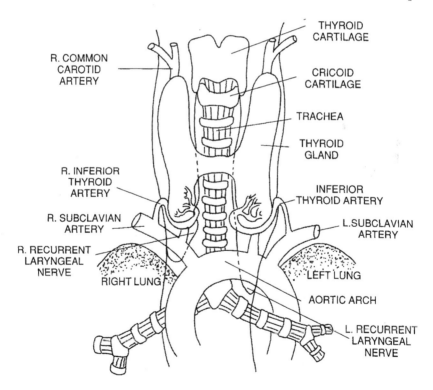

Figure 16.11 The course and relations of the recurrent laryngeal nerves in the thorax and neck.

cent of all laryngeal nerve palsies; damage to the right recurrent laryngeal nerve is much less common and damage to the superior laryngeal nerves and their branches is rare. The main causes of left recurrent laryngeal nerve trauma are lung or bronchial pathology, particularly bronchial carcinomas, because of the long course of the nerve across the left lung. Either recurrent laryngeal nerve may be damaged in the neck as a result of inadvertent injury during thyroid surgery when the inferior thyroid arteries are being isolated.

It ought to be straightforward to predict the consequences of this, or any other laryngeal nerve injury, but in practice the actual effects of laryngeal nerve damage can be quite variable. There are several reasons for this. It is often not clear in many cases whether the injury to a nerve is complete. In crush injuries to the recurrent laryngeal nerves, axons to a particular muscle or muscles may be preferentially affected, which is reflected in the associated functional deficit. The nerve supply to the posterior cricoarytenoid muscles which abduct the vocal folds are more vulnerable in these circumstances, for reasons which are not understood. With time there may be a partial and variable recovery of function. Finally, the nerve supply to the laryngeal muscles could be anomalous, especially if extensive anastomoses are present between the nerves.

A complete, total and permanent paralysis of one recurrent laryngeal nerve will paralyse all the ipsilateral intrinsic muscles of the larynx except the cricothyroid and the interarytenoid muscles which receive a bilateral innervation. The vocal fold on the injured side will be tensed by the unopposed action of cricothyroid and partially or completely adducted because of the weak, residual adductive action of the interarytenoid muscles. There would also be a sensory loss below the vocal folds. The position taken up by the affected vocal fold can vary quite widely. A partial recurrent laryngeal nerve injury generally affects the abductor muscles more than the adductors and this probably accounts for much of the variability observed in the position of the affected fold. Over time, the position adopted by a partially abducted fold may change to that of greater adduction so the time after the trauma at which an injury is assessed is also important. A partially adducted cord will result in breathlessness, particularly on exertion. It will result in a harsh, raspy hoarse voice which will also be weak. In many cases, the unimpaired side may make compensatory adjustments but usually some impairment in the voice and alteration in its quality will remain. Voice therapy can be very effective in assisting compensatory movements from the unaffected vocal fold. When compensation does not occur, the paralysed fold can be enlarged by injecting material such as fat, collagen or Teflon into the fold or by placing a prosthesis lateral to the fold. This is known as **thyroplasty**. After successful thyroplasty, the unaffected opposite fold meets the bulked out fold during adduction, thus enabling glottal closure.

Acute bilateral complete recurrent laryngeal nerve injuries cause severe stridor and difficulty in breathing as the consequence of severe restriction of the airway at the larynx. To restore adequate ventilation a tracheotomy may be required.

Damage to the superior laryngeal nerves or their branches is rare but when it occurs the usual result is hoarseness of the voice. The main reason for this is the loss of proprioceptive and mechanoreceptive feedback from the larynx. The cough reflex will also be affected.

A lesion that paralyses all laryngeal muscles including the cricothyroids suggests the possibility of a lesion to the vagus nerve close to its exit from the skull or a higher lesion in the brainstem affecting the vagal nuclei. The affected cord is completely paralysed and will take up a position halfway between abduction and adduction.

CHAPTER 17

Phonation

The main non-vital function of the larynx is the production of speech but it also produces sounds of emotion such as crying, distress or terror. As described in Chapter 1, speech production involves three distinct stages: the generation of an airstream; the conversion of airflow into a series of vibrations; and the modification of these basic vibrations by articulation. The larynx is capable of functioning in speech in all three of these processes. First, it acts as a source of sound through its ability to modulate the airstream by opening and closing the vocal folds within the laryngeal cavity. This is **phonation**. Second, the larynx can act as an airstream generator in its own right during the production of certain consonants known as glottal consonants. These sounds are not used in normal English but may be encountered in disordered speech, such as that produced by children with cleft palate, and in infant vocalization. Thirdly, the larynx can itself act as an articulator during the production of glottal stops.

Phonation

The most important function of the larynx during speech is to act as a sound source during phonation. Phonation is required for vowels and voiced consonants which together make up about two-thirds of the phonemes used in English. Several conditions have to be met before phonation can be produced. First, for any phoneme, there must be a flow of air from the lungs. Second, for voiced phonemes, the vocal folds must be adducted to some degree although it is not necessary to close the vocal folds completely. Third, the vocal folds need to be made sufficiently stiff so that they will vibrate in the exhaled airstream. A rubber band held in the hand produces no sound when plucked unless it is stretched.

Vocal fold vibration

A number of theories have been put forward to explain the mechanics of phonation during voice production. The majority of these theories are now of little more than historical interest as they have failed to gain support from the relevant anatomical or physiological evidence. The explanation that has now gained widespread acceptance for the mechanics of vocal fold vibration is the **aerodynamic-myoelastic theory** which accounts for vocal fold vibration as follows. At the onset of phonation during an expiration, the vocal folds are adducted. As they close, the flow of air produced by the expiration is interrupted as it can no longer escape through the glottis. This causes an increase in pressure, called the **subglottal pressure**, beneath the closed glottis. As expiration continues against the closed glottis, the subglottal pressure continues to rise until it is sufficient to overcome the muscular forces adducting the vocal folds and thus the vocal folds are forced open a little. This causes the release of a small amount of air through the narrow slit of the glottis into the supralaryngeal vocal tract. Consequently the subglottal pressure falls. The muscular forces adducting the vocal folds now exceed the force produced by the subglottal pressure, therefore the vocal folds begin to close. The closure of the vocal folds produced by the adductive force is aided by the **Bernoulli effect**. Air that passes through a constriction in a tube, such as that in the larynx caused by the adducted vocal folds, must increase its velocity if the same amount of air is to leave the constriction as enters it. This has the effect of lowering the pressure at the level of the constriction. In the particular case of the larynx, the vocal folds at the constriction are mobile; the effect of this reduction in pressure is to suck the folds together helping them to close more rapidly. Vocal fold closure is thus the result of the muscular force produced by the adductor muscles, the aerodynamic force resulting from the Bernoulli effect, and is also aided by the natural elastic recoil of the vocal folds themselves. Once the vocal folds have closed, there is a renewed build-up of pressure as expiration continues against a closed glottis allowing the phonatory cycle to be repeated. The cycle will continue either until the vocal folds are relaxed or until expiration ceases and there is no longer an airflow.

The exact time of each cycle determines the frequency. If you sing an A, the sixth note of the C major scale to which orchestras tune, your vocal folds vibrate at 440 times per second. This is obviously too fast for the unaided eye to see. Much of our knowledge about vocal fold behaviour is derived from laryngoscopic observations using a stroboscopic light source which emits pulses of light. The frequency of the light pulses can be varied until they coincide with the frequency of the vocal folds and appear to freeze the motion.

It is important to realize that sound production by the vocal folds is achieved in a completely different way to that of a tuning fork. When the prongs of a tuning fork are struck, the energy of the resulting vibration is transmitted directly to the molecules of air around in the form of rarefactions and compressions. In contrast, all that is occurring when a sound is produced by vibration of the vocal folds is that they are acting as valves and modulating an airflow already generated by the lungs. The direct transmission of the energy of vibration of the vocal folds to the air is not significant in phonation. The result of this valving of expiratory airflow by the larynx is the release of a series of small puffs of air into the supralaryngeal vocal tract, in other words, an airflow whose velocity changes periodically with time.

Although the opening and closing of the vocal folds involves a relatively rapid and apparently simple motion in a mediolateral direction, the details of the actual vibration are rather more complex. Part of the reason for this complexity lies in the structure of the vocal folds themselves which are not rigid but very mobile. The consequence of this is that different parts of the folds vibrate in different ways during the phonatory cycle. When the focal folds are forced open by the rise in subglottal pressure they do so from the bottom of the thickness of the adducting edge upwards until they separate at the top (Figure 17.1). The bottom parts of each fold thus vibrate out of phase with the top parts and reach maximum opening in advance of the top part of the folds. As the folds open they are also displaced upwards towards the vestibular folds. These complexities contribute to the frequency spectrum of vibration and are partly responsible for producing the harmonics (**formant frequencies**) that are present along with the **fundamental frequency** of vibration.

Another complexity of the phonatory cycle is in the degree of adduction needed to initiate phonation. In the preceding discussion, the assumption has been made that it is necessary that the vocal folds are closed completely along their entire length to initiate phonation. Direct observations of the larynx show that the vocal folds do not have to be fully closed to initiate vibration. Partial closure can be sufficient to constrict the airway enough to raise the subglottal pressure to initiate phonation before complete vocal fold closure.

The foregoing description of phonation also implies that vocal fold vibration occurs in a stereotypical and unvarying manner. This is certainly not the case. The larynx is an extremely versatile instrument and can make a wide range of adjustments to the way in which phonation occurs and voice is produced. Three auditory parameters of phonation can be distinguished: **pitch** or **frequency**; **loudness** or **intensity**; and **voice quality** or **timbre**. Each of these parameters can be varied within limits. However,

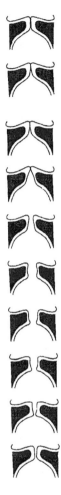

Figure 17.1 The movement of the vocal folds during one phonatory cycle starting from vocal fold closure. (Drawn after M. Hirano, *Otologia*, 21, Supplement 1, 1975.)

there are complex interactions between them, such that adjustments within the larynx to vary one parameter may result in alterations to either or both of the other two.

Mechanism of frequency control

The perceived pitch of phonation is a psychological (i.e. perceptual) correlate of the frequency, the number of vibrations per second. The perceived pitch rises as the frequency of vibration increases. The fundamental frequency of phonation, defined as the lowest frequency of the sine wave (S-shaped curve) that comprises the vibration, can be varied. The range of possible variation alters with the age and sex of the individual. Frequency is expressed in Hertz (Hz) which is a measure of the number of wave crests passing a given point each second (cycles per second). Typical ranges of fundamental frequency are 80–200 Hz for an adult male, 150–300 Hz for an adult female and 200–500 Hz in children corresponding to a range of 1–3 octaves for most people. Note that there is an extensive overlap in range between these three groups such that frequency alone can define neither the age nor sex of an individual.

The possible range of frequency in phonation produced by an individual is determined largely by the physical properties of their larynx as these dictate the most important determinants of the frequency range, the resting **length** and **thickness** of the vocal folds. The frequency range of phonation is skewed such that the modal frequency lies toward the upper end of the frequency range. This is because all speakers occasionally use very low frequencies of phonation that cannot be sustained for long periods. The most energy efficient and effective pitch range is centred about one quarter of an octave above the lowest frequency that can be produced. Another term often used in describing the frequency range of an individual is **habitual pitch**, the range of frequencies used by the speaker for the majority of the time. Pitch will move above and below this range for short times during normal speech. For example, when you express surprise or become animated, pitch tends to rise. Pitch tends to be lowered when you employ a soothing tone. People may change their habitual pitch in certain circumstances; lecturing or public speaking are good examples. A person may use an inappropriate habitual pitch that is too far removed from their optimal pitch; for example, a woman of medium build may use an unusually high light voice to convey an ultra-feminine or even childish persona. This, ultimately, will lead to vocal fatigue as the laryngeal muscles are used excessively and inefficiently.

The larynx can vary the frequency of phonation by making a wide range of adjustments to the vocal folds. The physical parameters of the vocal folds that can be changed are the **length, tension** and the **mass per unit length**. They are altered by movements of the laryngeal cartilages produced largely by the intrinsic muscles of the larynx and the contraction of muscles within the vocal folds themselves (see Chapter 16). The position of the arytenoid cartilages relative to the thyroid and/or cricoid cartilages either alter vocal fold length or open or close the glottis. Contraction of the muscles within the vocal folds changes their mass per unit length. Again, it must be emphasized that alteration in one parameter will also produce some change in the other parameters as well.

The analogy is often drawn between the vocal folds and the strings in musical instruments but there are certain difficulties with this analogy as strings do not behave the same as the vocal folds. A much better impression of vocal fold adjustments can be gained by looping a thick rubber band over your thumb and little finger. Stretch the rubber band until it is no longer lax, the same condition which must be met by the vocal folds prior to phonation. If the rubber band is now plucked, it will vibrate at low frequency. If the rubber band is lengthened by moving your thumb and little finger further apart, it will now vibrate with a higher frequency. However as the rubber band is elongated, it is also getting thinner (decreasing the mass per unit length) and the tension in it is also increased; the tension is felt as a pull on the fingers holding the rubber band.

What changes actually occur in real vocal folds to alter the frequency of vibration? Length is crucial in two respects. The resting length of the vocal folds is important which is why the male voice, in which the vocal folds are longer, has a lower modal frequency than the female voice. The range of frequencies possible in a female voice start from a higher baseline than male voices. It is easy to fall into the trap of thinking that if the vocal folds are shortened, the pitch will rise because this would make the length of male vocal folds more like female vocal folds. The frequency of vibration increases and pitch actually rises when the initial length is changed by *lengthening* the vocal folds. This is because as the vocal folds are lengthened, they become thinner. These changes may be accompanied by an increase in tension, just as in the stretched rubber band. The change in length of the vocal folds is thus a vital variable in determining the frequency of phonation. However, as described in Chapter 16, the maximum elongation of the vocal folds is only about 20 per cent of their initial resting length. Therefore, change in length alone cannot account for the normal range of frequency variation.

The **mass per unit length** of the vocal folds is the second important variable and will change as the length of the vocal folds alters. Essentially mass per unit length is a measure of the thickness of the vocal folds. Think of a stretched rubber band: 1 cm of unstretched band is thicker than 1 cm of stretched rubber band. An individual's vocal folds at rest will be a certain length and thickness determined by their genetic make up, their sex and age. The mass of tissue is fixed but will be spread more thinly if the vocal folds are elongated, so the amount of tissue per millimetre will be less. Thinner vocal folds are lighter and more elastic and will vibrate with a higher frequency than thick folds for the same subglottal pressure applied.

In addition, they are able to return to an adducted position faster, thus allowing a new phonatory cycle to begin more quickly. However, direct observations of the vocal folds by stroboscopic illumination suggest that, during normal conversation, the mass per unit length does not change by more than a factor of two. The range of frequency which can be obtained in speech cannot be accounted for by changes in mass per unit length alone as the frequency range varies more than this.

The third factor to take into account is **tension**. An increase in tension of the vocal folds will increase the frequency of vibration even without any change in length or mass per unit length. This could be achieved by fixing the thyroid and arytenoid attachments of the vocal folds and then contracting the vocalis muscle isometrically (see Chapter 3). Although it is very difficult to measure tension changes in the vocal folds, some change in tension almost certainly accompanies changes in the other two variables. However, at higher frequencies, pitch can still be increased even when the limits to which the vocal folds can be lengthened have been reached. Further increases in frequency are probably brought about by isometric muscular contraction in this part of the frequency range, thus increasing tension.

Investigations of the vocal folds during frequency changes generally show that the vocal folds behave in ways that would be expected. Thus, as vocal fold length increases, the frequency of vocal fold vibration is increased. This increase in length is accompanied by a change in shape of the vocal folds decreasing the mass per unit length.

The two main muscles believed to change the frequency of vocal fold vibration are the cricothyroid and thyroarytenoid muscles. The cricothyroids probably makes gross adjustments while the thyroarytenoids do the fine tuning. The **cricothyroid** muscles elongate the vocal folds by a combination of rotation and sliding at the cricothyroid joint produced by contraction of the two heads of each muscle. This can be verified quite easily by palpating the thyroid and cricoid cartilages in the neck (see Chapter 16) while singing or 'la-la-ing' an ascending scale. The cricoid arch is drawn upwards and forward towards the thyroid laminae. What cannot be felt is the lamina of the cricoid moving downwards and backwards taking with it the arytenoid cartilages and thus lengthening the vocal folds (see Figure 16.5). The cricothyroid muscles probably do not affect the tension of the vocal folds until approaching the limits of elongation.

The **thyroarytenoid muscles** oppose the action of the cricothyroid muscles. They decrease the distance between the thyroid laminae anteriorly and the arytenoid cartilages posteriorly, thus shortening the vocal folds. The lateral part of each muscle adducts and straightens the vocal fold. As with the cricothyroid muscles, contraction of the thyroarytenoid muscle is unlikely to alter tension within the vocal folds except at the limits of shortening. It is probable that increases in tension are produced as the result of contraction of the thyroarytenoid muscles against already contracting cricothyroid muscles. In addition, thyroarytenoid contraction will also increase the bulk, or mass per unit length, of the vocal folds which will also contribute to a change in pitch.

In addition, the **posterior cricoarytenoid** muscles may play a part through their secondary actions of altering vocal fold length from a thick, rounded profile to a thin, narrow band. At the same time the vocal folds undergo a progressive transition from a relaxed to a stiffer state. As pitch increases further, the vocal folds frequently fail to close completely as there is insufficient time for them to close before the onset of the next phonatory cycle. The consequence of this is an increasing tendency to breathiness in the voice at very high pitch.

The action of both cricothyroid and thyroarytenoid muscles requires that the arytenoid cartilages are stabilized on the cricoid cartilages, otherwise much of the effect of these two muscles in changing the length of the vocal folds would be offset through changes in the position of the arytenoid cartilages at the cricoarytenoid joint. This stabilization is carried out by the posterior cricoarytenoid muscle which is acting to maintain the length of the vocal folds against the shortening effect of the thyroarytenoid muscles. Its action of abducting the vocal folds also helps to offset the adductive action of the lateral part of the thyroarytenoid as it straightens the vocal folds.

For pitch to be lowered, there must be a reduction in vocal fold length, a fall in tension and an increase in mass per unit length. The natural elasticity of the larynx will assist in bringing about a reduction in pitch but this can only fall to the level of optimal or habitual pitch. Further reduction can only occur as the result of active mechanisms and the key muscles are probably the thyroarytenoids.

In summary, changes in pitch are brought about largely as the result of intrinsic adjustments within the larynx. The combined actions of the cricothyroid, thyroarytenoid and posterior cricoarytenoid muscles change the length, tension and mass per unit length of the vocal folds that are responsible, collectively, for altering the frequency of vibration. However, there are also external mechanisms that assist in pitch change, particularly alterations to the length of the supralaryngeal vocal tract through the actions of the suprahyoid and infrahyoid muscles (see Chapter 16).

Control of vocal intensity

Just as the frequency of vibration during phonation can be varied over a wide range, the intensity of phonation, and thus the perceived loudness of speech, may be altered considerably. Normal speech varies over a range of

30 decibels, a shout can reach 70 decibels and the trained voice may generate even higher intensities.

It is necessary to move more air to achieve higher intensities of speech. The intensity of the voice can be varied by mechanisms which operate beneath, within and above the larynx. Below the larynx, the intensity of speech can be varied by changing the amount of air delivered to the larynx and vocal tract during expiration (see Chapter 15). Within the larynx, more air can be released by changing the fraction of time that the glottis is closed. These two mechanisms are closely linked. Above the larynx, the shape of the vocal tract can be adjusted.

To move more air through the larynx during phonation, the relative duration of the opening and closing phases of the vocal folds during each phonatory cycle must be changed. As the intensity of phonation increases, the proportion of time during which the vocal folds are closing or closed in each phonatory cycle will fall. The **opening quotient** of the phonatory cycle is the time when the vocal folds are opening or open. In normal speech, the opening and closing phases of each cycle are approximately equal so that the opening quotient is about 50 per cent. Of the remaining 50 per cent, 35 per cent is spent in the closing phase with the vocal folds actually closed or adducted for 15 per cent of the time. As the opening quotient falls and the intensity increases, the time during which the vocal folds are open is reduced and the time spent with the folds actually closed increases. Because more air is exhaled against the closed glottis, the subglottal pressure will be raised. Each time subglottal pressure is doubled, intensity increases by 8 to 12 decibels. A subglottal pressure of only 2–3 cm H_2O will generate speech of low intensity but is generally 10–20 cm H_2O in conversational speech and can rise even higher.

This rise in subglottal pressure explains the changes in the phonatory cycle observed as intensity is increased. As the pressure rises, the vocal folds are blown apart with greater force and so open more quickly. The increased pressure differential means that the magnitude of the Bernoulli effect increases, making the vocal folds close more quickly. As the force with which the folds now meet in the midline increases, more energy has to be dissipated when the folds are forced together. The vocal folds have to remain closed for longer to ensure that this happens. The net effect of these changes is to release air at higher pressure into the vocal tract and hence to increase vocal intensity.

This increase in the closed phase is brought about by increased muscular effort. The lateral cricoarytenoid and interarytenoid muscles increase the adductive effort while greater tension in the vocal folds is produced by the combined contraction of the cricothyroid and thyroarytenoid muscles.

Raising the frequency and increasing vocal intensity have some mechanisms in common. This has several consequences. Although intensity and frequency can be varied independently, it can be difficult to increase one without the other; high intensity is often accompanied by a rise in pitch. A second consequence is that it can be difficult to generate high intensities when speaking at higher pitches. At high pitch, subglottal pressure will already be high, perhaps close to the maximum that can be generated, and increasing intensity in this situation cannot be achieved solely by laryngeal changes. Instead, the expiratory airflow has to be increased (see Chapter 15). The range of intensities that can be generated by an individual as they speak will be dependent upon frequency. The intensity range is at a minimum at the lowest pitches, reaching a maximum around 50–70 per cent of the frequency range before reducing again at higher pitches. Increasing loudness by using glottal tension alone to increase subglottal pressure is something that people with untrained voices are prone to do. The increased muscular activity eventually produces muscular fatigue and, in turn, vocal fatigue. The client then tries to compensate for vocal fatigue by increasing the force of adduction and subglottal pressure even more. If they persist in this practice, it can lead to various vocal fold pathologies as outlined in Chapter 16.

Above the larynx, the shape of the vocal tract can be adjusted to vary certain formants so that they coincide with harmonics of the laryngeal source. This can increase the resonant energy of these harmonics and has the effect of boosting intensity. The supralaryngeal vocal tract amplifies the laryngeal source in much the same way as a megaphone applied to the mouth passively boosts intensity when addressing a large crowd. Tactics to increase resonant energy are often employed with clients who have weak voices or need to project their voice in a large space. By setting up resonances in the nose and paranasal air sinuses (see Chapter 19), vocal intensity can be increased without having to strain the larynx unduly.

Voice quality

Voice quality is what makes an individual voice recognizable from any other. On one level voice quality is purely subjective which is why one person's favourite singer may jar on someone else. However, we can all usually agree that someone has a good voice even if we cannot say why. At another level, voice quality is more objective. When there is a change in voice quality of an individual, it is easily recognized. Even over a telephone it is usually possible to detect whether the other person has a cold or laryngitis. Changes in normal voice quality are often the first obvious sign of a voice problem. These can manifest, for example, as breathiness, hoarseness, lower than normal pitch or lower volume.

Voice quality may be defined to some extent by the frequencies present in a complex tone. Two different musical instruments, an oboe and a violin for example, are immediately recognizable for what they are even when playing exactly the same note. The fundamental frequency is the frequency of the given note but formants – vibrations in other frequencies – determine the characteristic of the overall sound. This is augmented by other factors such as resonance. It is the formants and other acoustic effects which differentiate a violin playing an A from an oboe playing the same note. Taking it one step further, the same characteristics distinguish a Stradivarius from a cheap beginner's violin even if played by the same virtuoso violinist.

It follows from this brief outline that voice quality is not determined by the characteristics of the vocal folds and their vibrations alone. Various features of the supralaryngeal vocal tract such as its length, area and volume ratios of different cavities to each other (e.g. mouth and pharynx) all contribute to an individual's voice quality.

As a final note of caution, the impression has been conveyed in this and the previous chapter, that the two vocal folds are always at the same horizontal level on either side of the larynx, that they vibrate in unison and vibration is symmetrical. Indeed, that is the situation under normal circumstances. However, various vocal fold pathologies, such as nodules, may produce asymmetric movements so that they vibrate out of phase with each other or do not open and close at the same time. These irregularities will cause a change in voice quality. Similarly, the horizontal levels of the two vocal folds relative to each other may be altered by trauma, laryngeal palsy or other neuromuscular disorders with consequent changes in voice quality.

CHAPTER 18

The face and jaws

The head contains many important structures pertinent to the practice of speech and language therapy. In particular, the oral and nasal cavities are involved in articulation of speech, and the pharynx, and its downward continuation, the oesophagus, are involved in swallowing; an understanding of normal swallowing mechanisms is fundamental to the understanding of dysphagia which is now an established part of the clinical repertoire of speech and language therapists. The mouth is considered in detail in Chapter 19 and swallowing is covered in Chapter 21. Because various abnormalities of development of the head can affect speech, the development and growth of this region is also covered in some detail in Chapter 20. This chapter serves to outline the structure of the head to orientate you before consideration of specific areas but also covers the structure of the face itself which is pertinent to various aspects of speech.

The form of the head and neck is determined by the underlying skeletal components which are the skull, hyoid bone, laryngeal and tracheal cartilages and cervical vertebrae. The **neurocranial** part of the skull houses the brain and the special senses of vision, hearing and balance. The **viscerocranial** parts of the skull form the entrance to the respiratory and gastrointestinal tracts through the nasal and oral cavities respectively. The viscerocranium also includes the **mandible**, the only mobile bone of the skull which articulates with the cranium at the **temporomandibular joint** enabling jaw movements to occur during mastication, swallowing and speech. The cervical vertebrae link the skull with the rest of the skeleton and the hyoid bone and laryngeal cartilages provide a skeletal framework for the larynx and pharynx in the anterior neck, already described in Chapter 16.

The blood supply of the head and neck is derived from the common carotid arteries and the vertebral arteries. The **common carotid arteries** divide into two major branches in the upper part of the neck. The **internal**

carotid arteries enter the skull to supply the brain (see Chapter 8) and eyes whereas the **external carotid arteries** branch extensively in the neck and face to supply virtually everything else (Figure 18.1). The superficial tissues of the face are supplied by the **facial arteries** which are branches of the external carotid arteries. In their course they give branches to the skin of the chin, lips, the external nose and anterior parts of the nasal cavities. The external carotid arteries pass through the parotid glands and each divides into two terminal branches within the substance of the gland. The **maxillary arteries** supply deep structures of the face and the other terminal branches, the **superficial temporal arteries**, run superficial to the zygomatic arch to supply the skin of the temporal region and the scalp. The **vertebral arteries**, so called because they pass through foramina in the cervical vertebrae for part of their course, are branches of the subclavian arteries and also supply the brain as described in Chapter 8.

The venous drainage of the head and neck is through the jugular veins (Figure 18.2). The **internal jugular veins** are large vessels formed at the base of the skull by the veins draining the brain as they leave the cranial cavity. They run alongside the internal and common carotid arteries and receive numerous tributaries from other tissues and organs of the face and neck as they pass down the neck. The smaller **external jugular veins** are formed from tributary veins draining the superficial face and scalp. These large vessels receive tributaries from the deep and superficial tissues of the face and scalp.

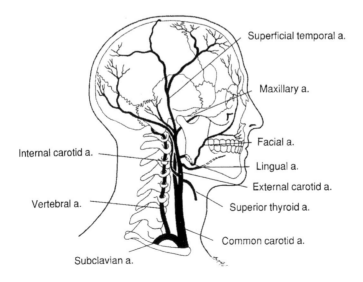

Figure 18.1 The carotid arteries and their branches.

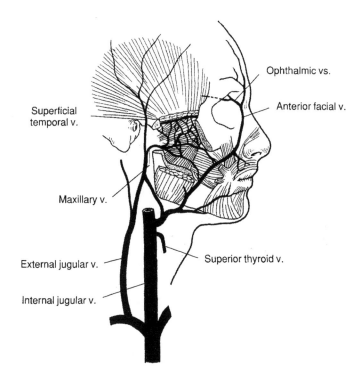

Figure 18.2 The venous drainage of the head and neck.

The head and neck is innervated by the **cranial nerves** and the cervical plexus. Some of these nerves have simple courses while others ramify extensively.

Various muscle groups involved in mastication, swallowing and speech are found in the head and neck. The **muscles of facial expression** are subcutaneous muscles in the face and scalp innervated by the facial nerve. As well as providing a variety of facial expressions, these muscles also play a part in mastication, swallowing and speech. The **muscles of mastication** attach the mandible to the cranium and can move it upwards, forwards, backwards and laterally. The **suprahyoid muscles** elevate the laryngeal skeleton and the **infrahyoid group**, which attach the laryngeal skeleton to the thoracic cage, depress the laryngeal skeleton. They are also involved in jaw movements. Two groups of muscles make up the bulk of the tongue: the **intrinsic muscles** alter its shape and the **extrinsic muscles**, which have attachments to adjacent bones, alter its position. The **muscles of the soft palate** move the soft palate during swallowing and speech. The **pharyngeal constrictor muscles** form the wall of the pharynx and contract from above downwards during swallowing. The palatine and pharyngeal muscles are mainly supplied through various branches of the vagus nerve.

The skull

To appreciate the appearance of the head and to understand the anatomy of various muscles and other structures some knowledge of the under-lying skeleton is necessary.

Viewed from the anterior aspect (Figure 18.3), the forehead is supported by the large dome-shaped **frontal bone**, which extends down as far as the **orbits**, or eye sockets, where it turns horizontally to form the roof of the orbits. The frontal bone contains the **frontal air sinuses**, two spaces continuous with the nasal cavities, which lie immediately above and medial to the superior orbital margins. The bridge of the nose is formed by the two **nasal bones** which, with the maxillae, surround the anterior openings of the nasal cavities. In life, the external nose is surrounded by the **nasal cartilages** which are lost during preparation of dried skulls thus creating openings into the nasal cavity much larger than the nostrils (Figure 18.3). The left and right **nasal cavities** are separated by a thin midline plate of bone, the **nasal septum**, which may deviate to one side or the other.

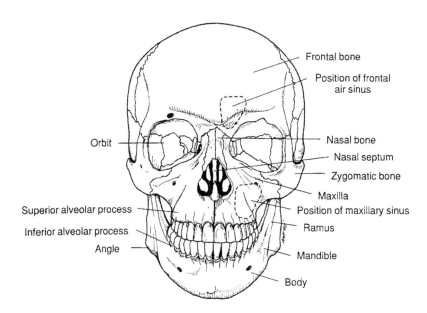

Figure 18.3 A frontal view of the skull.

The two **maxillary bones** form the bulk of the middle third of the facial skeleton between the orbits and the upper teeth (Figure 18.3). They form the upper jaws, partially surround the nasal cavities and form part of the floors of the orbital cavities. The left and right maxillae fuse beneath the anterior nasal aperture. At the inferior border of each maxilla, the **alveolar process** forms a U-shaped arch, which carries the upper teeth. The **maxillary air sinuses** lie within the bodies of each maxilla. The prominence of the cheeks is supported by the **zygomatic bones** lateral to each maxilla.

The **mandible** forms the lower jaw (Figure 18.4). It comprises a horizontal **body** and **alveolar process** supporting the mandibular teeth, and a vertical **ascending ramus** on each side. The body and ramus unite at the **angle** of the mandible. The superior aspect of each ramus is occupied by two bony processes, the triangular **coronoid process** anteriorly and the rounded **condyle** which forms the mandibular component of the temporomandibular joint on each side.

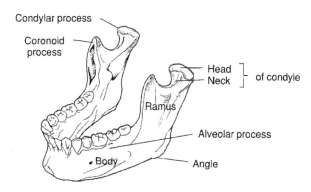

Figure 18.4 The mandible.

Seen from above, the greater part of the vault of the skull is formed by the paired **parietal** bones which are united at the midline **sagittal suture**. They are joined anteriorly to the frontal bone by the **coronal suture**. Posteriorly the parietal bones articulate with the occipital bone at the **lambdoid suture** which has the shape of an inverted V.

Viewed laterally, many of the bones forming the facial skeleton and those forming the vault of the skull can still be seen (Figure 18.5). In addition, the lower lateral aspect of each side of the skull part is formed by the greater wing of the **sphenoid** with the squamous **temporal** bone infilling between the frontal, parietal and occipital bones forming the vault of the skull. The **squamous temporal bones** form a large part of each side of the skull. The **mastoid process** is a large, thick, rounded process which extends downwards from the posterior part of each temporal bone.

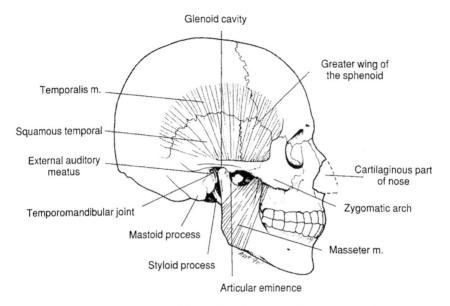

Glenoid cavity

Greater wing of
the sphenoid

Temporalis m.

Squamous temporal

External auditory
meatus

Cartilaginous part
of nose

Temporomandibular joint

Zygomatic arch

Mastoid process

Masseter m.

Styloid process

Articular eminence

Figure 18.5 The lateral aspect of the skull with the superficial muscles of mastication.

The zygomatic process extends anteriorly to join the zygomatic bone forming the **zygomatic arch**. The undersurface of each temporal bone posteriorly is hollowed to form the concave **glenoid fossa**, which forms the temporal surface of the **temporomandibular joint** and into which fits the condyle of the mandible. Just anteriorly there is a convex projection, the **articular eminence**, which also forms part of the temporomandibular joint. The **external auditory meatus** opens between the mastoid and zygomatic processes. The **styloid process** of the temporal bone is attached to the base of the skull but can be seen on a lateral view. It is a long, slender projection lying a short distance in front of the mastoid process.

The **infratemporal fossa** is a depression deep to the zygomatic arch and ramus of the mandible. The incomplete roof of the infratemporal fossa is formed by the greater wing of the sphenoid. The medial wall is formed by the **lateral pterygoid plate** of the sphenoid bone and the anterior wall by the maxilla (Figure 18.6).

The inferior aspect of the skull is best examined with the mandible removed (Figure 18.7). Anteriorly, the **hard palate** lies within the arch formed by the maxillary alveolar processes. It is formed by four bones, two large anterior **palatine processes** of the **maxilla**, and the posterior horizontal plates of the **palatine bones**. In adults, eight teeth are inserted into bony sockets of the alveolar processes of the maxillae on each side.

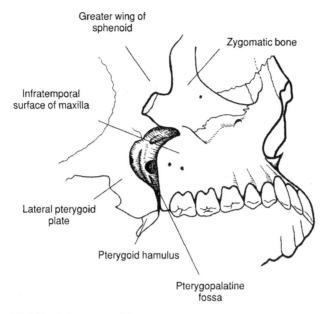

Figure 18.6 The infratemporal fossa.

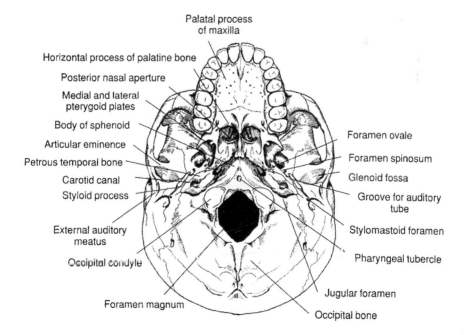

Figure 18.7 The inferior aspect of the skull.

The two **posterior nasal apertures** lie above the posterior margins of the hard palate. They are separated by the posterior border of the nasal septum and are bounded laterally by the backward projecting **medial pterygoid plates** of the sphenoid bone. The inferior end of each medial pterygoid plate projects downwards and laterally as a curved spike, the **pterygoid hamulus** (Figure 18.6). The larger **lateral pterygoid plates** are separated from the medial pterygoid plates by a V-shaped depression.

Immediately behind the posterior nasal apertures, the undersurface of the **body of the sphenoid** is visible. It is directly continuous with the inferior surface of the **occipital bone**, forming a broad median bar of bone which extends downwards and backwards to the **foramen magnum** which lies entirely within the occipital bone. A small midline elevation, the **pharyngeal tubercle**, is a short distance in front of the foramen magnum. Anterolaterally on either side of the foramen magnum are the two **occipital condyles**, which articulate with the first cervical vertebra. The large **jugular foramina** are lateral to each occipital condyle. The small, circular, **stylomastoid foramen** is midway between the styloid and mastoid processes. The wedge-shaped **petrous temporal bones** containing the middle and inner ear lie lateral to the body of the sphenoid between the infratemporal surface of the greater wing of the sphenoid and the occipital bone.

The surface anatomy of the face

The surface anatomy of the face is determined by the underlying bony structures and the superficial soft tissues which vary in depth and complexity. In many places, the bones are only covered by a thin layer of subcutaneous tissue and skin and are easily palpable whereas, in other areas, muscle and glandular tissue intervening between skin and bone alter the facial contours considerably.

Starting from above and progressing downwards, most of the cranial bones are subcutaneous (Figure 18.3). The forehead is subcutaneous and ends above the eyes at the prominent **supraorbital ridges** covered by the eyebrows. The orbital cavities are below the supraorbital ridges. The orbital cavities are completely filled by the eyes, a substantial amount of fat and the **extraocular muscles** but the margins of the orbits are subcutaneous and are easily palpated. The bridge of the nose between the orbital cavities and the pliable nasal cartilages are also palpable. The bones of the cheek are fairly prominent immediately below the orbits even in obese individuals but more inferiorly the cheek is filled out by a variable amount of subcutaneous fat. This **buccal fat pad** is more prominent in babies than in older children and adults. The alveolar parts of the maxilla housing the upper teeth can be felt through the upper lip. Likewise the chin and the lower teeth in the alveolar bone of the mandible can be palpated. Laterally, a prominent ridge of bone passing from the bones of the cheek to the external ear can be felt: this is the **zygomatic arch** formed from parts of the zygomatic and temporal bones. In front of the ear, the **temporo-mandibular joint** and **condyles** of the mandible may be felt, especially if the mouth is gently opened and closed. The lower border of the mandible extending backwards from the chin is subcutaneous as is the angle of the mandible. The ascending ramus of the mandible is largely covered by muscle. Behind the ear, the mastoid process of the temporal bone can be felt as a prominent lump of bone; this forms the upper attachment of the sternocleidomastoid muscle. Below the mandible, glandular tissue and fatty subcutaneous tissue lie superficially and smooth the skin contour as it passes from the lower border of the mandible down on to the neck.

Some of the larger muscles in the face can be made to stand out by clenching and relaxing the jaws; the **masseter** muscle passing from the zygomatic arch to the angle of the mandible can thus be felt and the **temporalis** muscle which lies over the temporal region of the skull from behind the orbital margins to above the ear can also be felt to contract if the teeth are clenched and relaxed.

Some of the arteries and veins supplying the head and neck are superficial. The **common carotid arteries** pass from the thorax into the neck deep to the sternocleidomastoid muscles to emerge from the cover of the muscle anteriorly at the level of the upper border of the thyroid cartilage (Figure 16.1). Their strong pulse may be felt here and this is the easiest place to feel for a pulse in an emergency. The external jugular vein crosses superficial to the sternocleidomastoid muscle and can be made to stand out by performing a Valsalva's manoeuvre by expiring forcibly with the glottis closed. As intrathoracic pressure rises, the vein becomes engorged with blood which cannot re-enter the thorax and the vein shows up (Figure 16.1). Some pathological conditions of the heart prevent free venous return and the vein will dilate. This may be especially noticeable as the patient changes posture from sitting up to lying down when the height of blood in the vein will increase.

The muscles of facial expression

The **muscles of facial expression** (Figure 18.8) are a large group of subcutaneous muscles which alter the contour of the face to produce different facial expressions. They are also involved in forming the shape of the lips during articulation of certain groups of phonemes and are used to keep food between the teeth during chewing.

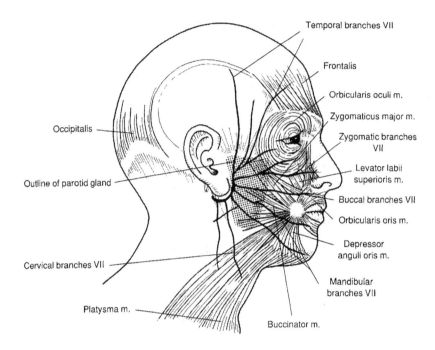

Figure 18.8 The muscles of facial expression and the distribution of the facial nerve on the face.

In the scalp, two pairs of thin flat muscles, one pair in the forehead and one overlying the occipital bone, are linked by a thin sheet of fibrous tissue; they move the scalp and wrinkle the skin of the forehead. Two circular muscles, the **orbicularis oculi**, lie in the subcutaneous tissue over the orbital margins and narrow or close the eye. Another circular muscle, the **orbicularis oris**, forms the major muscle within the lips. Several muscles in the cheek attach to and elevate the upper lip and corners of the mouth. The depressors of the lower lip pass from the chin into the lip. At the lateral margin of the lips, this muscle widens out and continues backwards as the **buccinator** muscle on each side forming the muscle of the cheek. The **platysma** muscles are thin subcutaneous muscles extending from the lower border of the mandible beneath the skin of the anterior triangles of the neck to reach the clavicle.

The facial nerve

The muscles of facial expression are innervated by the motor component of the **facial nerves**, the seventh cranial nerves. The facial nerves on each side enter the internal auditory meatus in the petrous temporal bone and follow a convoluted course through the middle ear (see Chapter 11). Within the middle ear, each facial nerve gives off parasympathetic nerves to the lacrimal, submandibular, sublingual and minor salivary glands of the same side and taste nerves to the tongue as well as the nerve to the stapedius muscle (see Chapter 22). Each nerve then travels from the middle ear through the facial canal in the temporal bone and emerges from the bone at the **stylomastoid foramen** deep to the mastoid process. The nerve on each side then enters the **parotid gland**, which occupies the space between the ramus of the mandible and the sternocleidomastoid muscle, and divides into five major divisions. These divisions may branch again within the substance of the parotid gland before the terminal branches emerge from the anterior aspect of the gland. The **temporal** branches innervate the muscles of the forehead. The **zygomatic** branches supply the muscles around the eye, particularly orbicularis oculi. The **buccal** branches run forward to innervate the buccinator muscle and the elevators of the upper lip. The **mandibular** branches travel along or below the mandible to supply the muscles of the lower lip. The **cervical** branches supply the platysma muscles.

Clinical anatomy of the facial nerve

Whatever the cause, damage to the facial nerve anywhere on its course from the brain to the parotid gland will result in complete ipsilateral facial palsy. The resulting **lower motor neuron lesion** (see Chapter 6) produces flaccid paralysis of the muscles. When the patient is at rest, very little abnormality may be noticeable but as soon as facial expression is attempted, only the unaffected side of the face will move actively (Figure 18.9); the other side may be moved passively by pull of muscles from the intact side but the intended expression will not be produced. If the muscles are not reinnervated, they will atrophy after two or three months resulting in loss of facial contour. If denervation persists, the muscle tissue is replaced by fibrous tissue which contracts as it forms; this mimics the effect of permanent contraction of the muscle and thus results in a permanent facial deformity which is disfiguring.

After emerging from the parotid gland, the multiple branches of each facial nerve lie very superficially, separated from the surface only by the skin, subcutaneous tissue and the flimsy muscles of facial expression. The nerves are therefore vulnerable to traumatic injuries of the face, particularly penetrating wounds. Their extensive distribution across the face also means that the facial nerve branches lie superficial to numerous other structures to which surgical access may be required; damage to the facial nerve is a potential hazard during maxillofacial surgery. In the case of

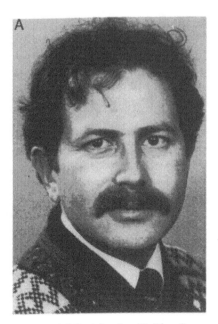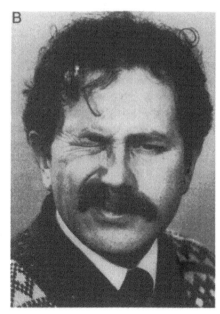

Figure 18.9 Facial palsy. (A) The client at rest. (B) The client attempting to close both eyes; note the eye does not close and the corner of the mouth does not turn up on the affected (left) side.

traumatic injury to nerve branches, nerve grafts can be attempted if the cut stumps of the nerve can be traced. Physiotherapy may also be of assistance in minimizing the deformity. During surgery of the face, the likelihood of facial nerve damage is minimized by avoiding the nerve completely. Good surgical access may be obtained to quite distant areas through incisions placed in the most cosmetically acceptable positions either above in the hairline over the temple or along skin creases in the neck. The nerve is enclosed in the surgical flap and may be safely turned aside. Some torsion may be placed on the nerves but this should only produce transitory paralysis of the muscles.

Damage to the buccal or mandibular branches of the facial nerve have the most profound effect on speech because these two nerves innervate the muscles of the upper and lower lips respectively. Damage to the entire facial nerve in its proximal course will also affect the lip muscles as well as the rest of the face. Inability to use the lips effectively means that production of any phoneme with a labial component will be affected, as will plosives and fricatives. If the muscles of the lower lip are denervated, it is difficult to retain saliva in the mouth and the client has a tendency to dribble which is embarrassing for them.

Other aspects of the clinical anatomy of the facial nerves have already been described in Chapter 11.

Lip movements during speech

Lip movements are essential for consonant articulation and lip rounding and spreading is important for vowel production. The movements of the lips may be independent but are also influenced by the position of the mandible. Lip movements can be divided into two broad categories. **Retrusive or protrusive movements** shorten or lengthen the vocal tract respectively and **lateral and vertical movements** alter the degree of constriction of the vocal tract.

Protrusive movements are achieved largely by contraction of the orbicularis oris muscles. This has the effect of lowering the formant frequencies and is used in production of some vowels such as /u/ as in (r<u>oo</u>f). A similar position is adopted for some consonants such as /ʃ/ as in <u>sh</u>oe or /ʒ/ as in trea<u>s</u>ure. Retrusion involves retraction and raising of the lower lip while the upper lip remains in place. This involves the muscles of the lower lip but also requires retrusion of the mandible (see below) and is used for labiodentals such as /f/ and /v/.

Lateral movements are brought about by the muscles of facial expression inserting into the angles of the mouth. This is the anatomical equivalent of phonetic spread lip vowels such as /i/. Vertical expansion is achieved by action of the elevators of the upper lip and depressors of the lower lip, the anatomical equivalent of rounded lip vowels in phonetic terminology such as /u/. Constriction is also necessary for some phonemes and is enacted by the orbicularis oris. The effect of lip position on vowel sounds can be verified by altering the lip configuration from spread to rounded while articulating /i/; the sound will change to /y/ as the lips are spread. A similar effect is achieved by altering lip position while saying /u/; spreading will change the vowel sound to a /ɰ/. The lips are described as having a neutral position for many vowels. This position is the one obtained by opening the lips by depressing the mandible without any movement of the lips by the lip musculature.

It follows from the above that any inability to move the lips properly, due to facial paralysis, is going to affect articulation of a wide variety of phonemes including many which involved concurrent movement of the lower jaw. Examples are /p/ /b/ /f/ /v/ /m/ /u/ and /i/.

Sensory innervation of the face

The skin of the face, in particular that surrounding the oral cavity, is an extremely important area of somatosensory reception and has a dense innervation from the **trigeminal nerve** (see Figure 11.4). The three divisions of the trigeminal nerve innervate discrete regions of skin through their cutaneous branches. The **ophthalmic** division innervates the skin from the upper eyelid as far back as the vertex of the skull. The **maxillary** division supplies skin from the lower eyelid down to the upper lip and laterally the cheek and temple. The **mandibular** division of the trigeminal nerve covers the skin of the lower lip, chin and the lower jaw as well as a large area which passes up in front of and above the ear. Structures deep to the cutaneous areas supplied by each division are supplied by the same division of the trigeminal nerve. For example, the palate lies deep to the skin supplied by the maxillary division and is supplied by other branches of the maxillary division. The ophthalmic and maxillary divisions of the trigeminal nerve are entirely sensory whereas the mandibular division contains both motor and sensory nerves. The motor nerves supply the muscles of mastication and some other muscles.

Loss of sensation from the lips as a consequence of injury to the maxillary or mandibular divisions of the trigeminal nerve means that the client cannot feel where their lips are as they contact other structures. Furthermore, proprioceptive information from the muscles of facial expression is through the trigeminal nerve so that positional sense is also lost thus compounding the problem. Sensory loss will thus affect lip movements and articulation. Anyone who has had dental treatment of lower teeth in which the lower lip is anaesthetized at the same time as the lower teeth will have experienced difficulties with articulation while the anaesthetic effect lasts. In this case, the effect of sensory loss is transient but after nerve injury the effect may be long lasting.

Mastication

The jaws, the temporomandibular joint and various muscle groups which move the jaws during mastication are fundamental to the understanding of various clinical aspects of speech and language therapy.

The temporomandibular joints

The temporomandibular joints are synovial joints formed between the heads of the mandibular condyles and the articular surfaces of the temporal bones (Figure 18.10). The two temporomandibular joints cannot execute movement independently of each other as they are joined by the mandible; as one joint moves the other joint must make some compensatory movement.

The **temporal articular surfaces** consist of the concave **glenoid cavity** anterior to the external auditory meatus and the convex **articular eminence**

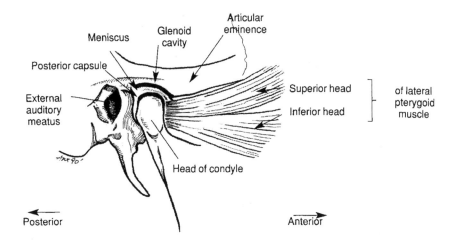

Figure 18.10 The temporomandibular joint.

anterior to the glenoid cavity. The two components form an S-shaped surface when viewed laterally. The articular surfaces of the **mandibular condyles** are approximately hemicylindrical anteroposteriorly. The convex heads of the condyles fit neatly into the concave glenoid cavity so that the joint is stable, but when the condyles move forward on to the articular eminences, the joint surfaces are poorly adapted and potentially unstable.

The joints, in common with all synovial joints (see Chapter 3), are surrounded by a capsule and non-articular surfaces within the capsule are lined with synovial membrane. The capsule is strengthened by **collateral ligaments** to prevent excessive backward movement of the condyles. The joint cavity of the temporomandibular joint is divided into two separate compartments by the fibrous **articular disc** or meniscus. The disc is quite thick anteriorly and posteriorly but is thinned down where it overlies the condyle.

Because of the shape of the articular surfaces and surrounding bone, movement of the joints is limited. Each condylar head may slide forward from the glenoid cavity on to the articular eminence or vice versa, or may rotate about a transverse axis through the condyles. Lateral movements of the mandible are produced by sliding only one condyle forward with some compensatory backward movement of the other condyle.

Muscles acting on the temporomandibular joint

Movements of the mandible are produced by the muscles of mastication, suprahyoid and infrahyoid muscles. The **muscles of mastication** have no function other than that of moving the mandible whereas the suprahyoid and infrahyoid muscles do have other actions; for this reason, the two latter groups are sometimes described as **accessory** muscles of mastication. The suprahyoid and infrahyoid muscles have already been described in Chapter 16.

Four pairs of muscles make up the **muscles of mastication** (Figure 18.11). The **masseter muscles** are powerful elevators of the mandible attaching to the zygomatic arch above and to the external surface of the angles of the mandible below. They close the mouth. The **temporalis**

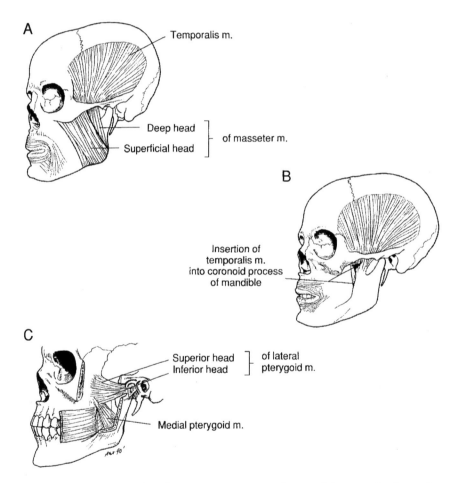

Figure 18.11 The muscles of mastication. (A) Lateral view of the superficial muscles. (B) With masseter removed. (C) With the superficial muscles and part of the mandible removed to show the deep muscles.

muscles are fan-shaped with extensive attachments to the temporal aspect of the skull from just behind the lateral orbital margin to above the ear. Each muscle passes down deep to the zygomatic arch to attach to the coronoid process of the mandible. Because of the extensive superior attachment and narrow inferior attachment of the muscle, anterior muscle fibres are vertical whereas the posterior fibres run horizontally. The vertical fibres elevate the mandible whereas the horizontal fibres retract it. The **medial pterygoid muscles** attach to the medial surface of the lateral pterygoid plates and run downwards and slightly backwards to attach to the medial aspects of the angles of the mandible. They are also elevators of the mandible. Elevation of the mandible can be achieved in any degree of protrusion.

The **lateral pterygoid muscles** run in a different direction from the other muscles of mastication, their fibres lying horizontally instead of vertically. Each lateral pterygoid muscle arises from the lateral surface of the lateral pterygoid plate and has two distinct parts. The large inferior part of each muscle attaches to the neck of the mandible and the smaller superior belly attaches to the disc of the temporomandibular joint. The inferior lateral pterygoid muscles protrude the mandible, drawing the condyles from the glenoid cavity on to the articular eminence. Because the eminence is convex, the head of the condyle will move downwards, thus producing a slight degree of opening of the mouth. The superior parts pull the articular discs forward as the lower part of the muscle protrudes the mandible. As the disc moves forward it may help to pack the space between the incongruent articular surfaces of the condyle and articular eminence, thus stabilizing the protruded mandible. If both lateral pterygoid muscles act together, the chin will protrude in the midline. If, however, only one lateral pterygoid muscle is used, the condyle on the same side is drawn forwards and the point of the chin deviates from the midline and is **laterally protruded** to the *opposite side*. At the same time, the other condyle must be restrained by action of the horizontal fibres of the temporalis muscle, the same muscle which would retract the mandible. The muscles of mastication are innervated by the **mandibular divisions** of the **trigeminal nerves**.

Opening the mouth requires the protrusive action of the lateral pterygoid muscles coupled with a downwards pull of the **suprahyoid muscles** operating from the hyoid bone. The hyoid must be fixed by the **infrahyoid muscles**, otherwise the hyoid bone would be elevated.

Movements of the temporomandibular joint during speech

The mandible is capable of an extremely wide range of movement and can be opened very wide or deviated markedly to either side of the midline. In conversational speech, the range of movement of the mandible is quite limited. The mouth is generally opened no more than 2 cms at maximum depending upon the utterance. Similarly the range of protrusion and retraction is small, generally less than 1 cm, sufficient to provide lip support for certain phonemes. Normally, there is no lateral deviation of the mandible during speech. If such deviation is detected, it is usually suggestive of underlying pathology or acquisition of peculiar habits of jaw movement. The underlying pathology may be of dental or neurological origin. A dental abscess under a tooth or a high filling, for example, will make the client deviate their jaw to avoid the offending tooth. Neurological damage to the motor nucleus of the trigeminal nerve in the brainstem will cause paresis (weakness) of the muscles of mastication on the affected side and the mandible will deviate to the affected side when a midline protrusion is attempted.

Movement of the lower jaw during speech determines not only the dimensions of the oral cavity but also influences the position of the lips and the tongue. Mandibular movements are therefore made during virtually any segment. Mandibular and tongue depression is used during production of low vowels, e.g. /ae/ as in father. A small degree of retraction is necessary for articulation of the labiodental phonemes /f/ and /v/ where the lower lip has to contact the upper teeth. Mandibular opening is also obvious during articulation of plosives /b/ and /p/ and fricatives, e.g. /f/ to release the stopping effect of the initial closed lip position.

The articulation of example phonemes in this chapter has centred on the anatomical structures involved in isolation. This is a somewhat artificial way of looking at things but is useful for understanding the contribution of individual components to specific segments. In reality, several articulators are used in most phonemes as will be realized from any phonetic analysis you have performed, not to mention voicing in the larynx for vowels and voiced consonants.

CHAPTER **19**

The mouth and nose

Speech and language therapists may have to examine the oral cavity during certain clinical procedures. It will help you either to examine a willing volunteer or to study your own mouth in a mirror to identify all the features visible in the mouth as described in the next section. This is a good introduction to the anatomy of the mouth and related structures.

The living mouth

The oral cavity consists of two portions, the oral vestibule and the oral cavity proper, although this distinction is rarely used in practice. The **vestibule** is a narrow, slit-like space which is limited externally by the lips and cheeks and internally by the teeth and alveolar processes, the parts of the maxillae and mandible housing the teeth (Figure 19.1). Note that in phonetics, the term *alveolar* refers specifically to the area immediately posterior to the upper anterior teeth and is therefore only a portion of the alveolar processes in the true anatomical sense. The groove between the lips and alveolar ridges is known as the **labial sulcus** and that between the cheeks and alveoli as the **buccal sulcus**. A small papilla is often visible in the vestibule opposite the crowns of the upper second molar teeth on each side and is the opening of the **parotid ducts**.

The **oral cavity** proper is enclosed by the lingual and palatal surfaces of the teeth and extends back to the **palatoglossal arches** (the anterior pillars of the fauces), which mark the junction between the mouth and the oropharynx (Figure 19.1). The **palatine tonsils** lie between the palatoglossal arches and the **palatopharyngeal arches** (posterior pillars of the fauces) and are quite variable in size. The majority of the floor of the mouth is occupied by the tongue while the remainder is formed by reflections of oral mucosa from the alveolar processes on to the ventral surface of the tongue forming the **lingual sulcus**. This region can be examined by asking the client to touch as far back on the hard palate with the tip of the

301

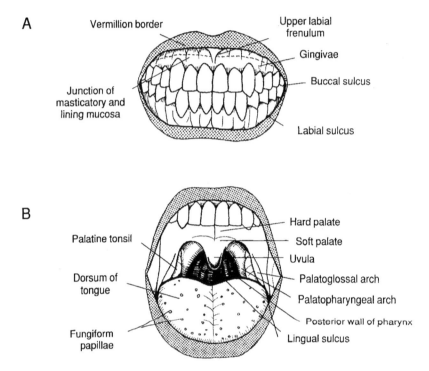

Figure 19.1 The mouth (A) with teeth intercuspated and (B) with the mouth open.

tongue as is comfortable (Figure 19.2). A thin crescent of mucosa, the **lingual frenum**, connects the ventral surface of the tongue to the floor of the mouth in the midline. Two small **sublingual papillae** are visible on the floor of the mouth on either side of the lower end of the frenum where the ducts of the submandibular salivary glands open into the oral cavity. Two prominent mucosal elevations, the **sublingual folds**, extend backwards and laterally from these papillae and cover the sublingual salivary glands. The roof of the oral cavity is formed by the **hard** and **soft palate**.

You should also be aware of the normal appearance of the mucosa lining the mouth. The **gingivae** (gums) surrounding the teeth are light pink in colour as is the mucosa covering the hard palate. The epithelium in these areas is quite thick and heavily keratinized to resist the abrasion of foodstuffs and therefore little of the underlying tissues shows through the surface layer. If you pull your lip away from your teeth, you will see an abrupt change in the mucosa just below the gingivae; the mucosa is reddish and becomes thinner so that blood vessels show through the

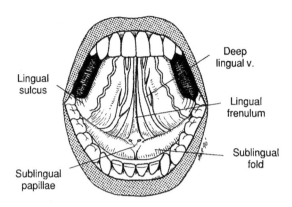

Figure 19.2 The floor of the mouth and the ventral surface of the tongue.

covering layer. This is also noticeable on the underside of the tongue where the deep lingual veins can be seen. The mucosa covering the dorsal (upper) surface of the tongue is very specialized to resist masticatory abrasion but also to house taste buds. The mucosa is formed into small projections called papillae (Figure 19.3). The most numerous papillae are small keratinized conical projections called **filiform papillae** which give the dorsal surface of the tongue its velvety appearance. Small pinkish button-like **fungiform papillae** containing taste buds are interspersed between the filiform papillae. A single transverse inverted V-shaped row of ten to twelve large papillae approximately 2 mm in diameter across the tongue are not visible without careful use of a dental mirror as they are so far back. These are the **circumvallate papillae** and also contain taste buds. The **dorsum** of the tongue usually displays an incomplete median furrow in the mucosa. In the roof of the mouth, the palatal mucosa anteriorly is pale pink in colour and a pale midline raphe is visible which terminates anteriorly at the **incisive papilla**. There are a variable number of prominent mucosal ridges, the **rugae** which extend lateral to the raphe anteriorly. Posteriorly, as the soft palate is approached, the mucosa becomes a deeper red in colour.

The teeth

Humans have two dentitions during their life. The teeth of the **primary** or **deciduous dentition** appear in the mouth between six months and two years after birth and some are retained until about the tenth year. The teeth of the **secondary** or **permanent dentition** erupt between six and twenty years and should last a lifetime. Between the ages of six and twelve,

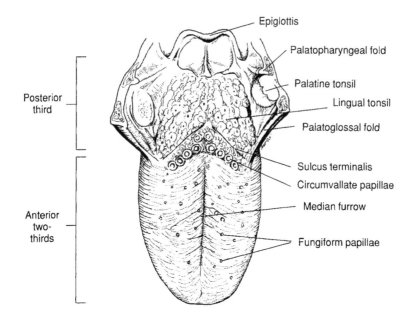

Figure 19.3 The dorsal surface of the tongue.

deciduous and permanent teeth are present in the mouth together: this is known as the **mixed dentition**.

There are different types of teeth within each dentition: incisors, canines and molars in the deciduous dentition and, in addition, premolars in the permanent dentition. **Incisors** are chisel-shaped teeth for cutting (incising) through food. **Canines** are conical teeth, originally designed for piercing or holding prey but now functioning as additional incisors. The posterior teeth, the **premolars** and **molars**, have broad crowns possessing conical projections known as **cusps**. Premolars have two cusps and molars have four or more cusps. These teeth are used for crushing and grinding food. Premolars, like the anterior teeth, are generally single rooted but molars are multirooted. The part of each tooth visible in the mouth is the **crown**. The **roots** are contained within bony tooth sockets and are therefore not visible on naked eye inspection of the mouth. The number of teeth present in the mouth will depend upon the age of the client and also on whether any teeth have been extracted because of dental caries or for cosmetic reasons.

For clinical purposes the dentition is divided into **quadrants** (Figure 19.4). Each maxillary (**upper**) and mandibular (**lower**) dental arch is divided into **left or right** quadrants, one on either side of the midline. In a full permanent dentition there should be 32 teeth, eight lying in each

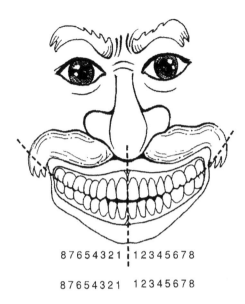

Figure 19.4 The quadrants of the mouth shown with a full permanent dentition.

quadrant. From the midline, each quadrant contains a central incisor, lateral incisor, canine, first premolar, second premolar, first molar, second molar and third molar (the wisdom tooth). In the deciduous dentition, there is a total of 20 teeth, with five in each quadrant. From the midline, these are a central incisor, lateral incisor, canine, first molar and second molar.

A shorthand reference system known as the **Zsigmond System** is commonly used to designate teeth during clinical examination and in written reports although there are other notation systems. In the Zsigmond System, the dentition is written out as a grid; each permanent tooth within a quadrant is given a number and each deciduous tooth is given a letter, as follows:

upper right quadrant	8 7 6 5 4 3 2 1	1 2 3 4 5 6 7 8	upper left quadrant
	E D C B A	A B C D E	
lower right quadrant	E D C B A	A B C D E	lower left quadrant
	8 7 6 5 4 3 2 1	1 2 3 4 5 6 7 8	

When looking at this grid note that it is written with respect to the **client's** left and right sides. Each tooth is designated by its number or letter enclosed in the appropriate grid. Thus the upper left deciduous second molar is written |E; the upper right permanent canine as 3|, the upper right deciduous lateral incisor as B|, and so on. This system is the most frequently used in the United Kingdom.

The surfaces of teeth have a terminology of their own. The outer surface adjacent to the lips is the **labial** surface, that adjacent to the cheek the **buccal** surface. The inner surfaces are known as the **palatal** surfaces in the maxillary dentition and the **lingual** surfaces in the mandibular dentition as they are adjacent to the palate and tongue respectively. The surfaces between two adjacent teeth in the same dental arch are the **mesial** surfaces facing the midline and the **distal** surfaces facing the back of the mouth. The sharp flat edges of the anterior teeth are the **incisal edges** and the broad surfaces with cusps on posterior teeth are the **occlusal** surfaces.

Developmental stages of the dentition

Detailed examination of the teeth and mouth is really the province of dentists but in many aspects of speech and language therapy practice you will be involved in combined clinics with orthodontists, maxillo-facial surgeons and ENT surgeons and should therefore be familiar with the terminology used to describe normal and abnormal aspects of the dentition. You can only see the teeth present in the mouth but it is often vital to obtain information about the teeth which are still developing in the jaws, which can be achieved by dental radiography. X-rays are partially absorbed by tissues containing heavy metal elements and as the teeth contain a significant percentage of calcium, as does bone, they will absorb the X-rays. A clinical radiograph is actually a negative so that soft tissues through which the X-rays pass appear black and those tissues which absorb X-rays appear white; the denser the tissue, the whiter they appear on the radiograph (Figure 19.5). Clinically, the major stages of tooth formation which can be detected by observation in the mouth or radiographically must be understood and related to their chronological sequence.

There are four important stages in the life history of developing teeth (Figure 19.5). **Calcification of the crown** is when the hard tissues, enamel and dentine, are first formed. This generally occurs several years before the tooth is visible in the mouth and can therefore tell the dentist that that particular tooth is developing normally. Before teeth calcify, the presence of the developing tooth is marked by a dark (radiolucent) area in the jaw bones. Completion of crown formation takes about three years for permanent teeth and between eight and twelve months for deciduous teeth. Examination of the progress in the formation of the

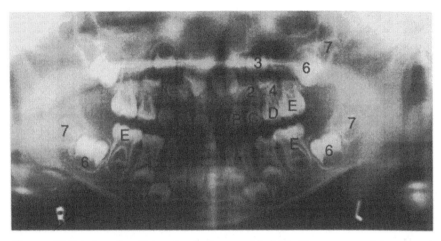

Figure 19.5 A dental radiograph of a 3 year old child. The crowns of the second permanent lower molars (7s) are just beginning to calcify, the lower first permanent molars (6s) have completed crown formation and the second deciduous lower molars (Es) are examples of fully developed teeth with roots fully formed. In the upper left quadrant, the permanent teeth are numbered and the primary teeth are lettered according to the Zsigmond system.

crown will tell the dentist whether the teeth are developing as predicted. The long process by which teeth move from their developmental position in the jaws into their functional position in the oral cavity is known as **eruption**. Each tooth appears in the oral cavity within a relatively restricted period and the teeth in each dentition appear in a particular sequence which is, unfortunately, not a simple front to back progression. The tooth roots, which take about twice as long as the crown to develop, can also be seen on radiographs and corroborate other evidence that the teeth are developing normally. A combination of oral examination and dental radiography enables the clinician to assess the development of the two dentitions and to determine if teeth are going to appear in their normal sequence at the normal time and in the correct location.

The sequence and timing of these stages is variable. Average timings are presented for the deciduous dentition in Table 19.1 and those for the permanent dentition in Table 19.2. The timing of these events varies considerably. Deciduous teeth may erupt more than six months on either side of the dates given in the tables and permanent teeth may erupt one year on either side of the given date. Mandibular teeth usually erupt about six months ahead of their maxillary counterparts and eruption is usually earlier in females than in males.

Table 19.1. Development of the deciduous dentition (in months)

Tooth	Age when calcification of crown starts	Age when crown complete	Age at eruption	Age when root complete
A	4/12 IUL*	3/12	6/12	18/12
B	4/12 IUL	3/12	6/12	18/12
C	5/12 IUL	9/12	18/12	30/12
D	5/12 IUL	6/12	12/12	24/12
E	6/12 IUL	12/12	24/12	36/12

*IUL = intrauterine life

Table 19.2. Development of the permanent dentition (in years)

Tooth	Order of eruption	Age when calcification of crown starts	Age when crown complete	Age at eruption	Age when root complete
1	2	1	4	7	10
2	3	2	5	8	11
3	6	2	5	11*	11*
4	4	3	6	9	12
5	5	4	7	10	13
6	1	Birth	3	6	9
7	7	6	9	12	15
8	8	12	15	18	21

* The eruption of permanent canines is delayed until their roots are almost complete.

Occlusion

Occlusion is the relationship between opposing teeth while they are in contact; this contact should produce a good functional relationship between the upper and lower teeth and also be aesthetically pleasing. **Orthodontics** is a branch of dentistry which deals with the treatment of malocclusion when one or both of these desirable conditions are not met.

Malocclusion caused by overcrowding can often be treated by extraction of permanent teeth to ensure adequate space is available for the remaining teeth or for those which have yet to erupt. The stage of growth and development of the child must be born in mind as natural growth may relieve the overcrowding by providing more room in the dental arches without any dental intervention. Teeth may be tilted, rotated or moved bodily by the use of forces applied by springs or rubber bands attached to removable or fixed orthodontic appliances applied to the teeth in an attempt to restore a functionally or aesthetically acceptable occlusion. It is not only the teeth but also the jaws, associated muscles and temporomandibular joints which need to be considered. In severe malocclusions, surgical augmentation or reduction of the relevant bones may be necessary before teeth are manipulated by orthodontic treatment since there are limits to the degree to which they can be moved.

When not in function, the mouth and lips are closed by the tonic contraction of the muscles of mastication and facial expression but the teeth are not in contact. This is known as the **postural** or **mandibular rest position**. There is a space of between 2 and 5 mm between the upper and lower teeth known as the **intercuspal** or **freeway space**. The intercuspal space varies considerably between individuals but is fairly constant for each person. The actual distance in an individual is influenced by a number of factors including head position, age, sleep and psychological state. Contraction of the muscles of mastication from the mandibular rest position will usually bring the teeth into intercuspal occlusion.

Characteristics of normal occlusion

The adult dentition should form a harmonious aesthetic and functional unit. An alteration in the position of the teeth or in occlusal function is called a **disturbance**. Disturbances which cause pathological alterations in the masticatory system are called **disorders**.

The most commonly used classification of occlusion is **Angle's classification** based on the relative positions of the maxillary and mandibular first molars. The majority of malocclusions are due to irregularities in the mesiodistal relationships of the maxillary and mandibular teeth in the intercuspal position (see below).

In a **normal intercuspal occlusion**, the mesial cusps of the maxillary first molars occlude between the mesial and distal cusps of the mandibular first molars, and thus the distal cusps of the maxillary first molars occlude with the distal cusps of the mandibular first molars and the mesial cusps of the mandibular second molars. It follows therefore that the teeth in each mandibular quadrant lie in a more mesial position in relation to their maxillary counterparts with the exception of the central incisors (Figure 19.6).

As the maxillary dental arch is wider than the mandibular arch, the buccal cusps of the maxillary molars and premolars occlude outside the buccal cusps of the mandibular posterior teeth. The palatal cusps of the maxillary molars and premolars occlude between the buccal and lingual cusps of the mandibular molars and premolars. The maxillary incisors and canines overhang their mandibular counterparts such that their palatal surfaces face the labial surfaces of the lower incisors and canines. The overhang is usually in the order of 2–3 mm and is called the **overbite** (Figure 19.7). **Overjet** describes the horizontal distance between labial surfaces of maxillary and mandibular incisors and is also usually in the order of 2–3 mm.

The classification of malocclusion

Malocclusions arise when the teeth occlude in a manner different from the normal occlusion described above.

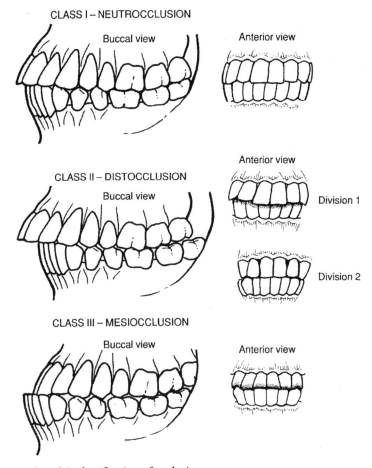

Figure 19.6 Angle's classification of occlusion.

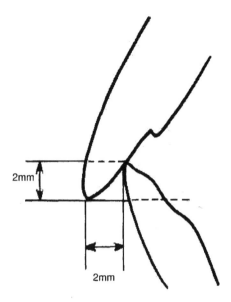

Figure 19.7 Overbite and overjet of anterior teeth.

The mandibular first molars may occupy one of three positions with respect to the maxillary first molars. These are neutral (as described above), distal or mesial. Malocclusions are divided into three broad classes known as **Angle's Class I** (neutrocclusion), **Angle's Class II** (distocclusion) and **Angle's Class III** (mesiocclusion). In clinical practice, there are almost infinite variations between these classes. Variations in tooth position may interfere with the occlusion of teeth in individual quadrants or segments of the dental arches without interfering with the overall arch relationship and may be encountered in any of the three main classifications.

Angle's Class I (neutrocclusion)

The majority of malocclusions detected in most populations fall into this category. Since the anteroposterior relationships of the dental arches are normal, the malocclusions found in Class I tend to be due to discrepancies between the length of the two dental arches and tooth size. If the arches are too small to accommodate the teeth, crowding occurs. Alternatively, if the teeth are disproportionately small compared with the dimensions of the dental arches, spacing results. The most frequent clinical signs in Class I malocclusions are crowding of the mandibular incisors and malposition of the canine teeth.

Angle's Class II (distocclusion)

In Angle's Class II the maxillary arch is further forward in relation to the mandibular arch than in a normal occlusion (Figure 19.6). The mandibular first molars thus lie distal to the maxillary first molars such that the mesial cusps of the maxillary first molars occlude between the mandibular second premolars and the mesial cusps of the mandibular first molars. The remaining premolars and molars are also in a distal relationship with their opposite numbers compared with a Class I occlusion.

Angle's Class II is subclassified into two divisions depending upon the position of the anterior teeth. In **Angle's Class II Division I**, the maxillary incisors are markedly proclined increasing the overjet beyond normal limits. There is often a tendency for the lower lip to rest behind the proclined maxillary incisors which further accentuates the protruded incisors. Because of the increased overjet, the mandibular incisors often tend to overerupt increasing the overbite. The maxillary arch is often V-shaped and therefore narrower than usual, being constricted particularly in the premolar region. Class II Division I malocclusions are often accompanied by imbalances in the dental bases (see below) and a short upper lip which produces inability to seal the lips. Clients with Class II Division 1 malocclusions are often habitual mouth breathers.

In **Angle's Class II Division II**, the maxillary central incisors are retroclined and crowded and the maxillary lateral incisors are proclined and overlap the central incisors. The maxillary arch is of normal width. The anteroposterior relationships of the arches are disturbed because the mandible is forced into a retruded position by tooth interference from the retroclined central incisors. There is no obvious skeletal base disharmony.

Angle's Class III (mesiocclusion)

In mesiocclusion, the mandibular molars lie mesial to the maxillary molars (Figure 19.6). The mesial cusps of the maxillary first molars occlude between the distal cusps of the mandibular first molars and the mesial cusps of the mandibular second molars. The rest of the dentition follows the same mesial relationship. In Class III malocclusions, the excessive mesial displacement is equal to at least the dimensions of a premolar tooth and is usually accompanied by skeletal anomalies: the mandible is large *relative* to the maxilla. The anterior teeth show a reverse or negative overjet such that the mandibular incisors occlude labial to the maxillary incisors. As a result of pressure from the lower lip, the mandibular incisors often show a lingual inclination. The maxillary arch may be constricted such that the buccal surfaces of the maxillary teeth occlude lingual to those of the mandibular teeth producing a crossbite.

Relationships of the dental bases

The positions of the dental arches with respect to each other and the sizes of the arches are governed by the positions and sizes of the supporting jaw bones. Those parts of the maxillae and mandible which lie above or below the teeth are known in orthodontic terms as the **dental bases**. The skeletal relationships of the dental bases are usually studied radiographically. The bases may be described as skeletal Class I (normal), skeletal class II (postnormal), and skeletal class III (prenormal) correspond with Angle's molar classification. In the postnormal relationship, the maxillae are large *relative* to the mandible whereas in the prenormal relationship the reverse applies. The term *relative* is important: for example, in skeletal Class III, a larger than normal mandible may be related to normal maxillae or alternatively, the mandible may be of normal size but related to small maxillae.

An important clinical guide to skeletal bone size and position is the facial profile between the nose and chin. In skeletal Class I, the facial profile is straight whereas in Class II varying degrees of convexity are present as a result of the protruding maxillae, a receding chin or a combination of both. In Class III, the profile is concave because of the prominent mandible and reduced maxillary size.

Intra-arch relationships of the teeth

While there may be discrepancies in the size and relationships of both the dental arches and their supporting skeletal bases, irregularities in position, number and form of teeth may also lead to malocclusion.

Teeth may be crowded or spaced if their combined mesiodistal diameters are larger or smaller than the corresponding arch length. The position of individual teeth in the horizontal plane may be altered by displacement, rotation or tilting. In the vertical plane, teeth may fail to erupt into occlusion or may overerupt beyond the occlusal plane. If teeth are missing from the dental arch due to extraction or congenital absence, the adjacent teeth will drift into the space until the stability of the occlusion is re-established. If, for example, the upper lateral incisors are congenitally absent the central incisors may drift laterally producing a central gap or **diastema**.

Disturbances of the occlusion

Disturbances may arise from primary malocclusions which include overcrowding, rotation or displacement of teeth from the dental arches. Increased overbite or overjet may produce altered incisor function and may deflect the mandible during closure. Lack of development of the alveolar processes in the posterior arch causes overclosure with reduction in vertical dimensions and failure of the posterior teeth to occlude: this is known as a **posterior open bite**. Overdevelopment of the posterior alveolar processes results in premature intercuspation of the posterior teeth leaving the anterior teeth with a reverse or negative overbite called an **anterior open bite**.

The establishment and maintenance of dental arch form

As teeth are erupting, the tongue tends to push them outwards whereas the muscles of facial expression push them inwards. The teeth eventually occupy a position where these two opposing forces are in equilibrium. Muscular imbalances can produce effects upon the teeth. Lip seal is determined by the length of the lips and position of the incisor teeth. If the lips are short, a gap is present and lip seal is only achieved with effort. In Class II Division I malocclusions, the lower lip is often positioned behind the maxillary incisors accentuating their proclination. In Class II Division II malocclusions, the jaw tends to be square and the lips are long. The tongue falls downwards and deprives the incisors of support such that the hyperactivity of the lips causes the upper central incisors to retrocline.

During suckling, the tongue is protruded against the anterior gum pads and makes rhythmic movements to force the milk into the pharynx. When solid food is taken, the tongue makes only momentary contact with the incisors before being drawn backwards across the hard palate. In some individuals, the infantile swallowing pattern persists to produce **tongue thrust swallowing**. Of atypical swallowers, 80 per cent have an anterior open bite and incisor proclination. Thumbsucking, frequent in young children, is usually discontinued after about the fourth year and any effects on the dentition produced during this time are usually reversible. If the habit persists, it may produce proclination of the maxillary anterior teeth, an anterior open bite and retroclination and crowding of the mandibular incisors.

Habitual mouthbreathing is usually associated with some form of nasopharyngeal obstruction and can induce dentofacial abnormalities. Because the suprahyoid muscles are continually active to depress the mandible to increase the efficiency of oral respiration, the tongue falls away from the palate. The unopposed pressure exerted by the muscles of facial expression leads to collapse of the maxillary arch producing a high palatal vault, crossbite, crowded and proclined incisors.

The effects of malocclusion on speech

The major speech problems associated with malocclusion relate to the position of the lips in relation to the teeth. In Class II malocclusions, it is often difficult to achieve lip seal or to bring the lower lip beneath the upper teeth with consequent difficulties in articulating plosives and labiodentals respectively. Clients will often adopt trick movements to overcome these shortcomings. Labiodentals will often be articulated by positioning the lower lip on the alveolar ridge – a 'labioalveolar' articulation. Similarly in Class III malocclusions, lip seal can be a problem and it is also difficult to retract the mandible sufficiently for accurate labiodental positioning. In this case, the client will often adopt a 'reverse labiodental' articulation by positioning the lower teeth against the upper lip when necessary. During or after orthodontic treatment, clients often need speech therapy intervention to 'unlearn' these trick movements and re-educate their articulators to use the conventional positions.

The tongue

The tongue is a mass of striated muscle covered by oral mucosa and much more extensive than it first appears. The **anterior two-thirds** lie within the oral cavity but even the full extent of this part of the tongue is not visible on intraoral examination. The **posterior third** of the tongue lies in the oropharynx and cannot be seen at all. This division is not based purely on location, but is an actual division marked by a V-shaped groove on the upper surface, the **sulcus terminalis**; the apex of the sulcus points backwards and may just be visible when the tongue is fully protruded (Figure 19.3). The division of the tongue into anterior two-thirds and posterior third is based on its embryological development (see Chapter 20). Behind the sulcus terminalis, the dorsum of the tongue is devoid of papillae and has a smooth nodular surface, produced by aggregates of lymphoid tissues, the **lingual tonsils**.

The muscles of the tongue

The lingual musculature can be divided into **extrinsic** and **intrinsic** groups. The extrinsic muscles are attached to various bony structures lying outside the body of the tongue. The intrinsic muscles, on the other hand, are entirely confined within the substance of the tongue. The muscles of the left and right sides are separated by a midline fibrous septum.

There are four pairs of extrinsic muscles attaching the tongue to the mandible, styloid process, hyoid bone and soft palate (Figure 19.8). The **genioglossus muscles** arise from the superior genial tubercles behind the midline of the mandible. Each large muscle is fan-shaped extending upwards and backwards into the tongue. The superior fibres enter the tip of the tongue, the middle fibres spread out into the dorsum of the tongue and the inferior fibres run backwards into the posterior third of the tongue. The

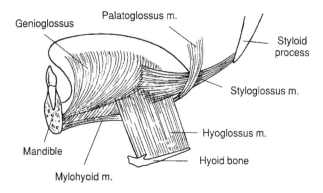

Figure 19.8 The extrinsic muscles of the tongue.

action of these muscles depends upon which fibre groups are brought into operation. Contraction of the posterior fibres protrudes the tongue. Contraction of the superior fibres pulls the tip of the tongue downwards towards the floor of the mouth. If superior and middle fibres contract, the tongue is depressed. The **styloglossus muscles** run from the tip of the styloid processes downwards and forwards on the lateral walls of the pharynx, between the superior and middle constrictors of the pharynx to the posterolateral margins of the tongue. The styloglossus muscles pull the tongue upwards and backwards and also elevate the lateral margins. The **hyoglossus muscles** attach to the superior surface of the hyoid bone. Each muscle enters the sides of the tongue and acts to pull the tongue downwards and backwards and to depress the lateral borders. The **palatoglossus muscles** are a component of both the tongue and the soft palate. They arise from the undersurface of the soft palate and pass downwards and forwards beneath the mucosa of the lateral wall of the pharynx forming the **palatoglossal arches** to insert into the sides of the tongue. The muscles have a dual action. If the soft palate is fixed by other muscles, the posterior third of the tongue is pulled upwards and backwards. If the soft palate is not fixed, the palatoglossus muscles pull the soft palate downwards on to the dorsum of the tongue. During either action, the palatoglossal arches are pulled together, thus narrowing the oropharyngeal isthmus.

The **intrinsic muscles** (Figure 19.9) lie entirely within the body of the tongue. They run in longitudinal, transverse and vertical bundles. The **vertical group** flatten and widen the tongue, the **transverse group** produce elongation and narrowing while the **superior** and **inferior longitudinal groups** turn the tip upwards or downwards respectively and also shorten the tongue.

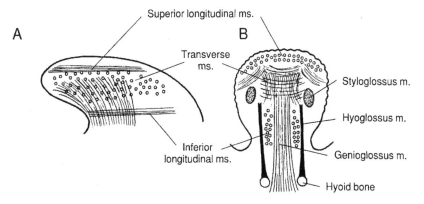

Figure 19.9 The intrinsic muscles of the tongue. (A) Longitudinal section. (B) Transverse section.

The intrinsic muscles reputedly modify the shape of the tongue whereas the extrinsic muscles alter its position but it is extremely difficult to move the tongue without altering its shape and, conversely, shape changes cannot occur without altering the position of the tongue to some extent. Moreover, change in shape in one part of the tongue inevitably causes a change in shape elsewhere. A rather revolting analogy is to think of having a large slug in your mouth: as one part moves and changes shape, the shape of the rest of the slug changes.

It is extremely difficult to delineate which muscles are used to achieve a given tongue position and hence a specific phoneme. It is relatively easy to predict the action of a muscle which has two bony attachments either side of an intervening joint but this just does not pertain for the tongue. The extrinsic muscles have one bony attachment so we can predict that contraction of that muscle will move the tongue towards that attachment as indicated above but the same cannot be done for the intrinsic muscles of the tongue. The intrinsic and extrinsic muscles interweave so it is likely that action of one muscle will distort another even when that muscle is not actively contracting. It is all but impossible to make electromyographic recordings from the tongue muscles without picking up signals from other muscles except near the attachments of the extrinsic muscles to their bony origin. Assigning roles to different tongue muscles in particular actions is therefore, at best, a 'best guess' or, at worst, mere speculation. However, it has been suggested that the extrinsic muscles of the tongue are responsible for gross positional changes for vowel production and that the intrinsic muscles are responsible for shape change and precision of articulation during consonant production.

The innervation of the tongue

The tongue is derived embryologically from several sources. The mucosa of the anterior two-thirds and posterior third of the tongue develop from the endoderm of different pharyngeal arches and therefore have a different sensory nerve supply (see Chapter 20). Furthermore, taste sensation is detected by different nerves from those serving somaesthetic sensation. The muscles of the tongue develop from yet another source and thus the motor innervation is distinct from the sensory innervation (Figure 19.10).

The somaesthetic sensory supply to the anterior two-thirds of the tongue is carried by the **lingual nerves**, branches of the mandibular division of the trigeminal nerve. Taste sensation from the anterior two-thirds of the tongue travels in the **chorda tympani** branches of the **facial nerve**. The lingual nerve and chorda tympani on each side run together until they separate just below the skull to enter the cranial cavity by different routes. The **glossopharyngeal nerves** serve both taste and somaesthetic sensation from the posterior two-thirds of the tongue. The **hypoglossal nerves** innervate all the intrinsic and extrinsic muscles of the tongue with the exception of the palatoglossus, which is embryologically a muscle of the soft palate and is innervated by the vagus nerve. The motor unit size of the tongue is small so that one axon innervates very few

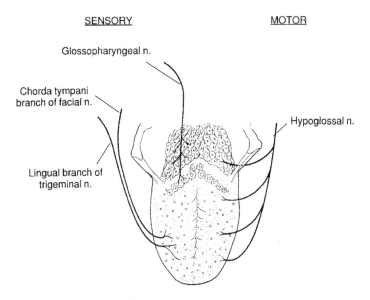

Figure 19.10 The innervation of the tongue.

muscle fibres enabling fine control of movement. Surprisingly, proprioceptive information from the tongue does not travel with any of the nerves mentioned above but travels instead through the cervical plexus formed from the upper cervical nerves.

The functions of the tongue

The tongue is an extremely important tactile organ and its powers for discrimination of size, shape and texture are highly developed. Any minor irregularity in the oral cavity such as a defective filling or a food fragment is easily detected; small alterations generally feel much larger than they really are. Taste receptors in the tongue and temperature receptors in the tongue, lips and oral mucosa protect the oral cavity and upper parts of the gastrointestinal tract from extremes of temperature and noxious, unpleasant-tasting substances. Swallowing only occurs when sensory information from the tongue indicates that the consistency, temperature and flavour of food is acceptable. The tongue forms food into a bolus and moves it into the oropharynx to be swallowed (see Chapter 21). The sensory function of the tongue and its motility enable the tongue to investigate, detect and remove food from most regions of the oral cavity and from between the teeth.

During mastication, the tongue plays an important role in placing food between the teeth. Much of the food which is displaced into the vestibule is returned between the dental arches or into the oral cavity by the contraction of the buccinator and orbicularis oris but precise movements of the tongue are essential for clearing the vestibule and lingual sulcus of small particles. Precision movements are also required for articulation of a number of phonemes during speech. Position is probably controlled by proprioceptive feedback through the muscle spindles of the tongue musculature but somatic sensory information is also important and speech is often temporarily disturbed following loss of sensation after anaesthesia of the lingual nerve during routine dental procedures.

The function of the tongue in speech

The tongue is used in the articulation of a wide variety of phonemes which include several consonants and all the vowel sounds. Phoneticians divide the tongue into several segments for classification of articulation of different phonemes but these bear little relationship to the anatomical divisions of the tongue (Figure 19.11). The tip of the tongue is the tip of the tongue and the blade is a short segment immediately posterior to the tip. The subsequent divisions are the front, centre and back. The segments from tip to back correspond to the anatomical anterior two-thirds of the tongue and the posterior third is called the root in phonetic terminology.

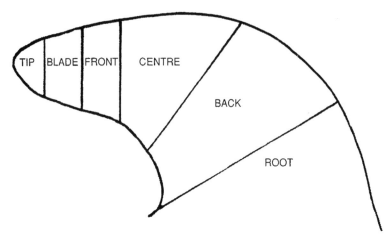

Figure 19.11 The phonetic divisions of the tongue.

Electropalatography is a technique for studying contact of the tongue with the palate including the alveolus. An upper denture base is constructed to fit the hard palate and contains an array of small sensors which are activated when the tongue contacts them. By coupling the sensors to an appropriate device, a record of tongue contact during articulation of specific phonemes can be made. This is a useful tool for diagnosis of abnormal tongue movements when records from a particular client are compared with records from normal speakers. Figure 19.12 illustrates the tongue contact for various consonants. In the majority, the tongue tip and blade are used to contact the alveolus or palate in various locations. The centre contacts the palate during articulation of /tʒ/ as in judge and /y/. Movement of the back of the tongue into contact with the raised soft palate is a **velar** movement in contrast to **velic** movement when the soft palate itself is moved. Examples of velopalatal phonemes are /k/ and /g/.

The position of the tongue in the oral cavity determines vowel sounds and is usually classified according to whether the tongue is raised or lowered (high or low vowels) and its position from front to back. Vowel sounds can thus be classified across the spectrum from high front to low back. For example, /i/ is a high front, /u/ a high back, /ae/ a low front, /a/ a low back vowel.

Clinical anatomy of the tongue

The lingual nerves, including the chorda tympani contributions from the facial nerve, run very close to the bone overlying the lingual aspect of the

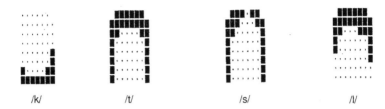

/k/   /t/   /s/   /l/

Figure 19.12 Electropalatograph recordings showing the contact of the tongue with the hard palate during articulation of, from left to right, /k/, /t/, /s/ and /l/. (Courtesy of Dr Sara Howard.)

mandibular third molars and are therefore susceptible to damage during surgical removal of impacted lower wisdom teeth. If the lingual nerve is damaged, somaesthetic and taste sensation is lost from the anterior two-thirds of the tongue on the affected side. Altered sensation occurs after about 10 per cent of mandibular third molar surgical extractions, but in most cases, is only transient; permanent damage occurs in less than 1 per cent of all cases. Loss of taste sensation is usually not too noticeable but some clients report an unpleasant metallic taste in the mouth. Loss of somatic sensation is, however, very disconcerting and uncomfortable for the patient. Because of loss of sensation, patients are often unaware of the position of the tongue and may bite it without realizing they have done so.

If one of the hypoglossal nerves is damaged, flaccid paralysis of the muscles of the tongue occurs on the affected side. If the tongue is protruded, it deviates to the injured side. Asking patients to stick out their tongues forcibly constitutes the clinical test for hypoglossal nerve function. Loss of sensory or motor function will also interfere with various oral functions such as speech, swallowing and mastication to greater or lesser degrees. Damage to the motor pathways affecting the nervous control of the tongue will produce dysarthria. Movement tends to be slowed and accuracy is poor. Tongue movements are therefore poorly coordinated with movements of other articulators, and positioning of the tongue when it eventually occurs is inaccurate.

Some children are born with a short lingual frenum, which results in **ankyloglossia** or tongue tie. The tongue does not show its usual range of mobility, especially in movements of the tip and blade, which affects not only linguodental sounds, but also many other phonemes involving the use of the tongue tip. **Macroglossia** is an abnormally large tongue. The tongue may be absolutely bigger and this occurs in **Down's syndrome**, for example. The tongue protrudes and affected individuals often artic-ulate by using linguolabial contact, not normally found in standard English usage.

Glossectomy, partial surgical removal of the tongue usually for oral cancer, is avoided if at all possible for obvious reasons. Treatment usually involves excision of the primary lesion if small followed by chemotherapy or local radiotherapy by implantation of radioactive crystals into the site of the lesion. Surprisingly, clients who have had a glossectomy are usually capable of a high degree of compensation by developing trick movements of the lips, jaws, pharynx and residual portion of the tongue to achieve reasonably clear articulation. However, some sounds, especially high front vowels are particularly difficult and may not be articulated as clearly as normal but some clients can even learn to compensate for this deficiency.

The palate

The roof of the oral cavity is formed by the bony **hard palate** anteriorly and the muscular **soft palate** which extends backwards from the free border of the bony palate towards the posterior pharyngeal wall and ends as the **uvula**, a small pendant protrusion. The normal appearance of the palate during intraoral examination has been described above.

The hard palate comprises the palatine processes of the maxillae anteriorly and the horizontal plates of the palatine bones posteriorly. These bones are continuous with the alveolar processes of the maxilla anteriorly and laterally. The bones are covered with oral mucosa which blends imperceptibly with the palatal alveolar mucosa and gingivae.

The soft palate extends from the posterior border of the bony palate and forms a movable partition between the oropharynx and nasopharynx. Note that the soft palate is not freely mobile from its attachment to the hard palate. The moveable part of the soft palate is about 2 mm posterior to the change from bone to connective tissue and is called the **vibrating line**; this may be demonstrated by asking the client to say 'Aaar'. The scaffold of the soft palate is the palatine aponeurosis of dense connective tissue, attached to the posterior margin of the bones of the hard palate. It is formed from tendons of one of the muscles of the soft plate and the other muscles attach to it. The lateral surfaces of the soft palate extend downwards and laterally as two prominent mucosal folds, the **palatoglossal** and **palatopharyngeal arches**. The palatoglossus and palatopharyngeus muscles run beneath these folds to pass into the posterior third of the tongue and pharynx respectively.

The muscles of the soft palate

There are four pairs of muscles moving the soft palate (Figure 19.13). Two pairs enter the soft palate from above, whereas the second pair enter from below. The vestigial musculus uvulae forms the bulk of the uvula.

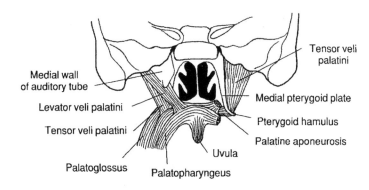

Figure 19.13 The muscles of the soft palate viewed posteriorly.

The **tensor veli palatini** muscles arise between the pterygoid plates and the adjacent medial walls of the auditory tubes. The fibres converge as they descend, forming a narrow tendon which passes medially around the pterygoid hamulus of each medial pterygoid plate. The tendons pierce the buccinator muscles and the fibres fan out into the soft palate to form the palatine aponeurosis with the tendon of the muscle of the opposite side. The tensor veli palatini muscles, as their name suggests, tense the soft palate. Because of their attachment to the auditory tube, these muscles also open the tube to equalize pressure on the tympanic membrane. The **levator veli palatini** muscles arise from the lateral surface of the carti-laginous auditory tubes and from the lower surface of the adjacent petrous temporal bones. They attach to the palatine aponeurosis and elevate the soft palate also opening the auditory tube.

The **palatopharyngeus** muscles originate from the palatine aponeu-rosis near the posterior margins of the hard palate. They run downwards and backwards beneath the mucosa of the lateral pharyngeal wall forming the palatopharyngeal arches posterior to the palatine tonsils. In the pharynx, each muscle is attached to the pharyngeal wall and to the posterior border of the thyroid cartilage. These muscles are pharyngeal elevators, pulling the wall of the pharynx upwards. The **palatoglossus** muscles have already been described with the extrinsic muscles of the tongue (see above).

The majority of the palatal muscles are innervated by the **pharyngeal branches** of the **vagus nerves**. These nerves contribute to the **pharyngeal plexus**, a fine nervous network which surrounds the pharyngeal wall and comprises motor (vagus), sensory (glossopharyngeal) and autonomic nerves. The tensor veli palatini muscles are supplied by the mandibular division of the trigeminal nerve. The sensory supply to the hard and soft palate is derived from the maxillary divisions of the trigeminal nerves.

Functions of the palate in speech

The soft palate plays important roles in swallowing and speech. When relaxed, the soft palate hangs down and the inferior surface of the soft palate contacts the posterior third of the tongue. This default position of the soft palate allows air to pass from the nasal cavities into the lower respiratory system during ventilation; this position is also adopted to allow exhaled air into the nasal cavity during articulation of nasal phonemes /m/ /n/ and /ŋ/. The soft palate is raised to seal off the nasopharynx from the oropharynx during swallowing or speech. Raising and tensing the soft palate prevents food from entering the nasal cavities during swallowing. Adopting the same position during speech prevents air from entering the nose during articulation of all phonemes except nasals. When the soft palate is raised during swallowing to prevent food entering the nasopharynx, the levator and tensor muscles are both used to form a rigid barrier. However, when the palate is raised during speech (**velic closure**), only the levators appear to be used. A raised soft palate is sufficient to deflect the air stream through the mouth and does not need to be tensed. This also has the advantage that the soft palate can be returned to its default dependent position much more quickly if it only has to be depressed and not relaxed as well.

Velic closure is probably not simply a matter of elevation of the soft palate but also involves some forward movement of the posterior pharyngeal wall (**velopharyngeal closure**). This can be impaired in children with cleft palate where the soft palate may be too short to form an effective seal. Similarly in dysarthric clients where the nerve supply to the palatine muscles is affected by damage to the central nervous motor pathways, velopharyngeal closure is often slowed or impaired. If velopharyngeal closure is inefficient, air will leak into the nasal cavity and non-nasal sounds will acquire a nasal component (**hypernasality**). If velic movements are poorly coordinated with other aspects of articulation, nasal phonemes may not have the nasal component (**hyponasality**). Often hypernasality and hyponasality occur together.

The salivary glands

There are three pairs of **major salivary glands** which are external to the oral cavity and empty their saliva into the mouth through long ducts. **Minor salivary glands** are small aggregates of salivary tissue scattered in the oral mucosa lining the lips, cheeks, hard and soft palate and the tongue with short ducts entering the mouth through the covering mucosa. Salivary glands produce two types of saliva. **Serous saliva** is watery but contains some digestive enzymes whereas **mucous saliva** contains mucins which make it viscous so that it is an efficient lubricant.

Saliva has many functions: some are obvious but others not so. First, saliva acts as a **lubricant** for all oral functions such as mastication, swallowing and speech. Second, it is vitally important to maintain oral hygiene. The major constituent of saliva of either type is water which washes debris from the teeth and oral mucosa. Saliva also contains various antibacterial agents. It also contains inorganic ions, particularly bicarbonate, which act as a **buffer** to prevent the build up of acid. The pH of the mouth is neutral (pH 7.2) and if the pH falls to below pH 5.5 by accumulation of acid then the calcified tissues of the teeth – enamel and dentine – can be dissolved, resulting in dental caries. When we eat, food sticks to our teeth and the residue is colonized by bacteria which metabolize the food for their own use but produce acid as they do so. Salivary bicarbonate neutralizes the acid, which breaks down into water – adding to the saliva – and carbon dioxide – which can be exhaled – thus ensuring that the pH returns to normal after we have eaten. The digestive enzymes in saliva are inefficient as they only have a short time to act before food enters the stomach where these enzymes are inactivated. Nevertheless, they do help break down some food debris on the teeth.

The **parotid glands** (Figure 19.14) are large serous glands filling the space between the ramus of the mandible and the sternocleidomastoid muscle and extend beyond the space both deeply and superficially to

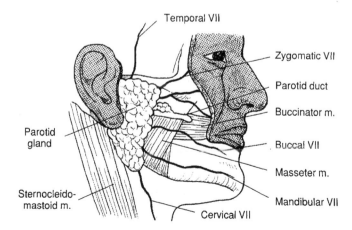

Figure 19.14 The parotid gland and facial nerve.

overlap these structures. Each gland extends up as far as the zygomatic arch and down as far as the angle of the mandible although their size is quite variable. The **parotid duct** passes forward from the upper anterior aspect of each gland superficial to the masseter muscle about a finger's breadth below the zygomatic arch. It turns medially at the anterior border of masseter to pierce the buccinator muscle and enter the oral cavity opposite the upper second molar tooth. The duct is easily palpable on the face as a cord-like structure if the teeth are clenched to make the masseter stand out. The gland is enclosed in a tough fibrous connective tissue capsule, the **parotid fascia**.

The **submandibular glands** (Figure 19.15) lie, as their name suggests, under the mandible and contain a mixture of serous and mucous cells. Each gland has a superficial and deep part. The superficial part of the gland lies in a slight depression on the medial side of the posterior part of the lower border of the mandible. The superficial lobe of the gland is continuous around the posterior free edge of the mylohyoid muscle forming the floor of the mouth with the deep lobe beneath the oral mucosa in the floor of the mouth. The submandibular duct passes forward from the deep lobe along the floor of the mouth to open into the oral cavity at the sublingual papillae under the tongue (Figure 19.2).

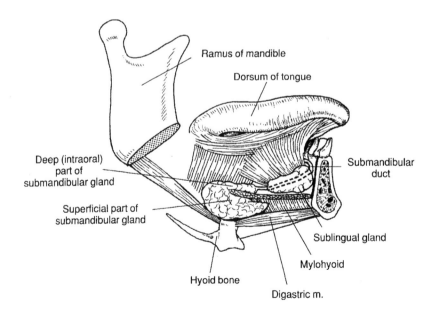

Figure 19.15 The submandibular and sublingual glands.

The **sublingual glands** (Figure 19.15) are the third pair of major glands and lie wholly within the oral cavity under the mucosa of the floor of the mouth alongside the submandibular ducts on either side of the tongue. Multiple ducts open into the oral cavity along the sublingual fold or into the submandibular ducts. The sublingual glands are entirely mucus-secreting.

Clinical anatomy of the salivary glands

The normal functioning of the major and minor salivary glands are integral to the health of the oral cavity. Saliva is extremely important for physiological maintenance of oral hygiene through its cleansing actions and its regulation of intraoral pH. It is also the lubricant for all major oral functions including swallowing and speech. Failure of secretion of these glands produces a dry mouth (**xerostomia**) which is itself an unpleasant condition but also leads to other diseases of the oral cavity, particularly infective ones, because of the lack of cleansing and buffering action of saliva. As well as difficulty with oral function, clients usually experience rampant dental caries and periodontal disease. They often have recurrent attacks of **oral thrush**, a fungal infection caused by opportunist organisms taking advantage of the disturbed oral pH.

The salivary glands may be affected by obstructive conditions, such as narrowing of the duct exits due to irritations from an ill-fitting denture or blockage by salivary calculi, small stones formed by precipitation of calcium and phosphate in saliva. **Mumps** is a viral infection of the salivary glands; they swell and become very painful due to the connective tissue capsules surrounding them, limiting their expansion. An autoimmune disease known as **Sjogren's syndrome** mainly affects middle-aged women; they also have dry eyes and rheumatoid arthritis, and this triad of symptoms is diagnostic. Radiotherapy for cancer of the head and neck frequently damages the salivary glands. However, in the majority of clients showing signs of xerostomia the causes are apparently less dramatic although their effects are not. Apparently innocuous activities such as mouth breathing may reduce saliva. Anxiety and stress also tend to reduce salivary output but the major cause is drug interaction with the autonomic nerve supply regulating salivary output.

Salivary glands receive both a sympathetic and parasympathetic supply from the autonomic nervous system. Postganglionic sympathetic nerves to structures in the head and neck originate from the ganglia of the **cervical sympathetic chain** and are distributed along blood vessels to their target organs. Parasympathetic secretomotor nerves travel with their parent nerves to the vicinity of the target organ. The parotid glands are supplied by the **glossopharyngeal nerves** and the submandibular and sublingual glands are innervated by secretomotor nerves from the **facial nerve** travelling in the **chorda tympani**. The facial nerve is also the source of postganglionic nerves to the **lacrimal glands** which secrete tears, a serous fluid which protects the conjunctiva covering the anterior aspect of the eyeball from infection. This is why dry eye may be seen alongside xerostomia.

The effects of autonomic stimulation on salivary secretion are not clear-cut. Even in the absence of nervous stimulation, there is a resting secretion of saliva. Parasympathetic activation stimulates production of a copious watery secretion of saliva. Sympathetic stimulation produces a small flow of thick saliva rich in mucins; the client will experience 'dry mouth' despite the continued secretion of very thick saliva.

Drugs which mimic the action of the sympathetic nervous system (**sympatheticomimetics**) are the major cause of xerostomia as an unwanted side-effect. Such drugs include antidepressants including mild sedatives and tranquillizers, anticonvulsants, antipsychotics, antihypertensives (to lower blood pressure) and antiarythmics (to regulate abnormal heart beat), antihistamines, decongestants and expectorants, anticancer drugs, antiparasitics and antispasmodics (used to prevent diarrhoea). This list is formidably long! It is essential during taking a case history (not just for suspected xerostomia) to ascertain what, if any, drugs and medicines your client is taking as it can affect their condition in unexpected ways and may compromise your treatment plan. At present SLTs in the UK have no powers to prescribe or alter the client's medication, so you must *always* consult the client's medical practitioner before making any comment to the client about their drug regime.

The nasal cavities

The nasal cavities are the entrance to the respiratory tract and function to warm, humidify and cleanse incoming air (see Chapter 14).

The bridge of the nose is formed by the two **nasal bones** which with the **maxillae** surround an opening known as the **anterior nasal aperture**. The rest of the nose on the face is formed by the **external nasal cartilages**. The nostrils open downwards on to the face. The nose is divided throughout its length into the left and right **nasal cavities** by a thin vertical plate of bone, the **nasal septum**, which may deviate to one side or the other. The lateral wall of each nasal cavity has three downwardly curving bony plates, the **superior, middle** and **inferior conchae**, projecting into the cavities to increase their surface area (Figure 19.16). The three conchae divide each lateral wall into four recesses. The uppermost recess is the **sphenoethmoidal recess** and the three lower ones are known as the **superior, middle** and **inferior meati**. The **inferior meatus**, below the inferior concha, contains the opening of the **nasolacrimal** duct which drains tears from the orbit to the nasal cavity. The nasal cavities are continuous posteriorly with the pharynx.

The paranasal air sinuses

The paranasal air sinuses are paired, bilateral air-filled intra-bony cavities, frequently of unequal size, within the maxillary, frontal, sphenoid and ethmoid bones. They are lined with respiratory epithelium, producing mucus which passes through openings in the lateral walls of the nose into the nasal cavities by the action of cilia on the epithelial surface. The openings of the air sinuses into the meati are illustrated in Figure 19.16.

The **maxillary sinuses** lie within the bodies of the maxillae (see Figure 5.2). Each sinus is roughly pyramidal with the base forming the lateral wall of the nose and the apex extending into the zygomatic process of the maxilla and frequently into the zygomatic bones. Its roof is the orbital plate of the maxilla and forms the floor of the orbit. The floor of the sinus is narrow, extending around the roots of the upper premolar and molar teeth in the alveolar process of the maxilla. Each maxillary sinus opening lies high up on its medial wall and drains into the middle meatus. The paired **frontal sinuses** occupy the frontal bone above the orbital margin and may extend posteriorly above the roof of the orbit (Figure 19.16). They are roughly triangular in shape and usually asymmetrically separated by a bony septum which is rarely in the midline. They drain through a duct which passes down from the floor of the sinus into the middle meatus.

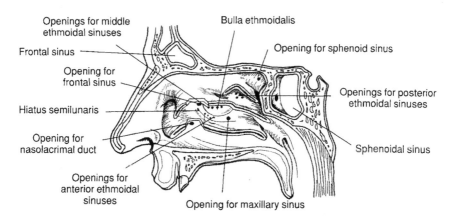

Figure 19.16 The lateral nasal wall showing the openings of the paranasal air sinuses and the location of the frontal and sphenoidal air sinuses.

The **sphenoidal sinuses** lie in the body of the sphenoid bone with a bony septum separating right and left sinuses (Figure 19.16) and open into the sphenoethmoidal recess. The **ethmoidal sinuses** or air cells are a group of small intercommunicating cavities in the ethmoid bone between the nose and the medial wall of the orbit (Figure 5.2). They are divided into anterior, middle and posterior groups. The anterior and middle groups drain into the middle meatus and the superior group drains the superior meatus respectively.

The sinuses lie outside the main airstream and therefore are not as susceptible to dehydration as is the nasal mucosa itself. Thus a supply of mucus is guaranteed under most conditions. The air-filled sinuses, along with other cavities such as the oral cavity and pharynx, add resonance to the voice, a quality which is clearly diminished when there is an upper respiratory tract infection affecting the nose and sinuses.

CHAPTER 20

Development and growth of the face and jaws

The morphology of mature tissues and organs depends upon the developmental processes which produce them and apparent illogicalities in anatomical structure can often be explained by their development. Clinically, developmental abnormalities are not uncommon. Although many of them can now be detected and corrected as a result of improved prenatal monitoring and postnatal surgery, practitioners must always bear in mind the persistent effects that some abnormalities may have on the well-being of the client. Many abnormalities have their origins very early in embryonic development; an understanding of these events as well as the development of specific areas pertinent to the practice of Speech and Language Therapy is therefore necessary.

Early embryology

Fertilization generally occurs about the middle of the menstrual cycle (approximately 14 days before the next menstrual period) and is the union of the haploid chromosomes carried in the male spermatozoon with those in the nucleus of the ovum, the female germ cell (see Chapter 2). After fertilization, events proceed remarkably rapidly. The fertilized ovum undergoes a series of rapid cell divisions to produce a ball of cells. This ball then hollows out to form a cluster of cells at one end which will form the **embryo**. This cell cluster is surrounded by an outer layer of cells which form the **placenta** by which the developing embryo is attached to the maternal circulation in the second week of pregnancy. After **implantation** of this complex in the uterine lining, during which placenta formation occurs, the embryo passes through various clearly recognizable stages.

At first only two distinct layers of cells can be recognized in the embryo, the **ectoderm** and **endoderm**. At this early stage various membranes form around the embryo, enclosing fluid in which the embryonic cell mass is bathed. Towards the end of the second week of pregnancy, a third embryonic

331

layer, the **mesoderm**, differentiates during the stage known as **gastrulation** to convert the two-layered embryo into a three-layered form. The rudimentary **nervous system** then develops during **neuralation** and with it a fourth layer of germ cells, the **neural crest** or **ectomesenchymal cells**. These events take about two and a half weeks from fertilization and this period is known as the **pre-embryonic period**. In the subsequent five and a half weeks, the **embryonic period**, the four **primitive germ layers** interact with each other in various combinations to produce the rudiments of all the body systems and organs. As these embryonic tissues begin to differentiate, they group together into identical **segments** along the craniocaudal axis of the embryo. As development proceeds, some of these segments remain distinct whereas others merge to form the limbs. The external form of the human embryo is almost completely achieved eight weeks after conception while, internally, the rudiments of all organs and systems have been laid down. Some organs develop so completely in this short period that they are indistinguishable except in size from their mature form whereas others are still rudimentary. The latter continue to differentiate and develop throughout the remaining seven months of intrauterine life, the **fetal period**, but the major activity for most organs during the rest of gestation is growth.

The most active period for formation of new tissues and organs is the first eight weeks post-conception. For two of these weeks until the first missed period, pregnancy may not even be suspected and confirmation may take an additional two weeks during which half the embryonic period has passed. During these four weeks, considerable embryonic development will have taken place but it is at this time that the embryo is most susceptible to damage by environmental factors. Two examples will illustrate the potential dangers of drug treatment and exposure to infection during the early stages of pregnancy. Thalidomide, a drug designed to relieve morning sickness in early pregnancy, turned out to be teratogenic (literally, 'monster-forming'). Women who took this drug over a very limited period gave birth to babies with serious limb malformations. Many drugs are contraindicated during pregnancy. A woman contracting rubella (German measles) during early pregnancy may experience nothing more than a high fever. Nevertheless, the developing ears of the embryo may be seriously malformed, resulting in deafness. The risk of potential damage may be minimized by immunization of young teenage girls against rubella.

The cellular basis of differentiation and development

The fertilized ovum is **totipotent**: it can produce all the diverse cell types found in the mature organism. Embryonic cells pass through a series of cell divisions becoming more specialized as they do so. As development proceeds, the types of cells which can arise from a single parent cell becomes gradually restricted. Cells which have become restricted in their expression are **pluripotent**. Eventually, cells become so highly specialized that they are capable of producing only a single cell type following division and thus become **unipotent**.

As cells become specialized to form the basic tissues, differential expression of selected genes results in the intracellular production of proteins, which in turn confer particular structural and functional characteristics on the cells (see Chapter 2). Thus, while all cells have the potential to produce all the proteins of the body, increased specialization is determined by regulation of the expression of genes. For example, as muscle cells become specialized for contraction, they produce and organize large amounts of actin and myosin in their cytoplasm. Likewise, salivary cells synthesize mucins for secretion as they become specialized for protection. Although both cell types have features in common, it is the quantity and quality of protein products which confer specificity.

The embryonic germ layers

After the pre-embryonic stage, four germ layers can be recognized in the embryo: **ectoderm**, **endoderm**, **mesoderm** and **neural crest** or **ectomesenchyme** tissue. The cells in each embryonic germ layer are pluripotential: the fate of cells is restricted to certain categories even at this early stage (Figure 20.1). Combinations of cells from different germ layers contribute to the development of different organs and systems. Ectodermal cells produce the outer layers of skin, hair and related glands as well as forming the central nervous system during neuralation. Mesodermal cells form connective tissue. Muscle, bone, cartilage, blood cells, the heart and blood vessels and the supporting fibrous framework of virtually all tissues and organs fall into this category. Endodermally-derived cells form the epithelial lining of the respiratory tract and the gastrointestinal tract. Ectomesenchyme gives rise to various elements which are widely scattered in the body but its principal derivatives are the sensory and autonomic parts of the peripheral nervous system. In the head and neck, neural crest tissue substitutes for mesoderm to produce all connective tissues except muscle which is derived from mesoderm.

Most organs and tissues contain cells derived from two or more germ layers. For example, the lining of the respiratory tract consists of an endodermal epithelium and a deeper mesodermally-derived connective tissue layer innervated by nerves derived from neural crest tissue. Thus the development of the specific cell types found in the organ systems involves the interaction of at least two of the primitive germ layers. The process of

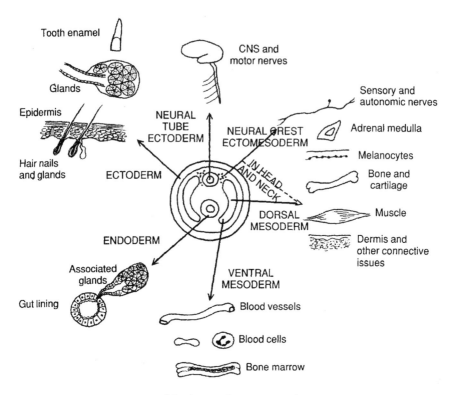

Figure 20.1 The derivations of the four embryonic germ layers.

induction is the mechanism by which one cell type can influence the developmental potential of other cells; these interactions are sometimes called epithelio-mesenchymal interactions.

The cells which arise from the successive divisions of the fertilized ovum have a surprisingly limited repertoire of behaviour and it is the regulation and coordination of this repertoire which leads to the formation of complex multicellular organisms (Figure 20.2). The behaviour of embryonic cells is not radically different from that of mature cells and similar traits are regulated by similar mechanisms.

Cell division plays an important role in the differentiation and development of embryonic tissues and continues to do so throughout subsequent fetal and postnatal growth. As organs and tissues mature, a homeostatic balance is achieved between cell replication and cell loss (see Chapter 2). **Programmed cell death** (or **apoptosis**) is also important in the formation of some organs and tissues. For instance, the cells in the luminal part of glandular ducts die and the epithelial cells covering some embryonic outgrowths die at specified times to allow the underlying

EMBRYONIC CELL

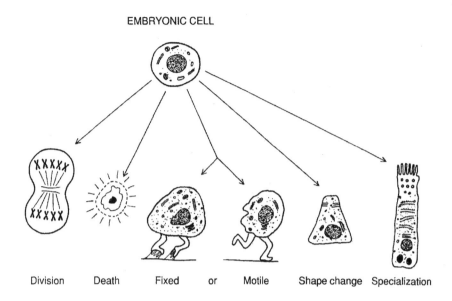

Division   Death   Fixed   or   Motile   Shape change   Specialization

Figure 20.2 The repertoire of embryonic cells.

mesodermal tissues to fuse. **Cell motility** and the **migration** of whole populations enables cells produced in one area to populate other regions. Thus embryonic gland cells proliferate and migrate into the underlying mesoderm from their origin in the ectoderm. Selective cohesion of these cells prevents them from straying from their proper location. Changes in **cell shape** help determine the morphology of particular tissues and organs. For example, columnar cells can be converted into wedge-shaped cells due to contraction of cytoskeletal components at one end of the cell; if this process is repeated throughout a sheet of epithelium, it will be converted into a tube.

The expression of the limited repertoire of developing cells is ultimately controlled through the expression of selected genes for a specific period of time. The genes can be switched on by controls within the cell or controls delivered by another cell through inductive interactions between embryonic cells. The expression of genes in an orderly sequence to produce the necessary cell behaviour in the right place at the right time produces the complete organism.

Neuralation

The formation of the central nervous system is a very significant event in the development of the embryo. Inductive interactions come into play with the dorsal mesoderm inducing changes in the overlying dorsal ectoderm (Figure 20.3). Cuboidal ectodermal cells either side of the midline of the dorsal surface of the embryo are transformed into wedge-shaped cells. As these shape changes become more emphasized across the ectodermal sheet, the sheet rolls up from either side of the midline to form two ridges which eventually make contact and merge to form the **neural tube** running along the midline from head to tail. The complete neural tube is separated from the parent ectoderm to lie within the mesoderm (Figure 20.3). Shortly after completion of the tube, the cranial end expands to form the **brain vesicles** from which the brain will develop (Figure 20.4). The most anterior vesicle is the **prosencephelon** which becomes subdivided into the **telencephalon** from which the forebrain (the cerebral hemispheres) develop; the cavity forming the vesicles remains in the mature brain as the lateral and third ventricles. A mass of

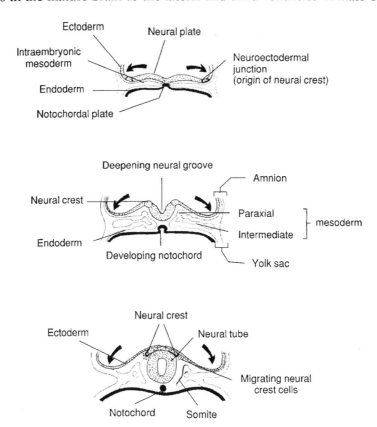

Figure 20.3 Progressive stages in the formation of the neural tube and neural crest.

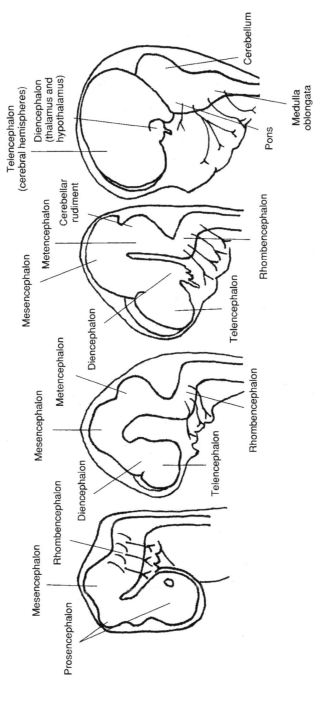

Figure 20.4 Development of the brain vesicles.

cells in the floor of the lateral ventricles develops into the basal ganglia. The **diencephalon** is the posterior part of the prosencephalon and cell masses in its wall develop into the thalamus and hypothalamus. Next is the **mesencephalon** which grows slowly compared to the other areas and forms the midbrain; the cavity survives to maturity to become the cerebral aqueduct. The most posterior brain vesicle is the **rhombencephalon** which forms the hindbrain (the pons and medulla oblongata) and the cerebellum. The rhombencephalon shows a series of transverse surface elevations called the **rhombomeres** shortly after it has formed; the rhombomeres have a profound influence on the development of the head and neck (see below). The neural tube posterior to the rhombencephalon becomes the spinal cord and the ventral cells differentiate into motor neurons innervating muscles.

As the neural tube separates from the dorsal ectoderm, the **neural crest** is formed by cells migrating from the dorsolateral area of the neural tube (Figure 20.3). They are known as **ectomesenchyme** because these cells derive from ectoderm but share some of the characteristics of both ectoderm and mesoderm. The **neural crest** contributes to a wide variety of structures and tissues. It forms the sensory and autonomic components of the peripheral nervous system, the adrenal medulla and pigment cells in the skin – melanocytes. Neural crest tissue replaces conventional mesoderm in the head and neck and in that region forms all the connective tissue elements normally derived from mesoderm with the exception of muscle. As well as these derivatives, neural crest also appears to play a significant part in the formation of other organs, possibly by induction. Some congenital birth defects affect many disparate organs and systems: for example, **di George syndrome**, characterized by malformation of the heart and absence of the thymus, important in the development of immunity, is believed to result from faulty development and migration of ectomesenchyme which therefore fails to induce changes in other tissues.

Segmentation of the embryo

The extensive mesoderm on either side of the newly formed neural tube increases in density to form a block of tissue along the length of the tube. This separates into smaller pieces which demarcate the **somites** (body segments). Somite formation begins in the cervical region and proceeds posteriorly resulting in a number of paired blocks of mesodermal tissue arranged along the dorsal midline axis of the embryo. Within each somite, further differentiation can be seen (Figure 20.5). The mesoderm destined to form skeletal elements, **sclerotomes**, can be distinguished from

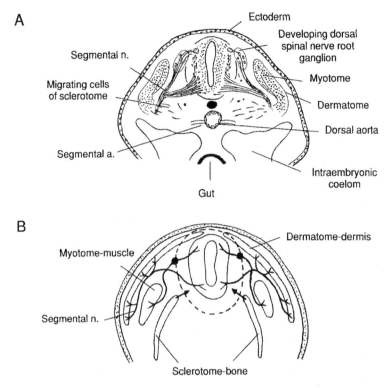

Figure 20.5 Segmentation of the embryo. (A) The internal features of a segment. (B) Further internal differentiation of a segment.

myotomes, which form muscle, and **dermatomes**, which form the dermis of the skin. In addition to the somites in each segment, there is also a segmental nerve and artery arising from corresponding segments of the spinal cord and aorta respectively. In simple animals, the segmentation is preserved as they develop further, each part of the body looking identical. In more complex animals, the segmental pattern is obscured to some extent by limb development as the derivatives of several adjacent segments merge and blend. The repetition of each segment can still be appreciated, for example, in the human thorax where disposition of vertebrae, ribs, neurovascular bundles and muscles is the same except in minor anatomical detail. Even if the segmental pattern is lost, tissues derived from the same segment remain connected even when extensive migration has occurred. The common nerve supply of structures in different locations indicates a common segmental origin. For instance, the skin of the shoulder and the diaphragm are both derived from the fourth cervical somites: both are innervated by nerves derived from that segment. The phrenic nerves to the diaphragm pass the length of the thorax from the neck to reach the muscle, indicating the route of migration of the muscle of the diaphragm during its development.

Formation of embryonic shape

Growth of the embryo is not uniform and the precocious development of some areas results in shape changes (Figure 20.6). Growth of the brain vesicles expands the head region and accentuates the fold at the neck. This folding pushes the developing heart area back beneath the head into the

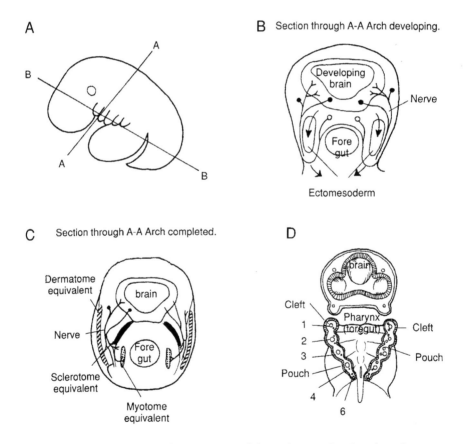

Figure 20.6 (A) The external appearance of the embryonic head at 4 weeks. (B) A section through a pharyngeal arch in the plane A-A showing the internal features of the arch. (C) Further differentiation of the arch. (D) The arches sectioned in plane B-B showing the pharyngeal clefts and pouches.

thoracic region. The endoderm thus becomes enclosed between the neural tube and cardiogenic area to form the foregut. As well as the upper portion of the gut itself, the foregut also gives rise to the lower part of the respiratory tract. An outpouching from the ventral foregut becomes the trachea and lungs. Similarly, a tail fold at the posterior end of the embryo encloses the hind portion of the endoderm to form the hind gut. These enclosed areas are formed into tubes by a combination of cell shape changes and lateral growth of the embryo which causes more pronounced curvature in the transverse axis.

Formation of the pharyngeal arches

In the cervical region of the embryo, the back of the primitive mouth cavity is continuous with the upper part of the foregut, the eventual pharynx and oesophagus. In this region mesoderm is very sparse, but neural crest tissue grows from the rhombencephalic region and migrates between the foregut tube and the ectoderm in six paired bands to form structures known as the **pharyngeal** (or branchial) **arches** (Figure 20.6). Neural crest tissue migrates laterally from the rhombomeres in the rhomben-cephalon along specific pathways such that the cells from each rhombomere do not mix; each pharyngeal arch thus becomes populated with ectomesenchyme from specific rhombomeres. The ingrowing neural crest tissue is accompanied by arteries from the primitive aorta and by nerves arising from the brainstem. As the ectomesenchymal cells migrate they create six bilateral bars of tissue around the foregut tube which eventually fuse with their opposite number in the midline to complete each arch. Between adjacent arches, the ectoderm and endoderm are almost in contact. Indeed, in animals which develop gill slits, the two layers eventually perforate. Nothing quite so dramatic occurs in human development although for some time, little intervening tissue is found at the sites of these potential gill slits, producing deep **pharyngeal clefts** on the external surface and **pharyngeal pouches** in the internal pharyngeal wall. In the arches themselves, the ectomesenchyme differentiates into connective tissue precursors, analogous to those formed in the somitic mesoderm. The pharyngeal arches play a significant role in the development of the craniofacial complex (see below).

Derivatives of the pharyngeal arches

Each pair of arches consists of an **ectomesenchymal** core covered by **ectoderm** externally and lined by **endoderm** internally (Figure 20.7). Within the ectomesenchymal core, separate tissue blocks can be recognized which eventually give rise to muscle, dermis and skeletal components. In addition, an artery and a nerve runs along each arch. The

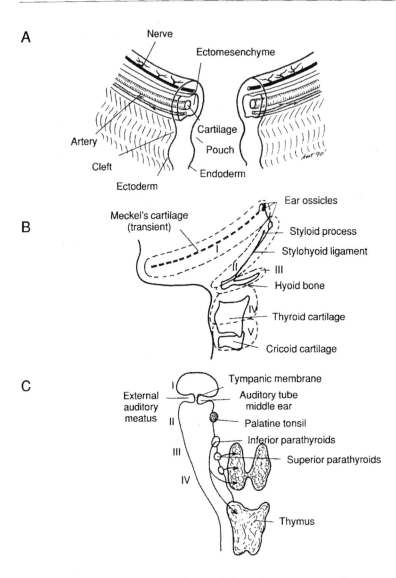

Figure 20.7 The pharyngeal arches and their derivatives. (A) The structure of the pharyngeal arches. (B) The skeletal derivatives. (C) The pharyngeal pouches and clefts.

fate of the muscular and dermal components and the nerve are inextricably linked as the muscles and mucosa carry their nerve supply with them wherever they migrate. The fate of blood vessels and skeletal ectomesenchyme is not so clearly defined.

The **muscles of mastication** are derived from the first (**mandibular**) arch along with the anterior belly of the digastric, mylohyoid and tensor veli palatini muscles. All of these muscles are supplied by the **mandibular division** of the trigeminal nerve, the nerve of the first arch. The covering ectoderm and lining endoderm become the skin overlying the mandible and the oral mucosa of the floor of the mouth and tongue and are similarly innervated. Muscle from the second (**hyoid**) arch migrates cranially to become the **muscles of facial expression** taking with them the nerve of the second arch, the **facial nerve**. Only one insignificant muscle is derived from the third (**glossopharyngeal**) arch but a considerable area of lingual and pharyngeal mucosa derives from this arch and hence is innervated by the **glossopharyngeal nerve**. The lower three arches never become clearly recognizable external features in the human embryo and the precise derivatives of each arch are uncertain. Nevertheless, the muscles of the larynx, pharynx and palate derive from these arches and are innervated by the pharyngeal and laryngeal branches of the **vagus nerve** which innervate the lower arches.

The skeletal components of each pharyngeal arch are cartilaginous initially although some components are converted to bone later in development. A transitory cartilage, **Meckel's cartilage**, arises in the first arch but is resorbed as the mandibular bone develops. The posterior tip of Meckel's cartilage remains and forms two of the ear ossicles, the **malleus** and **incus**. The remaining ossicle, the **stapes**, is formed from part of the second arch cartilage. The skeletal elements derived from the lower arches are the styloid process, hyoid bone and laryngeal cartilages. The styloid process ossifies in the second arch cartilage and the **hyoid bone** is formed from contributions from the second and third arch cartilage. The **laryngeal cartilages** are derivatives of the cartilages of the lower arches.

Most of the arteries are transitory structures and the contribution of these embryonic arteries to the mature cardiovascular system, if any, is not obvious. The third arch arteries become the subclavian arteries and the left fourth arch artery forms the aortic arch which accounts for the difference in levels at which the recurrent laryngeal nerves branch from the vagus nerves on each side.

The **clefts** and **pouches** which are formed between adjacent arches also contribute something to the adult form. The first cleft remains and is progressively deepened to form the **external auditory meatus** by outgrowth of the mandibular arch above and second arch below as they form the auricle. The second arch ectoderm extends caudally to overgrow and obliterate the clefts of the lower arch. Internally, the first and second pouches combine to form the tubotympanic recess which becomes the **middle ear** and **auditory tube**. Part of this recess is invaded by lymphoid tissue later in development to form the **pharyngeal tonsil**. The lower pouches differentiate into parathyroid tissue and the thymus.

Developmental anomalies of the pharyngeal arches

Like any other components of the embryo, the pharyngeal arches can be affected by developmental disturbances of various sorts. A group of syndromes are characterized as **first arch deformities** because the major effect is on derivatives of the mandibular arch and its associated structures. It is difficult to be categorical about the many syndromes which fall into this category because they are comparatively rare and show a wide range of defects often in structures derived from other parts of the developing embryo. Nevertheless, some common characteristics can be found. The mandible is usually under-developed (**micrognathia**); this leads to dental malocclusion (see Chapter 19) and problems with creating lip seals which in turn affects the articulation of various phonemes such as bilabial and labiodental sounds. If the lower jaw is narrow, this prevents the tongue descending into the floor of the mouth at the correct time which, in turn, prevents palatal fusion resulting in cleft palate (see below). The posterior part of the first arch cartilage develops into the malleus and incus: if these fail to develop or are malformed, there is usually some degree of conductive deafness (see Chapter 23). The external ear is usually malformed and may show bizarre forms: epithelial tags, extra bits of external ear, are often present. Surprisingly, the nerves and muscles are very rarely affected.

Two examples of first arch deformities will serve to illustrate some of the common features and also the wide range of signs and symptoms which may be associated with them. **Mandibulofacial dysostosis** (Treacher-Collins syndrome) manifests as hypoplasia of the mandible and also the zygomatic bones, dental malocclusion and deformed external ears. Children born with **Pierre-Robin syndrome** exhibit extreme mandibular hypoplasia, cleft palate and defects of the eye and ear; in the early stages they also tend to respiratory distress because the tongue is displaced backwards interfering with the airway. In some other manifestations of first arch disorders, the external auditory meatus fails to develop with obvious effects on hearing.

Further development

The impression created thus far is of an orderly series of events following on one from the other and this is the case in the early embryonic stages as the germ layers and the neural tube form. Once these basic tissues have differentiated, the formation of different organs and systems proceeds at different rates; some may be quite advanced before others even begin to form. Four weeks' post-conception, a primitive circulatory system centred on the cardiogenic area is established, the heart itself begins to develop within the cardiogenic area and the gut tube is formed as the configuration of the embryo changes and its curvature becomes more pronounced. While the formation of these well-defined systems is occurring, the muscles and skeletal components of the locomotor system are differentiating within the somites and similar processes in the pharyngeal arches produce the corresponding components in the head and neck.

Thus, within four weeks, the major components of the nervous system are formed, the gastrointestinal tract is mapped out, the cardiovascular system has developed extensively and the body segments have differentiated along with the pharyngeal arches of the lower face and neck. In the second half of the embryonic period, these various systems develop more fully and the rudiments of specific bones, muscles and blood vessels are formed. Externally the embryo becomes human in appearance with the development of the limbs and the external features of the face.

Some of the major events in the formation of the embryo are given in Table 20.1 to place events in their relative time scale.

Table 20.1

First week post-conception
Rapid division of fertilized ovum; cells in contact with uterine wall.

Second week
Implantation; formation of placenta; bilaminar embryo.

Third week
Mesoderm and cardiogenic area form; neural tube formation starts; head fold and tail fold begin to enclose endoderm.

Fourth week
Neural tube closes; primary brain vesicles arise; limb buds appear; heart present as a tube; pharyngeal arches complete; outgrowth of foregut to form lower respiratory tract.

Fifth week
Further development of the brain and peripheral nerves; lung buds appear; heart is divided internally.

Sixth week
Bone formation starts.

Seventh week
Heart formation is complete; skeletal muscle differentiates; external features of embryo established.

Craniofacial development

By the time the craniofacial complex begins its development, the embryo has reached the stage of development described above for the fourth week post-fertilization. The folding of the head and tail has taken place, segmentation is in progress and limb development has begun. The central nervous system has developed precociously, producing a prominent head fold (Figure 20.8). The **pharyngeal arches** now develop as ectomesodermal neural crest tissue invades the cervical region between the ectoderm and the foregut endoderm. As the pharyngeal arches grow around the foregut, they protrude considerably beyond the buccopharyngeal membrane creating a slit between the upper aspect of the first pharyngeal arch and the ectoderm covering the developing brain. This slit is called the primitive mouth cavity or **stomodeum** and the buccopharyngeal membrane forms its posterior wall (Figure 20.9). As well as invading the cervical area to form the pharyngeal arches, ectomesoderm also invades between the developing brain and the covering ectoderm to form a bulge above the stomodeum known as the **frontonasal process** (Figure 20.9).

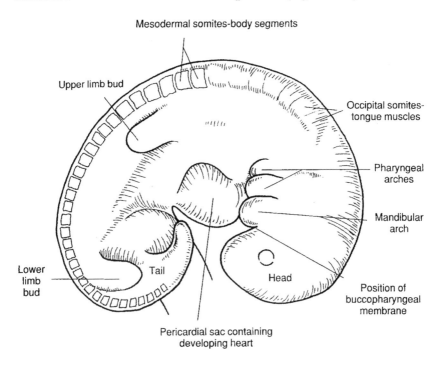

Figure 20.8 The external appearance of the embryo at three and a half weeks' postconception.

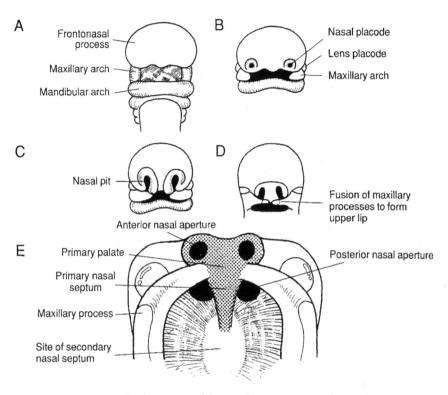

Figure 20.9 (A)–(D) The formation of the nasal pits, primary palate and nasal septum and upper lip. (E) The primary palate and primary nasal septum from the oral aspect.

From these seemingly unpromising beginnings, the contours of the face are formed and separate oral and nasal cavities are produced in somewhat less than a month. Because of this compressed timescale, many things happen simultaneously which if described together can be difficult to follow. An outline of craniofacial development is presented first followed by more detailed consideration of some of the individual events.

Development of the nasal cavities begins first and partial separation of the oral and nasal cavities is achieved by the **primary palate** shortly afterwards. Simultaneously, the tongue develops in the floor of the mouth and occupies virtually all of the oronasal cavities. The **maxillary arches**, which form the cheeks and upper lips, also develop at this time. The separation of the nasal cavities from each other and from the oral cavities is completed by outgrowths from the maxillary arches. The **tectoseptal processes** complete the nasal septum and the **palatal processes** complete the palate. These processes fuse with each other to separate the various cavities and similar fusions take place externally to form the features of the face. Differential growth of the brain and eyes exerts pressure on the more slowly developing face to mould its external contours. Differentiation of ectomesenchymal tissues into bone and muscle completes the structure of the different regions of the craniofacial complex.

Formation of the primary nasal cavities

At the beginning of the fifth week *in utero*, ectodermal thickenings appear on the frontonasal process. One pair of thickenings, the **nasal placodes**, arise anteriorly and a second pair, the **lens placodes**, arise laterally (Figure 20.9). The nasal placodes come to lie very deeply in the frontonasal process by continued proliferation of neural crest tissue in the frontonasal processes and any active erosion of the underlying ectomesoderm by the nasal placodes; they eventually differentiate into olfactory epithelium. The invagination of the nasal placodes into the frontonasal process produces two pronounced pits on its inferior aspect which are the **primitive nasal cavities**. The tissue separating the two grooves is the **primary nasal septum** and this extends horizontally at its inferior border as the **primary palate** which separates the primary nasal cavities from the stomodeum. The primary nasal cavities open into the stomodeum posteriorly.

The maxillary arches

As the primary nasal cavities form, the stomodeum is transformed from a slit to a cavity by the addition of side walls. These are formed by the **maxillary arches**, which arise as outgrowths from the posterosuperior aspects of the mandibular arches (Figure 20.9). The maxillary arches grow forward between the mandibular arches and the frontonasal process. As their forward growth continues, the upper aspect of each maxillary arch meets the tissues around the nasal pits. This part of the frontonasal process is thus subject to pressure from either side by the encroaching maxillary processes and by the enlarging lens placode lying further laterally. The result is that the area between the primary nasal cavities is pushed into prominence, beginning to form the contour of the external nose.

The maxillary processes were once thought to compress the section of the frontonasal process enclosed between them to form the philtrum while the maxillary processes formed the lateral 'cupid's bow' of the upper lip. It now appears that the maxillary processes grow forward to pass in front of the primary palate formed by the frontonasal process to meet in the midline. The maxillary processes thus form the entire upper lip. As the orbicularis orbis muscle differentiates within the lips a muscle-deficient area is left centrally which becomes the philtrum.

Formation of the secondary nasal septum

The next stage of orofacial development is the completion of the partition of the oral and nasal cavities and of the two nasal cavities (Figure 20.10). A process from the upper medial aspect of each maxillary process grows between the inferior aspect of the developing brain and the roof of the stomodeum to form the tectoseptal processes. The two processes fuse in the midline and grow down behind the primary nasal septum to form the **secondary nasal septum** to complete the separation of the two nasal cavities from each other.

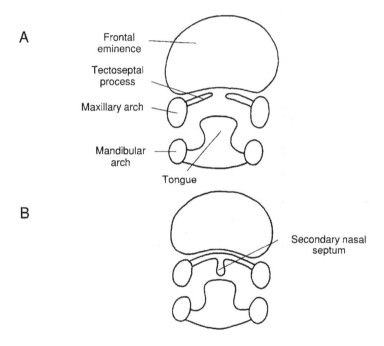

A

Frontal eminence

Tectoseptal process

Maxillary arch

Mandibular arch

Tongue

B

Secondary nasal septum

Figure 20.10 The formation of the secondary nasal septum.

Formation of the tongue

The tongue has an important influence on subsequent events leading to the separation of the oral and nasal cavities. The mucosa of the tongue develops from the ventral endoderm of the foregut lining the anterior internal aspects of the pharyngeal arches (Figure 20.11). These endodermal outpouchings are subsequently invaded by muscle.

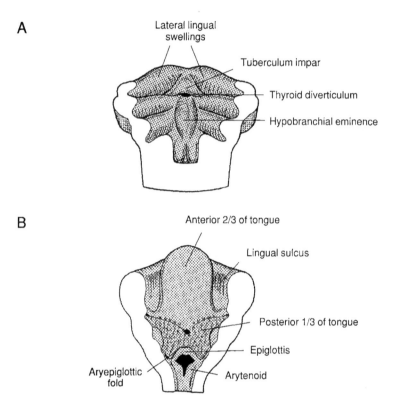

Figure 20.11 The development of the tongue. (A) The processes contributing to the mucosa of the dorsum of the tongue. (B) Their contribution to the mature tongue.

Tongue development begins very early, even before the pharyngeal arches have fused anteriorly. A small swelling, the **tuberculum impar** or **median tongue bud**, at the level of the second arch, is the first part of the tongue to develop. A pair of swellings, the **lateral lingual swellings**, develop from the endoderm overlying the first arch in the floor of the stomodeum shortly afterwards. As they enlarge, they fuse with the tuberculum impar. Somewhat later, another swelling, the **hypobranchial eminence**, appears behind the anterior structures at the level of the third arch and is separated from them by a pronounced groove, the **sulcus terminalis**. In the adult, the groove still persists as the sulcus terminalis between the anterior two-thirds and posterior one-third of the tongue (see Chapter 19).

Muscle derived from the **occipital myotomes**, which are additional segments just above the cervical somites, invades the tongue early in the second month of development. Developing muscle cells stream into the floor of the mouth and invade the endodermal outpouchings to form the muscles of the tongue so that the tongue fills the oronasal cavity (Figure 20.10). The endoderm differentiates into the specialized gustatory mucosa of the tongue. The occipital myotomes bring their nerve supply, the hypoglossal nerves, with them.

The complex derivation of the tongue explains its correspondingly complex innervation from so many different sources (see Figure 19.10). The anterior epithelium developing over the first arch is innervated by nerves from that arch, the mandibular division of the trigeminal. Likewise, the derivation of posterior epithelium of the tongue from the third arch explains its innervation by the glossopharyngeal nerve which is the neural element of that arch. The muscles are innervated by the hypoglossal nerves.

Formation of the secondary palate

About six weeks' post-fertilization, medially-directed outgrowths known as the **palatal shelves** arise from the lower medial aspect of each maxillary process (Figure 20.12). Because the developing tongue is so large and the mandibular arch comparatively narrow at this stage, the tongue occupies the whole of the oronasal cavities and deflects the palatal shelves downwards on either side of the tongue.

By eight weeks, the mandibular arch enlarges considerably, allowing the tongue to drop into the floor of the mouth between the body of the forming mandible. The mandible and tongue also move forward to align with the growing maxillary arch, thus vacating the upper part of the oronasal cavity. At this point, the palatal shelves abruptly change their orientation from vertical to horizontal and meet each other in the midline. Their anterior edges meet the posterior edge of the primary palate to complete the roof of the mouth.

Palatal elevation – the movement of the shelves from the vertical to the horizontal – was thought until recently to be due to the release of restraint imposed by the tongue as the tongue dropped clear of the shelves. Recent experimental evidence has shown that depression of the tongue before the normal time does not result in palatal shelf elevation. However, elevation occurs extremely rapidly at the appropriate time suggesting that factors within the shelves determine elevation. Glycosaminoglycans (GAGs) accumulate in the extracellular matrix of the ectomesenchyme of the shelves just before palatal elevation takes place; GAGs are hydrophilic and attract water which renders the shelves turgid and prompts their elevation.

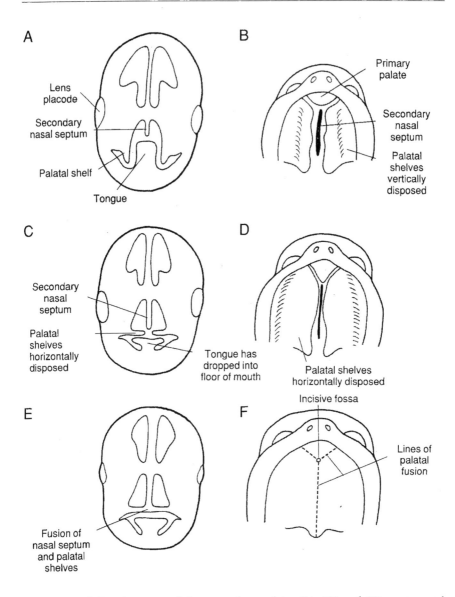

Figure 20.12 Development of the secondary palate. (A), (C) and (E) are coronal sections and (B), (D) and (F) show the sequence of events viewed from the oral aspect.

By the time palatal shelf elevation has occurred, the secondary nasal septum has elongated sufficiently for the three processes to converge at the midline of the palate. Nevertheless, the processes are still separated from each other and adjacent processes by small gaps and must fuse before partition of the various cavities is complete. Fusion entails contact of the ectodermal covering of the processes followed by its removal to allow the ectomesenchymal cores to merge. The ectodermal covering forming the medial edge epithelium carries attachment molecules on its surface. These will only attach to like molecules and the cells covering the palatal and tectoseptal processes will not adhere to epithelium in other parts of the oral cavity. If the fusing processes are misaligned, the epithelium covering each one will not adhere. Adhesion is vital because once it occurs, the medial edge epithelium breaks down and dies by apoptosis to allow fusion of the underlying ectomesenchyme to occur. The epithelium on the oral side of the shelves differentiates into oral epithelium and that on the nasal side differentiates into respiratory epithelium. The cause of programmed epithelial cell death is not fully understood but its timing is determined by the underlying ectomesoderm.

Palatal fusion begins about ten weeks post-conception midway along the junction of the palatal processes and spreads anteriorly and posteriorly to complete fusion of the two palatine shelves with each other and with the primary palate. The palatine shelves also fuse with the downgrowing secondary nasal septum. Almost as soon as palatal elevation has taken place, bone formation begins in the lateral parts of the palate and spreads medially. Posteriorly, however, the palate is invaded by developing muscle from the adjacent fourth pharyngeal arch which differentiate to form most of the muscles of the soft palate.

External changes in the orofacial complex

Over the four weeks during which palate formation takes place, much occurs externally. The brain and the eyes grow precociously, pushing the frontonasal process and other parts of the orofacial complex towards the midline initiating some of the facial contours. Most significantly, the eyes move during this time to lie anteriorly as they are displaced forward due to brain development. Where the different processes meet externally, fusion similar to that described in the palate takes place although no adjustment of position of the processes relative to each other is necessary; fusion occurs by epithelial breakdown. Fusion of the upper border of the maxillary processes and the lateral border of the frontonasal process takes place along a line running from the medial canthus of the eye down between the junction of the nose and cheek and between the philtrum and lateral part of the lip. Similarly, the lower border of the maxillary processes and upper border of the mandibular processes fuse except where the lips differentiate.

Abnormalities of facial development

Failure of coordinated growth of the different processes forming the orofacial complex results in inappropriate fusion or even failure of fusion of processes (Figure 20.13). This produces a **cleft** with some measure of deformity of the facial contours. Similarly, failure of ectodermal breakdown leads to persistent clefts between adjacent correctly aligned processes. Similar abnormalities occur after failure of palatal shelf elevation.

The persistent clefts lie along the lines of potential fusion between the embryonic processes and the abnormalities are named according to their location. By far the commonest defects are clefts of the lips and palate. At one extreme, this may be a bilateral facial cleft running down from the medial canthus of the eye along the lines of fusion of the maxillary and frontonasal processes, between the philtrum and lateral parts of the upper lip, across the alveolar ridges approximately between the lateral incisor and canine teeth, between the junction of the primary palate and palatal shelves and finally down the midline of the palate to the uvula. At the other extreme, cleft palate may be nothing more than a few minute canals lined by epithelium (oronasal fistulae) along the palatal fusion lines where ectodermal breakdown is incomplete. The extent of cleft lip and palate may be anywhere between these extremes and, anteriorly, may be

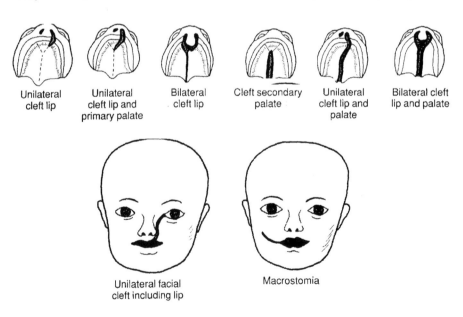

Unilateral cleft lip

Unilateral cleft lip and primary palate

Bilateral cleft lip

Cleft secondary palate

Unilateral cleft lip and palate

Bilateral cleft lip and palate

Unilateral facial cleft including lip

Macrostomia

Figure 20.13 Clefts of the palate, lips and face.

unilateral or bilateral. Apart from the disfigurement resulting from these abnormalities, failure of partition of the nasal and oral cavities produces difficulties in suckling, mastication and swallowing as food finds its way into the nasal cavities. Difficulties with speech also arise. Isolated facial clefts between the maxillary and frontonasal processes are surprisingly rare and are usually associated with cleft lip and palate. Failure of fusion of the maxillary and mandibular processes results in an enlarged mouth, a condition known as **macrostomia**. Conversely, sometimes fusion proceeds too far producing a small mouth or **microstomia**.

Cleft palate alone occurs in one in every 2500 live births and has a greater incidence in females. **Combined cleft lip and palate** is more frequent, with estimates varying between 1 in 800 and 1 in 1000 live births; combined defects are commoner in males. There is no clear-cut genetic pattern to facial abnormalities although the risk is increased significantly in subsequent children born to the same parents of an affected child. If, on the other hand, one parent was born with a cleft deformity, the chances of offspring having a deformity rise to between 1 in 6 and 1 in 8. Recent studies of familial cleft palate indicate that a portion of the X chromosome could be responsible for the underlying genetic defect. Clefts are also found in various other rare genetic abnormalities where the cleft is but one of the manifestations.

The treatment of cleft palate is complex and takes a considerable time. The sooner the treatment is started, the better the prognosis. Cleft deformities should be detected as part of extensive neonatal screening procedures so that treatment can be started almost immediately. As soon as possible after the cleft deformity is detected, orthodontic appliances are fitted to bring the cleft together. Primary repair of cleft lip is usually undertaken about three months postnatally. At about two years of age, palatal repair is carried out by using flaps cut from the nasal mucosa above and the lateral parts of the palatal mucosa below to bridge the gaps and form a soft tissue repair. The soft palate is usually repaired later by suturing a flap of mucosa taken from the posterior pharynx across the defect. Bony defects which still persist can be repaired in early adolescence by the insertion of bone grafts. Surgical and orthodontic treatment is usually required to correct the severe dental malocclusions which occur as a result of the palatal clefts. Treatment starting soon after birth often continues until adulthood.

The development and growth of the skull and jaws

As soon as the somite stage of the embryo is completed, skeletal elements begin to differentiate in various areas of the craniofacial complex and their subsequent development and growth takes place as the differentiation of soft tissues proceed.

The skull may be considered as three interdependent parts, known as the neurocranium, viscerocranium and basicranium. The **neurocranium** comprises the curved bones housing the brain. The **viscerocranium** is the bones forming the facial skeleton around the nasal cavities and roof of the mouth, often referred to in surgical terms as **the middle third of the face**; the mandible is also part of the viscerocranium. The **basicranium** (or chondrocranium) is formed by the complex bones which form the floor of the cranial cavities. The viscerocranium, the bones of the facial skeleton, derives from the ectomesenchyme of the pharyngeal arches. The development and growth of the skull and jaw bones is intimately linked to the tissues and organs they enclose which constitute functional matrices. A **functional matrix** is a tissue, organ or space which determines the detailed shape of a particular bone by influencing its growth and subsequent maintenance. Some of the larger functional matrices are in their turn influenced by more general factors affecting bone and tissue growth.

Influences on growth

Growth of different constituents of the body is not uniform. The general growth pattern exhibited by the external configuration of the trunk and limbs and followed by most organs and viscera is called the **somatic growth pattern** (Figure 20.14). There is rapid growth after birth which levels off until the pubertal growth spurt about 12–14 years of age. In contrast, the central nervous system and special senses follow the **neural growth pattern**. They grow at a precocious rate and complete most of their growth by about six or seven years.

Genetic determination and timing of growth underlie these growth patterns but they are subject to modification by a variety of general factors such as hormonal influences, nutritional status, disease and socio-economic factors. These general factors tend to affect overall growth. Thus, delay in sex hormone secretion, and hence puberty, will slow somatic growth. Functional matrices, on the other hand, have limited local effects.

Because the underlying tissues have a profound influence on the overlying bones, the bones of the skull will grow at different rates; those overlying the brain and surrounding the eyes will follow the neural growth pattern and those of the viscerocranium will follow the somatic growth pattern. The basicranium grows at an intermediate rate to coordinate the growth of the neurocranium and viscerocranium. It is these different growth rates which explain the relative proportions of the head in babies,

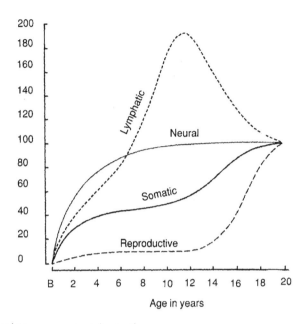

Figure 20.14 Human postnatal growth curves.

children, juveniles and adults. All babies appear to have huge appealing
eyes, big heads and tiny faces. The neurocranium has grown to about 60
per cent of its adult size at birth whereas the viscerocranium has
achieved only about 40 per cent of its adult size; about half the height of
the skull is neurocranium and half is viscerocranium. The proportions
change during infancy as the facial skeleton grows to support the teeth
and the growth of the brain ceases. By the age of ten, the neurocranium
has grown to about 95 per cent of its adult size and the viscerocranium to
about 65 per cent; the viscerocranium therefore accounts for a propor-
tionately larger percentage of facial height. This continues throughout
puberty until adult proportions are achieved on maturity when the neurocranium accounts for about one-third of skull height and the
viscerocranium for about two-thirds. The growth of the skull and jaws also
affects the size of the mouth and position of the tongue and soft palate and
therefore influences the range of potential articulatory movements in
infancy.

Development of the neurocranium

The brain and the eyes are the chief functional matrices influencing the
neurocranium. These structures follow the neural growth pattern and are

quite large by birth and almost adult size by the tenth year. Bone formation begins at ossification centres more or less in the middle of the adult bone. Bone grows outwards from the ossification centres until the bones contact each other at the sites where sutures are formed. Where more than two bones contribute to the sutures, spacing tends to be wider leaving large areas of fibrous tissue between the bones called **fontanelles** (Figure 20.15). The **anterior fontanelle** lies at the junction between the frontal and parietal bones; the **posterior fontanelle** is formed where the parietal and occipital bones meet. The paired **anterolateral** and **postero-lateral fontanelles** lie at the meeting of the various bones forming the lateral walls of the skull. Sutures contain osteogenic cells within the fibrous tissue separating the bones which can differentiate to form bone. The impetus for growth appears to be the tensing of the suture as the bones are forced apart by expansion of the underlying brain and eyes. Unlike the close interdigitation of the mature bones, the sutures are straight-edged at birth which allows the bones to move relative to each other during birth itself. Shortly after birth, the bones begin to interdigitate and the fontanelles decrease in area. The posterior and anterolateral fontanelles close within three months of birth and the lateral fontanelles after a year whereas the anterior fontanelle persists until well into the second year of life.

The role of the brain as a functional matrix is dramatically demonstrated in such conditions as **hydrocephaly** where accumulation of excess cerebrospinal fluid in the ventricles of the brain causes excessive expansion of the brain. The neurocranium is enlarged and the bones are extremely thin in such cases. Conversely, **microcephaly** or **anencephaly**,

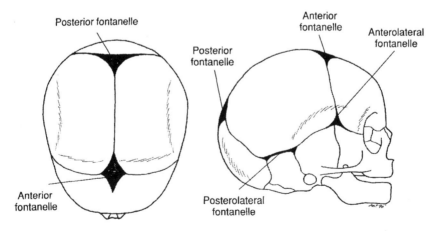

Figure 20.15 The fontanelles of the neurocranium.

in which the forebrain fails to develop properly, result in a cranial vault of greatly reduced size giving the appearance of a flat skull behind the facial skeleton.

Development of the basicranium

The **nasal capsule** is a complex cartilage which develops around the forming nasal cavities but is not fully developed until about three months post-conception. The **otic capsule** forms around the developing ear and the petrous temporal bone develops from it. The cartilaginous bones of the basicranium predominantly follow the neural growth pattern but continue enlarging after seven years to accommodate the growing nose and facial skeleton anteriorly and the nasopharynx in the midzone. Cartilaginous joints form between individual bones and are growth sites for the basicranium. The growth capacity of these joints appears to be largely independent of functional matrices. Many of these joints are transient but some persist, notably the joint between the body of the sphenoid and the occipital bone, where growth continues until 12–14 years of age. Growth in width of the basicranium occurs in the early postnatal years to coordinate with neural growth and takes place mainly at sutures placed laterally between neurocranium and basicranium. Deficiency in cartilaginous growth produces a small basicranium in comparison to the neurocranium and viscerocranium. As a result, the basicranium is shorter than normal and the middle third of the face is not as prominent as the forehead and mandible, producing a typical dish-shaped face as seen, for example, in achondroplasiac dwarfs.

Development of the viscerocranium

The eyes, frontal lobes and adjoining neurocranium follow the neural growth pattern and cause lateral expansion of the upper facial skeleton. Eye growth also has the effect of pushing the maxilla downwards. The developing teeth begin to grow significantly around the fourth month post-conception and act as a functional matrix for the lower parts of the maxilla and palatine bones, in particular causing the palate to deepen and the alveolar ridges to develop. As the maxillary sinuses begin to develop as outgrowths of the nasal cavities around five months' post-conception, a significant amount of internal resorption takes place. The brain also influences longitudinal growth of the mid-facial bones by carrying them forward as the frontal bone of the brain enlarges the anterior cranial fossa.

By birth, the precocious neurocranial growth makes the middle third of the face look relatively small compared with its adult dimensions: in particular, the face lacks height. However, the action of two functional matrices soon alter these proportions. The deciduous teeth develop and erupt soon after birth (see Chapter 19), promoting growth of the alveolar ridges as well as adding the bulk of their crowns to facial height. In addition, the maxillary sinuses continue to enlarge by stimulating internal resorption of the maxillary and zygomatic bones, which is compensated for by external deposition thus adding to facial height. By the age of ten, neural influences on the facial skeleton have more or less ceased but dental and general influences continue. Eruption of the permanent dentition stimulates further growth of the maxilla and the pubertal growth spurt affecting all the facial bones promotes further growth, allowing room for eruption of the second and third molar teeth during early and late puberty respectively

The mandible

At birth, the configuration of the mandible is quite different from the adult morphology. The chin is not prominent, the alveolar portion is scant and the angle of ramus to the body is obtuse, with the condylar head pointing backwards (Figure 20.16). The shape is modified into the adult form by the action of several functional matrices. Activity in the muscles of mastication and suprahyoid muscles plays a significant part prenatally: jaw movement can be detected in the fetus about five months' *in utero*. The temporomandibular joint also acts as a functional matrix in the condylar area. The teeth form the matrix for the alveolar ridge. In addition, the spaces of the oral cavity and oropharynx play some part as does the all-pervading influence of the brain.

As the teeth of the deciduous dentition erupt and complete their development in the first three postnatal years, the alveolar processes of the mandible increase in size adding bone to the mandible and also increasing total facial height. As the teeth of both jaws erupt and establish occlusion, adjustments are made to the angle between the body and ramus to maintain the appropriate occlusal plane by reducing the obliquity of the angle. As the deciduous dentition becomes functional, dietary changes are introduced which require more muscular effort stimulating hypertrophy of muscles which hence exert more force on their areas of attachment. Growth in width of the mandible is most pronounced early in life to enable the condyles to keep pace with the glenoid cavities on the temporal bone as they are pushed apart by the developing brain. Changes in width are restricted to the ramus and condylar parts of the mandible. The anterior dental arches show comparatively little change, probably because of the constant size of the teeth. The pubertal growth spurt promotes general growth of the viscerocranium including the mandible and

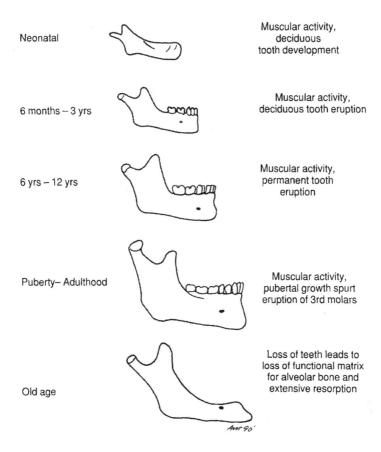

Figure 20.16 The postnatal growth of the mandible and changes in edentulous individuals.

attached muscles which leads to increased activity of the functional matrices. This growth allows space for eruption of the second and third molars as length of the mandible increases.

Influences of craniofacial growth on the oral cavity

Acquisition of language and speech is a complex topic outside the scope of this book. However, some aspects of craniofacial growth do influence the development of speech but this is an area which is significantly under-researched. By 18 months, a child should have acquired the rudiments of speech and should be able to utter several words and be beginning to string them together into phrases. It appears that consonants articulated at the back of the mouth are mastered first whereas vowels are acquired from front to back. There are several anatomical reasons for this pattern.

In a newborn infant, the larynx is very high compared to its adult position (see Chapter 16). The cricoid cartilage is about the level of the third cervical vertebra and the hyoid bone is high up under the tongue. As a result, the large tongue is also high filling the oral cavity and protruding to rest on the lower lip. The tongue is also in contact with the soft palate posteriorly which limits the range of depression of the soft palate. Because of the size of the tongue, babies are obligate nose breathers as the oral cavity is all but occluded by the tongue. It is only during crying, and to a lesser extent during suckling, that the mouth is opened but even then the only area in which the tongue can change its position significantly is in the oropharyngeal region. Crying, often regarded as a necessary evil by parents, is in fact beneficial to development of speech because, during crying, respiration assumes a more speech-like pattern with rapid inspiration and prolonged expiration.

At about three months of age, the baby should be able to hold its head up unsupported. This is due to increasing strength in the neck muscles and their action alters the curvature of the cervical part of the vertebral column. Prenatally and for the first three months the whole vertebral column is concave anteriorly. As the baby acquires head support, the cervical part of the column becomes concave posteriorly which may, in part, account for the descent of the larynx to nearer its adult position in relation to the cervical vertebrae.

From about 4 months' postnatally, the facial skeleton increases in height corresponding with the eruption of the deciduous teeth beginning at about six months (see Chapter 19). The tongue thus has more room to manoeuvre. Some vowel sounds can be recognized and some posterior velar consonants may also be discerned. As the deciduous teeth continue to erupt the mandible and maxillae increase in height and the palate assumes its vaulted shape producing even more room for tongue movement. As the child acquires its deciduous teeth, its diet changes from liquid to semi-solids and solid food. The muscles of facial expression are vital for efficient suckling but as the role of food intake is assumed by the muscles of mastication, the muscles of facial expression are emancipated from their purely feeding role and can therefore be used more for facial expression and articulation.

Abnormalities of visceral craniofacial growth

Craniofacial growth abnormalities may arise at any time during the embryological development and subsequent growth of the face. The aetiology of most conditions is unknown but may relate to malpositioning and maldevelopment of neural crest tissue although some craniofacial malformations are genetically linked or are manifestations of systemic defects in bone formation.

Malformations of the middle third of the face include **mandibulofacial dysostosis** (Treacher-Collins Syndrome), in which the zygomatic bones are abnormally small or absent producing sunken cheeks, **Down's Syndrome**, in which the nasal bones and maxillae are reduced in size producing a saddle nose and narrow face, and **hypertelorism**, in which the interocular distance is abnormally wide.

Changes in the skull and jaws after cessation of growth

A careful distinction should be made between changes which result from the ageing process directly and those which occur as a consequence of pathologies which produce their main effects in later life. The loss of teeth and, hence, functional matrices supporting the alveolar components of the jaws was almost inevitable in middle and old age decades ago, but now there is no reason why teeth should not be preserved throughout life and the profile of the facial contours maintained. However, there are some age changes in bone in general which apply equally to the skull and mandible. **Osteoporosis**, loss and thinning of bone, occurs in old age but may be related to hormonal changes as it is particularly prevalent in post-menopausal women. Osteoporosis predisposes to fractures in the elderly in normally robust bones like the femur but can affect all bones. Disuse atrophy of bones may also occur in old age as a general decrease in activity of many elderly people takes place, but it is less marked in the skull and jaws because sedentary and bedridden people still eat.

Although dental health is improving markedly, many people still lose their teeth at a relatively early age. In such edentulous patients, characteristic changes occur in the tooth-bearing bones (Figure 20.16). Alveolar bone is also lost altering the profile of the bones. Consequent upon the loss of alveolar bone, the mandibular profile returns to something like its neonatal appearance. The alveolar profile is lost in the incisive area resulting in a prominent chin beneath sunken-in lips, and the angle of the mandible becomes more obtuse as occlusal height is lost. Alveolar bone in the maxilla is lost resulting in a shallower palatal vault but is not as marked as bone loss in the mandible.

These changes present problems and a challenge for the provision of well-fitting and stable dentures as there is very little ridge to fit a denture upon. For example, in lower dentures margins may well encroach on to muscular tissue, particularly the mylohyoid and temporalis muscles, resulting in either soreness of the intervening mucosa or displacement of the denture during mandibular movements and swallowing. Ill fitting dentures are not conducive to accurate articulation as they tend to move.

CHAPTER 21

The anatomy and physiology of swallowing

Swallowing is a very complex activity which is part voluntary and part reflex. It involves virtually all the muscle groups in the head and neck and their associated nerve supplies from the cranial nerves described in earlier chapters. Food is chewed and broken down in the mouth to a suitable consistency and then manipulated to form a bolus which is propelled into the pharynx by the action of the tongue. The bolus passes through the pharynx and oesophagus into the stomach by the action of muscles in their walls. To ensure that food is routed correctly and does not enter the nasopharynx or larynx, protective reflexes accompany the main actions of swallowing. Other reflexes can operate to expel food from these areas should it enter them inadvertently. Because swallowing is such a complex process, it can be disrupted by a number of disease processes; abnormal swallowing activity is **dysphagia**, a problem which is assuming greater significance in certain areas of speech and language therapy practice.

The structure and function of many of the components of the face, jaws, and mouth involved in swallowing have already been described in Chapters 18 and 19.

The pharynx

The pharynx is a midline tube partially surrounded by muscles and is about 15 cm long. It begins posterior to the nasal cavities and becomes continuous with the oesophagus posterior to the level of the cricoid cartilage. The pharynx lies between the cervical vertebrae posteriorly and the nasal and oral cavities and the larynx anteriorly. The lateral and posterior walls of the pharynx comprise muscles lined by mucosa. Because the respiratory and gastrointestinal tracts share a common pathway through the pharynx, the lining mucosa is covered by stratified squamous epithelium except in the nasopharynx where the lining epithelium is respiratory epithelium. The muscular layer is arranged into

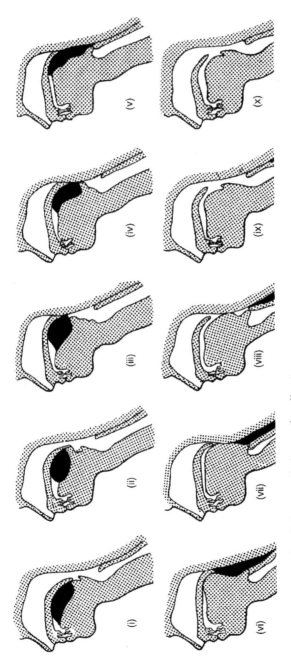

Figure 21.1 The oral and pharyngeal phases of swallowing.

an inner circular group, the **pharyngeal constrictors**, and an outer longitudinal group which is not very pronounced. The constrictor muscles contract in a continuous wave from above downwards (Figure 20.1), increasing pressure on the food bolus and propelling it through the pharynx into the oesophagus. The longitudinal muscles attach to the base of the skull and palate and blend into the circular muscles. They assist in elevation of the pharynx. The pharynx also plays a role in articulation. Its diameter can be varied by muscular constriction and its length adjusted by activity of the suprahyoid muscles. These changes alter the size of this part of the supravocal tract and therefore alter pitch and resonance.

For descriptive purposes, the pharynx is divided into three regions although these are functionally continuous. The three regions are designated the **nasopharynx**, **oropharynx** and **laryngopharynx** from above downwards and are related anteriorly to the nasal cavities, oral cavity and larynx respectively (Figure 21.2). The junction of the nasopharynx and oropharynx is demarcated by an imaginary horizontal line where the elevated soft palate meets the posterior pharyngeal wall at the pharyngeal isthmus. The junction of the oropharynx and laryngopharynx is an imaginary line through the tip of the epiglottis.

The nasopharynx lies behind the nasal cavities and functionally is part of the respiratory tract. The backward sloping roof of the nasopharynx is

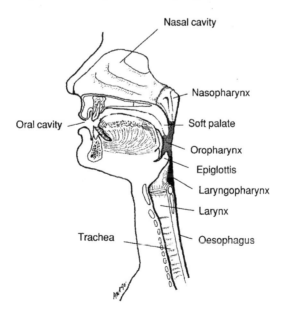

Figure 21.2 The divisions of the pharynx.

formed by the sphenoid and occipital bones forming the base of the skull. The **pharyngeal tonsil** is of variable size lying in the mucosa covering the roof and posterior wall. The anterior parts of each lateral wall are formed by the medial pterygoid plates and the upper posterior parts of the lateral walls are formed by a sheet of connective tissue (the pharyngobasilar fascia). The cartilaginous **auditory tubes** open into the nasopharynx by piercing the fascia on either side producing the tubal elevations on the lateral walls. The levator and tensor muscles of the soft palate are attached to the cartilage (see Chapter 19). The lower lateral and posterior walls of the nasopharynx are formed by the superior constrictor muscles.

The oropharynx lies behind the oral cavity and the pharyngeal part (posterior third) of the tongue. The anterior limit of the oropharynx is marked by the palatoglossal folds. The lateral and posterior walls of the oropharynx are muscular and are formed by the superior and inferior constrictor muscles. The palatine tonsils lie in the space between the palatoglossal and palatopharyngeal folds (see Figure 19.1). The mucosa of the tongue is reflected on to the anterior surface of the epiglottis as the single median and two lateral glossoepiglottic folds. The depressions between these folds are the **valleculae**.

The laryngopharynx extends from a plane passing through the tip of the epiglottis down to the oesophageal entrance at the level of the inferior border of the cricoid cartilage. The laryngeal inlet faces upwards and backwards opening into the upper anterior wall of the laryngopharynx. The lower anterior wall is formed by the posterior wall of the larynx. The **piriform recesses** lie on either side of the laryngeal inlet and extend from the base of the epiglottis to the cricoid cartilages in the space between the thyroid cartilage and posterior laryngeal wall. They are enclosed between the laminae of the thyroid cartilages laterally and medially by the outer surfaces of the cricoid and arytenoid cartilages. The middle and inferior constrictor muscles form the lateral and posterior walls of the laryngopharynx.

The muscles of the pharynx

The **pharyngeal constrictor muscles** are three pairs of circularly orientated muscles which are deficient anteriorly and fit into each other rather like a series of cones (Figure 21.3). They are all attached posteriorly to a vertical fibrous band, the pharyngeal raphe, which extends from the pharyngeal tubercle on the inferior surface of the occipital bone down the posterior midline of the pharynx to blend with the fibrous covering of the oesophagus.

The **superior constrictor muscles** on each side curve anteriorly from the pharyngeal raphe to become continuous with the buccinator muscles

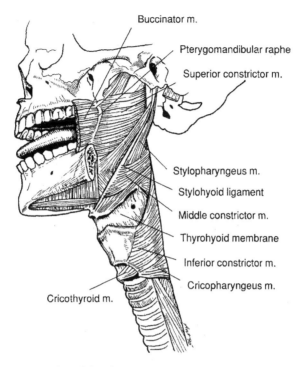

Figure 21.3 The muscles of the pharynx.

between the medial pterygoid plates and the mandible. They are also attached anteriorly to the lower border of the medial pterygoid plates. The **middle constrictor muscles** pass from the pharyngeal raphe and converge anteriorly to form a narrow attachment to the stylohyoid ligaments and the upper border of the hyoid bone, partially overlapping the inferior parts of the superior constrictors. The **inferior constrictor muscles** insert anteriorly into the lateral surfaces of the thyroid cartilage at the oblique ridge and the cricoid cartilage. The upper muscle fibres curve downwards laterally enclosing the lower parts of the middle constrictors to the thyroid and cricoid cartilages. The lower fibres run horizontally from the cricoid cartilage and become continuous with the upper circular muscles of the oesophagus. These muscle fibres are often designated as the **cricopharyngeus muscle** which may function as a sphincter between the pharynx and oesophagus to prevent air ingestion during respiration.

The longitudinal muscles of the pharynx (Figure 21.3) are the **stylopharyngeus** and **palatopharyngeus** muscles. The stylopharyngeus muscles arise from the styloid processes and run downwards to blend with the lateral pharyngeal walls. The palatopharyngeus muscles arise from the undersurface of the soft palate and have already been described in Chapter 19. Both muscles work in concert with the suprahyoid muscles to elevate the pharynx during swallowing and speech.

Pharyngeal innervation

Motor nerves from the pharyngeal branches of the **vagus nerves** and sensory branches from the **glossopharyngeal nerves**, together with autonomic nerves supplying mucous glands in the pharyngeal mucosa, form an extensive **pharyngeal plexus** in the walls of the pharynx. The vagal branches innervate the constrictor muscles and the glossopharyngeal components provide sensory innervation of the oropharyngeal and laryngopharyngeal mucosa.

The auditory tubes

The **auditory tubes**, also known as the **Eustachian** or **pharyngotympanic tubes**, connect the middle ear with the nasopharynx (Figure 21.4). Each tube exits the middle ears as a narrow bony canal in the petrous temporal bone. As they leave the bone, the medial two-thirds of each tube is enclosed by cartilage beneath a bony roof. The cartilage produces the **tubal elevation** where the auditory tubes open into the nasopharynx (Figure 21.2). The tensor and levator veli palatini muscles are attached to the cartilages anteriorly and posteriorly respectively. The auditory tubes are lined with respiratory epithelium containing mucous glands.

The auditory tubes allow air to enter the middle ear cavities so that air pressure on each side of the tympanic membrane separating the outer and middle ear can be equalized to prevent distortion or even rupture of the eardrum by excess pressure differentials. Air enters the auditory tubes when they are opened by the pull of the levator and tensor veli palatini muscles as they elevate the soft palate during swallowing. Unpleasant and often painful pressure differentials often build up during air travel as aircraft ascend and descend. The pressure may be relieved by swallowing. When cleft palate affects the soft palate (see Chapter 20), the palatal muscles do not have a firm attachment to the palate and therefore cannot exert an efficient pull on the auditory tube which therefore do not open fully. Pressure is not equalized across the tympanic membrane and mucus does not drain from the middle ear, leading to repeated infections of the middle ear (**glue ear**). Enlargement of tonsillar tissue in the vicinity of the auditory tube openings can also reduce drainage from the middle ear, also resulting in glue ear. The incidence of glue ear can be minimized by placement of a grommet into the tympanic membrane which allows air into and fluid out of the middle ear. More recently, laser surgery has been

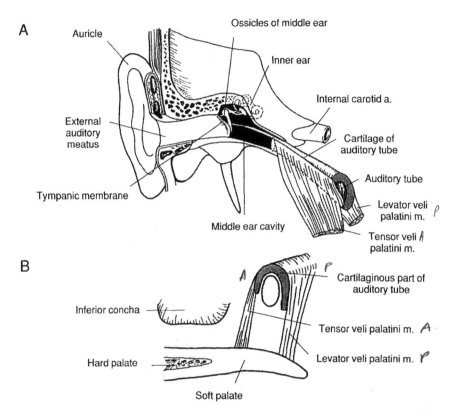

Figure 21.4 The auditory tube. (A) A coronal section showing the structure of the auditory tube. (B) Muscular attachments to the auditory tube.

used to create a minute hole in the tympanic membrane to serve the same function. The auditory tubes are potential conduits for cross infection from the nasopharynx to the middle ear and it is not uncommon for upper respiratory tract infections to produce inflammation of the middle ear (**otitis media**) via this route.

Oropharyngeal tonsillar tissue

There are several aggregates of lymphoid tissue (tonsils) in the pharynx to protect the lower gastrointestinal and respiratory tracts from pathogenic organisms (Figure 21.5). Tonsillar tissue forms an incomplete ring around the entrance to the oropharynx. The **lingual tonsils** lie beneath the mucosa of the posterior third of the tongue and form the base of the ring. The paired **palatine tonsils** lie in the depression between the palatoglossal and palatopharyngeal arches and make up the sides of the

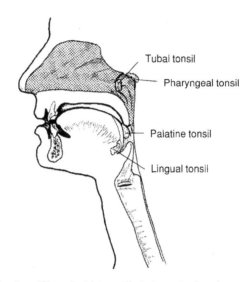

Tubal tonsil

Pharyngeal tonsil

Palatine tonsil

Lingual tonsil

Figure 21.5 Distribution of lymphoid (tonsillar) tissue in the pharynx.

ring. The ring, sometimes called Waldeyer's tonsillar ring, is completed by the **pharyngeal tonsil** in the roof and posterior wall of the nasopharynx. The **tubal tonsils** are inconsistent nodules around the pharyngeal openings of the auditory tubes. The mucosa covering the tonsils extends deeply into the lymphoid tissue as tonsillar crypts which gives the tonsillar surface a pitted appearance. The tonsils, particularly the pharyngeal and palatine tonsils, often become infected and enlarged (**tonsillitis**). As well as pain and discomfort, the enlarged tissue can interfere with function, especially elevation of the soft palate. Enlarged pharyngeal tonsils (**adenoids**) prevent complete closure of the soft palate against the posterior pharyngeal wall, which allows air to escape into the nose producing **hypernasality** during speech. Enlarged pharyngeal tonsils can also virtually occlude the nasopharynx, forcing the client to breathe through the mouth and producing **hyponasality** during speech as air does not enter the nose during articulation of nasal consonants. Enlargement of the tubal tonsils may block the auditory tubes leading to glue ear. Because children are still developing immunity to foreign antigens, lymphoid tissues are very active; prepubertally, tonsils are about twice their adult size so that pathological enlargement of what is already a significant tissue mass has a much more profound effect in children than adult tonsillitis. Surgical removal (tonsillectomy) of the palatine and/or pharyngeal tonsils may be undertaken if infection is persistent.

The oesophagus

The oesophagus is a muscular tube continuous with the laryngopharynx above at the level of the cricoid cartilage (Figure 21.6). It has a short cervical course behind the trachea before passing into the thorax where it lies on the posterior wall approximately in the midline. It enters the abdominal cavity by piercing the diaphragm and enters the stomach almost immediately. The oesophagus is lined by stratified squamous epithelium to resist abrasion by foodstuffs during swallowing. The lumen of the oesophagus is very narrow unless dilated by the presence of food and is further constricted by the cricopharyngeus muscle superiorly and the diaphragm inferiorly; the diaphragmatic constriction is called the **cardiac sphincter**. The oesophagus is also constricted where it passes posterior to the left main bronchus in the thorax and the left atrium of the heart. These narrower areas are of clinical importance as they may impede the passage of a gastroscope and they are the most likely areas to be damaged if corrosive fluids are accidentally swallowed. Left atrial enlargement may also constrict the oesophagus. The oesophagus is innervated by parasympathetic nerves from the vagus nerves and sympathetic branches from the thoracic sympathetic nerves.

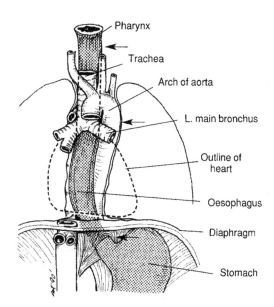

Figure 21.6 The course and relations of the oesophagus. Arrows indicate sites of constriction of the oesophagus.

Swallowing

When food has been broken up and rendered to a consistency suitable for swallowing by adequate mastication and mixing with saliva, the food is formed into a pellet, the **bolus**, of suitable size for swallowing by the action of the tongue against the hard palate. The bolus is propelled backwards from the mouth into the oropharynx by action of the tongue. As the food touches certain trigger spots in the oropharynx, a sequence of reflex muscle activities is initiated and the food is propelled through the lower pharynx and oesophagus into the stomach. To prevent accidental entry of food into the nasopharynx, the soft palate is elevated. Similarly, the larynx is elevated, the rima glottis closed and respiration briefly suspended to prevent food entering the larynx and lower respiratory tract. These actions direct the bolus along the correct route through the pharynx and ensure the airway is protected throughout.

Traditionally, for ease of description, swallowing is separated into **oral**, **pharyngeal** and **oesophageal phases** according to the position of the bolus in the gastrointestinal tract. In reality, swallowing is a continuous process and segregation into phases is not particularly accurate. It takes about a second to propel food from the mouth into the oropharynx and less than a second for the food to traverse the pharynx and enter the oesophagus where it takes another second or two to reach the stomach. It is unclear what initiates swallowing but it may be a combination of the completion of a certain number of masticatory cycles and the sensory feedback from the oral cavity about the consistency of food. The latter is certainly important because, in the same individual, the amount of mastication required varies considerably with initial food consistency.

The oral phase of swallowing is often subdivided into the oral preparatory phase and the oral phase. The **oral preparatory phase** is the preparation of food into the bolus by mastication and mixing with saliva. During this phase, which varies considerably in length according to the consistency of food, lip seal is maintained by the muscles of facial expression and mastication. The lip and buccinator muscles are used to remove food from the oral vestibule and return it between the teeth. The oral cavity is also sealed posteriorly by active depression of the soft palate against the back of the tongue. The tongue tip is used to collect food into a bolus against the teeth and hard palate. All these actions are voluntary.

The **oral phase** is initiated by elevation of the tongue tip and blade against the hard palate which begins to push the bolus backwards. The sides of the tongue are also raised to form a groove to direct the food into the pharynx. A prerequisite for swallowing is mandibular elevation although the mouth does not have to be closed completely. However, it is notoriously difficult to swallow with the mouth open as any experience of prolonged dental treatment will confirm. Mandibular elevation enables the suprahyoid muscles to act from a fixed mandible to move the hyoid bone rather than the mandible. Raising the hyoid bone facilitates the upward movement of the tongue against the hard palate. It also draws the laryngeal inlet up beneath the posterior pharyngeal part of the tongue (Figure 21.1). As the tongue obliterates the oral cavity and forces the bolus to the back of the mouth until it contacts the palatoglossal folds (the **faucal arches**), the posterior part of the tongue is depressed to form a chute into the oropharynx. Both the extrinsic and intrinsic muscles of the tongue are used to perform its complex movements during the oral phase. At the same time the soft palate is elevated to close off the nasopharynx and direct the bolus into the oropharynx. The oral phase of swallowing is also voluntary and takes about a second.

It is often thought that movement of food from the mouth into the pharynx is voluntary until the bolus has passed the faucal arches. However, it may be truer to say that the action is reflex but the individual is conscious of certain aspects of swallowing as it occurs, such as compression of the bolus between the tongue and hard palate, but is unaware of palatal and laryngeal movements occurring simultaneously. Thus it may not be possible to prevent swallowing once initiated, but it may be possible to delay initiation of swallowing. The converse applies in some instances when swallowing requires considerable effort, such as when trying to swallow a large tablet.

Irrespective of whether the oral phase is voluntary or reflex, contact of food with certain areas of the oropharynx stimulates a chain of reflex contractions in the muscles of the pharynx and oesophagus. By applying topical anaesthetics to various regions of the mouth and pharynx it has been shown that, in the majority of people, the reflex stage of swallowing is triggered by food contact with the mucosa overlying the posterior pharyngeal wall, innervated by the glossopharyngeal nerve, or the faucal arches. The reflex activity is coordinated in the brainstem (see below). Even if some of the muscles involved are denervated, they simply fail to contract but the next muscles in the sequence will still contract at the right time.

The initiation of reflex activity is the beginning of the **pharyngeal phase** of swallowing (Figure 21.1). Sequential contraction of the pharyngeal constrictor muscles moves the bolus rapidly through the pharynx. At the same time, the larynx and pharynx are elevated beneath the epiglottis. The hyoid bone is also drawn forward by the geniohyoid muscles, thus dilating the oropharynx. As the bolus moves into the oropharynx it contacts the epiglottis, forcing the elastic cartilage backwards over the laryngeal inlet as the larynx rises to meet the epiglottis. Because of the upward convexity of the epiglottis, food is diverted laterally into the piriform recesses either side of the laryngeal entrance. The positioning of the epiglottis to protect the larynx is passive but other active movements also prevent food entering the lower respiratory tract. Respiration is temporarily suspended to prevent inhalation of food, the laryngeal entrance is narrowed by contraction of the aryepiglottic muscles, and the elevation of the hyoid bone by the suprahyoid muscles moves the laryngeal entrance into a more vertical orientation. Despite these actions, the laryngeal entrance is not closed completely and it is still possible for food to enter the larynx. As a final protective mechanism, the vocal and vestibular folds are strongly adducted by the interarytenoid muscles completely closing the rima glottis and blocking the airway. Any food entering the larynx will thus be arrested by the folds and expelled by the cough reflex (see below). In reality, the mechanisms operating to protect the airway occur from below upwards: respiration is suspended, the vocal and vestibular folds close, then the laryngeal entrance is narrowed.

Forceful contraction of the cricopharyngeus muscle initiates the passage of the bolus through the oesophagus, the **oesophageal phase** of swallowing. Coordination of activity of the pharyngeal and oesophageal muscles is controlled through the vagal nuclei in the brainstem. Surgical resection of part of the oesophagus, in cases of oesophageal cancer, for example, results in delay between contraction of the muscles above the resection and the intact muscles below since the vagal nuclei are still programmed to make the missing portions contract. Because respiration is suspended, the diaphragm is relaxed allowing free passage of the bolus from the thoracic into the abdominal part of the oesophagus and into the stomach. As respiration is resumed, the diaphragm contracts exerting a sphincteric action on the oesophagus to prevent reflux of the stomach contents into the lower oesophagus. The oesophageal phase takes about two seconds.

Swallowing of fluids is somewhat different from swallowing solids. Although passage of fluids from the mouth through the pharynx into the oesophagus is similar, once fluids enter the oesophagus, they descend by gravity. Although their presence in the oesophagus stimulates a wave of contraction, the fluids actually reach the stomach ahead of the contractile wave.

Protective reflexes

Several important reflexes protect the lower airway and gastrointestinal tract from the effect of foreign bodies or ingestion of potentially toxic foodstuffs.

The **gag reflex** occurs if a swallowing reflex is elicited but the stimulating material cannot be swallowed. Instead of swallowing, the mouth is opened and the posterior part of the tongue is elevated in an attempt to expel the offending material. In addition, the vertical muscles of the pharynx and superior constrictors also contract to help expel the material. The soft palate is also elevated to prevent material entering the nasopharynx. Some clients have extremely sensitive afferent arcs to their gag reflexes, making intraoral examination quite difficult: in these circumstances, the application of a short acting topical anaesthetic may be beneficial to client and clinician. It is difficult to explain why stimulation of the same afferent reflex arcs stimulate swallowing in one instance and gagging in another. There is no obvious explanation, but it may be to do with the fact that the mouth is usually closed during swallowing and open during gagging. It has been suggested that it is the sudden application of material to the posterior pharyngeal wall that evokes a gag reflex rather than the continuous progression of material from lips along the tongue and into the pharynx as occurs in the oral preparatory and oral phases of swallowing.

Vomiting is the forceful ejection of the stomach contents by sudden contraction of the muscles of the anterior abdominal wall which forces the stomach contents through the cardiac sphincter. It is a very complex reflex, and the stimuli for vomiting are not as obvious as they may seem. In some instances, vomiting occurs almost immediately after ingestion of harmful substances but it may be delayed for a considerable time. The complex activities such as retching which precede and accompany vomiting as well as the muscular activity expelling the stomach contents are coordinated by a group of neurons in the brainstem. Unlike most other reflexes, vomiting is not depressed either by sleep or general anaesthesia and can still occur in both circumstances. Because the gag and cough reflexes are depressed or absent under these conditions, it is not uncommon for vomit to be aspirated with the result that the client either asphyxiates due to respiratory tract obstruction or suffers lung damage and infections such as pneumonia. Anyone who is unconscious and may vomit should be placed in the recovery position lying prone with their head turned to one side, provided they can be moved without exacerbation of other injuries. If vomiting ensues, vomit will drain from the mouth and the risk of its inhalation is minimized.

The **cough reflex** is also important in protection of the lower airway if foodstuffs accidentally enter the larynx. The cough reflex has been described in Chapter 15.

Nervous control of swallowing

Swallowing may be voluntarily initiated or may occur reflexly in response stimulation of the pharyngeal mucosa by, for example, accumulated saliva in the mouth. Voluntary initiation requires higher areas of the brain but reflex swallowing does not. In reality, only about 25 per cent of daily swallows are directly related to eating and drinking and voluntarily initiated.

Voluntary initiation of swallowing involves bilateral areas of the prefrontal cortex just anterior to the face area of the lower parts of the primary motor cortices (Figure 21.7). Stimulation of this area, sometimes referred to as the **frontal swallowing centre**, produces swallowing activity in voluntary muscles around the mouth, the tongue and pharynx. Most of the oral musculature is represented symmetrically in both hemispheres whereas representation of pharyngeal and oesophageal

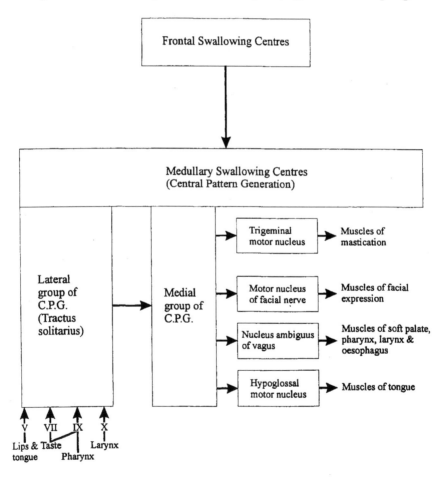

Figure 21.7 The neural control of swallowing.

muscles is asymmetrical. This asymmetry determines which hemisphere is dominant for swallowing; in most subjects this bears no obvious relationship to handedness. Neurons of the frontal swallowing centre project through various descending pathways to the brainstem to the so-called **medullary swallowing centre** or **central pattern generator (CPG)**. There is some evidence that the frontal swallowing centre is somatotopically organized such that different parts of this area influence the medullary swallowing centre at different phases of the swallowing cycle. If the cortex is examined by MRI as swallowing is initiated passively, for example, by introducing water into the client's mouth, several cortical areas become active. Areas involved in sensory and motor processing of swallowing include the facial areas of the sensory and motor cortices, the prefrontal cortices, the frontal opercular area of Broca's area and the insular cortex, as well as areas involved in attention and affective behaviour such as the parietal and temporal association cortices. Activation of these areas is bilateral in most cases, but activity in the premotor and frontal opercular cortex and insula shows marked lateralization.

The **central pattern generator** comprises two groups of neurons related to the cranial nerve nuclei associated with the nerves most involved in swallowing. Sensory inputs from the trigeminal, glossopharyngeal, and vagus nerves innervating the mouth, pharynx and larynx respectively converge on to the **nucleus of the tractus solitarius** on each side, the site where taste sensation also terminates. This nucleus and the surrounding reticular formation form the **lateral group of the CPG**: each receives inputs from peripheral sensory receptors and the frontal swallowing centres and triggers and organizes the swallowing motor sequence by connections with the **medial group** of neurons in the CPG. The major nucleus with motor output for swallowing is the **nucleus ambiguus**, controlling muscles of the palate, pharynx and larynx; the medial group comprises this nucleus on each side and the adjacent reticular formation. This bilaterally represented group distributes excitatory stimuli to different motor neuron pools via the trigeminal, facial and hypoglossal nuclei and nucleus ambiguus so that the corresponding muscles of the jaws, face, tongue and soft palate, pharynx, larynx and oesophagus act in the correct spatiotemporal sequence. Not all activity in the CPG is stimulatory; there are strong inhibitory signals preventing contraction of muscles not required for a particular phase of swallowing.

Dysphagia

It should now be appreciated that normal swallowing, after voluntary or reflex initiation, involves the coordinated action of various muscle groups in precise sequence. It is not surprising that it does not take much to disrupt the complex mechanisms required to swallow, including those reflex activities designed to protect the lower airway.

Any degree of abnormal swallowing behaviour is termed **dysphagia**. Dysphagia may be **obstructive** or **pathophysiological**. Obstructive dysphagia may be **intrinsic**, due to obstructions within the pharynx or oesophagus such as carcinoma, or **extrinsic** due to other structures occluding the food passage; such things as aortic aneurysm, enlargement of lymph nodes in the thorax secondary to bronchial carcinoma or left atrial enlargement in heart disease may cause extrinsic obstructions. Obstructive dysphagia can usually be treated surgically and is not strictly within the province of speech and language therapy; it is the pathophysiological causes of dysphagia which are your concern. A formidably long list of diseases can account for dysphagia of pathophysiological aetiology but essentially they fall into two groups, neurological diseases and injuries and xerostomia.

Xerostomia (dry mouth) may be a direct result of diseases affecting the salivary glands but are usually due to side effects of various drugs (see Chapter 19); in the latter case, xerostomia can often be alleviated or minimized by a change of drug regime.

Any **neurological disease or injury** which affects the frontal swallowing centres or the CPG and the interconnecting nerve pathways directly, the cranial nerve nuclei regulating activity of muscles involved in swallowing, or other structures and pathways involved in regulation of muscular activity such as the cerebellum and basal ganglia may produce some degree of dysphagia as well as other characteristic signs and symptoms. In acute care, CVA is probably the most frequent diagnosis in clients referred for investigation of dysphagia; multiple sclerosis, Parkinson's disease, brain tumours and head trauma are other common diagnoses. Dysphagia is an almost inevitable consequence of chronic neurodegenerative diseases such as motor neuron disease, Parkinson's disease, cerebellar ataxia or chorea.

Dysphagia has severe consequences. Socially, inability to swallow leads to embarrassment and frustration and consequent avoidance of situations associated with the social aspects of eating and drinking. More seriously, malnutrition and dehydration will occur with consequent deterioration in the client's general health and resistance to infections. Dysphagia is often complicated by **aspiration** of foodstuffs into the lower airway with possible asphyxiation or, more likely, lung infections such as pneumonia which may prove terminal. Aspiration is obviously potentially life-threatening. Under normal circumstances, aspiration of foodstuffs into the laryngeal vestibule (**penetration** or supraglottal aspiration) would invoke a cough reflex. Subglottal aspiration (**aspiration**) of foodstuffs is comparatively rare during normal swallowing because of the protective mechanisms operating but is a frequent occurrence in dysphagic clients. If there are no signs such as coughing or throat clearing to show that food has been aspirated, this is referred to as **silent aspiration**. Silent aspiration is most dangerous and is most prevalent when dysphagics attempt to swallow liquids.

Investigation of dysphagia

The major priorities for any client with swallowing difficulty are to maintain adequate levels of nutrition and hydration and to minimize the risk of compromise of the airway by aspiration. Even when the clients are receiving nutrition via nasogastric tube or similar means, there may still be a risk of aspiration from build up of saliva within the mouth. This can be controlled to some extent by anticholinergic drugs but this often results in production of thick, sticky saliva which is difficult to clear and may cause choking attacks.

There are essentially two reasons for investigating swallowing behaviour. First, the client may report difficulty with swallowing or signs of dysphagia may have been observed by other health care professionals or carers. Second, swallowing function should be examined if the presenting disease is known to be likely to cause dysphagia. There are three commonly used methods for investigating swallowing behaviour; one may be carried out at the bedside but the other two require specialized equipment and personnel.

Bedside assessment begins, of course, with a case history which may involve family or carers if the degree of debility in the client is severe. It should include information on nutritional status, weight loss and the state of dentition, whether natural or prosthetic, as well as the results of any neurological assessments carried out. Dysphonia (see Chapter 17) should also be investigated as a clue to the ability or otherwise to adduct the vocal folds and thus protect the lower airway. The client may then be given a measured volume of cold water to drink; the time taken to drink it and the number of swallows are measured. Small sips over a prolonged time may indicate self-compensation to avoid aspiration. Coughing, 'wet voice' and breathlessness are all indications of aspiration. Further tests may be carried out by observing the client swallowing small volumes of semi-solids or solid food. Such tests have become more refined and can now involve direct measurement using equipment such as pressure detectors, movement transducers or Doppler probes attached to the neck. These devices enable accurate measurement of pressure changes within the pharynx, transit times in different phases of the swallowing cycle and swallowing capacity.

Fibre optic nasoendoscopy evaluation of swallows (FEES) is now being used more routinely. The endoscope is placed transnasally with the tip placed initially behind the uvula then lowered to the level of the epiglottis. FEES gives no information about the oral or oesophageal phases of swallowing but can reveal delay in the initiation of the pharyngeal phase. However, as soon as the larynx is elevated, further observation is obscured. FEES can, however, detect food residue in the valleculae or piriform recesses which are indicators of dysphagia.

Videofluoroscopy, a specialized type of radiography, is used for more detailed investigations and is the most comprehensive and accurate method of assessment of dysphagia. The client is given thin or thick liquid barium sulphate or barium-sulphate-coated soft-solid bolus to swallow and radiographic recordings from anterior and lateral views of the swallowing action are made over a series of swallows. The radiographs are analysed for various factors some of which require qualitative visual observation (e.g. food residues in the pharynx after swallowing is completed) while others require detailed quantitative analysis (e.g. timing and duration of each phase of swallowing).

Two examples of neurological disease, CVA (stroke) and Parkinson's disease will illustrate some aspects of dysphagia and reinforce some of the aspects of regulation of swallowing and dysphagia described above.

CVA

CVA, as emphasized in Chapter 8, may occur anywhere within the vascular supply to the brain and normal function will be disrupted depending on the brain areas damaged by the vascular lesion. Estimates vary but about 40 per cent of clients with a unilateral CVA in the cerebral hemispheres exhibit dysphagia. Surprisingly, they show a reasonably rapid recovery of normal swallowing, usually within weeks of the initial lesion. The bilateral representation of swallowing in the cerebral cortex underlies the recovery. The severity of symptoms depends on whether the swallowing-dominant hemisphere is affected but as swallowing dominance obeys no general rule, it is unlikely that the dominant side will have been identified beforehand. Both dysphagics and non-dysphagics show reduced pharyngeal responses to transcranial magnetic stimulation of the affected hemisphere but non-dysphagics have a much higher response to stimulation of the unaffected hemisphere in the muscles controlled by the frontal swallowing centres. Although there is some dispute about the site and side of lesions most likely to produce dysphagia, there is some evidence that right-sided lesions of the anterior circulation (the anterior and middle cerebral arteries) most often lead to dysphagia with aspiration. Should dysphagia occur, the degree and speed of recovery appears to depend on the reorganization of the unaffected non-dominant hemisphere; the representation of pharyngeal muscles in the unaffected hemisphere increases with time.

It is also not clear why some clients aspirate while others do not. In many clients, sensory function appears to be intact so they should be able to sense the presence of foreign material in the larynx. It is probably more likely due to poor hyolaryngeal movements which mean that the laryngeal entrance is not as well protected and/or that there is a delay between the end of the oral phase and onset of the pharyngeal phase of swallowing. This delay is particularly significant when swallowing liquids as the liquid will already be entering the pharynx before the protective reflexes become operative. Pooling of material in the pharynx observed by videofluoroscopy is a strong indicator of the likelihood of silent aspiration; in normal subjects there is no pharyngeal residue after swallowing.

It should be borne in mind that CVA clients will exhibit many other signs and symptoms, especially during the early stages, and these may complicate testing and diagnosis. For example, left CVA clients often show a degree of '**apraxia of swallowing**', another manifestation of oral apraxia (see Chapter 13) in which movements of the tongue, jaws and lips to command is lost but spontaneous movement is retained.

Brainstem strokes are comparatively rare compared with cerebral hemisphere CVA but if located in the area of the CPG swallowing is very likely to be adversely affected. Wallenberg syndrome (also called lateral medullary syndrome) is a result of CVA in the posterior inferior cerebellar artery which supplies the CPG area of the brainstem as well as the cerebellum (see Chapter 8). This may produce complete inability to swallow if the stroke affects both sides of the brainstem. There is, however, good recovery from dysphagia if aspiration is prevented in the early stages with 80 per cent of clients able to resume full oral nutrition. The reasons for this are not understood.

Parkinson's disease

While the prognosis for dysphagic stroke clients might appear to be reasonably good, in most cases of neurodegenerative disease, dysphagia is an almost inevitable consequence. In many cases, pneumonia is the actual cause of death, possibly as a result of complications following aspiration of foodstuffs.

In Parkinson's disease, about 50 per cent of clients in the early stages have dysphagic signs if examined for them, but generally do not report them and show few overt signs of feeding difficulty. As the disease progresses the incidence of dysphagia rises rapidly to 90 per cent. However, subglottic aspiration only occurs in the later, more severe, stages of the disease. As might be expected from a disease affecting the substantia nigra, a component of the basal ganglia which produces muscular rigidity and hypokinesia (see Chapter 10), there are profound effects on the oral and pharyngeal muscles. These lead to difficulty of tongue control and, in turn, to poor bolus transport from mouth to pharynx. The oral and pharyngeal phases of swallowing are often dissociated and therefore uncoordinated. If there is a pharyngeal constrictor paralysis, then food is likely to pool in the pharynx and the chances of aspiration are therefore increased. This is likely to be silent aspiration in the later stages, the client neither experiencing any difficulty with swallowing nor coughing when aspiration does occur.

The nature of dysphagia and its likely direct and indirect consequences on the general health of the client means that this is an area of speech and language therapy where a team approach is of utmost importance. Input from dietitians, physiotherapists, occupational therapists, pharmacists, radiographers, ENT and neurology consultants and possibly dentists as well as speech and language therapists may all be required to work towards a successful outcome.

CHAPTER 22

The ear and hearing

The ear picks up sound waves carried by air to its outer part, amplifies them in the middle part and converts the energy into electrical activity in its inner part. This electrical activity transmits the sensations through the auditory pathways to the auditory areas of the brain where it is perceived as sound. Here, sounds are decoded and interpreted. En route, the ear and the auditory pathways help to determine the loudness, pitch, quality and direction of sounds, as well as when they start and stop. It is therefore necessary to know the basic physics of sound to understand how the ear works.

The physics of sound

Sound waves are changes in air pressure generated by a sound source. When you bang a drum, the drumskin is depressed some distance into the drum and then rebounds. As it does so, it compresses the air molecules closer together so that the air pressure immediately above the drumskin increases. The drumskin will then move back down into the drum leaving a slight depression hence more room for the air molecules to spread out; air pressure will therefore drop. As the drumskin rebounds again the whole cycle will be repeated in a manner similar to the vocal folds during phonation described in Chapter 16. This will go on while the drumskin oscillates back and forth until the drumskin stops vibrating, either by placing a hand on the drumskin which brings the sound to an abrupt halt or by the inherent stiffness of the drumskin. In the latter case, vibrations will slowly decrease in amplitude until they fade away: this is **damped oscillation** (Figure 22.1). The alternate bands of compressed and rarefied air travel outwards from the sound source. If we could stand at the side and watch them pass, we would see the equivalent of a barcode, alternating black lines of compression and white space of rarefaction. If we were mathematical and counted the number of air molecules in each fraction of air passing by then plotted them against time on a graph, the result would be a wavy line of regular alternating peaks and troughs: this is a **sine wave** (Figure 22.1). The number of peaks passing by each

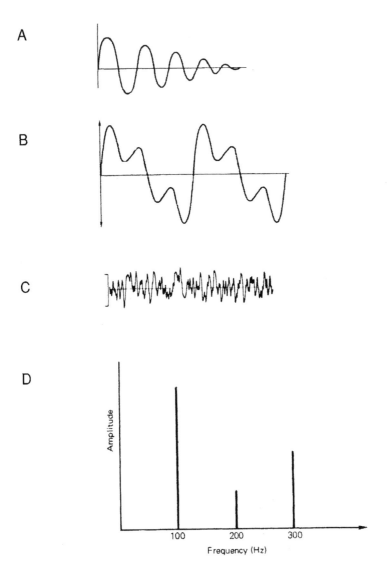

Figure 22.1 Sound waves. (A) A sinusoidal waveform with damping. (B) A complex periodic waveform. (C) Aperiodic waveform. (D) Spectral analysis of a complex waveform.

second, the number of cycles per second, is the **frequency** measured in Hertz (**Hz**) which determines pitch. The difference between the highest and lowest parts of the sine wave is the **amplitude** – measured in decibels (**dB**) – and is perceived as loudness. The decibel scale is a logarithmic scale, so a 40 dB sound has a pressure level 100 times that of a 20 dB sound. The human ear can receive sounds up to about 100 dB without discomfort or damage. At this level the pressure on the eardrum is about 1 000 000 greater than the pressure of the faintest detectable sounds at about 10–20 dB, the loudness of a whisper. The decibel scale is a relative scale and is measured relative to a known pressure. For measuring changes in **sound pressure level** a standard reference value is used. To satisfy your curiosity, it is 0.00002 Pascals. Strictly speaking, decibel measurements should therefore be written as dBSPL (decibels of sound pressure level) as dB without the SPL does not give the reference scale. In the rest of this chapter, assume SPL after any dB reference.

A single sine wave at one exact pitch can only be generated electronically. Any natural sound source is complex, consisting of a **fundamental frequency**, the lowest frequency of vibration, and several **harmonic frequencies** produced from resonating vibrations induced by the fundamental frequency. The harmonics are what tells us that middle C with a frequency of 261 Hz is being played on a trumpet or sung; harmonics are generated in a trumpet in the brass tubing and in the voice by the pharynx, oral and nasal cavities. Harmonics are multiples or fractions of the fundamental frequency so that for middle C, there will be harmonics at 522 Hz, 1044 Hz and so on. As well as harmonic vibrations, there are vibrations which are not simple multiples of the fundamental frequency: these are **overtones** which also determine the characteristics of a particular sound. When the harmonics and overtones are added to the fundamental frequency, the waveform is no longer a simple sinusoidal curve but a **complex waveform** (Figure 22.1). If the harmonics are in phase with the fundamental frequency, in other words, they happen at the same time or with a regular delay, the resulting waveform will still show regular variations in amplitude; this is a **periodic waveform**. If they are significantly out of phase, the amplitude will change rapidly, and these sounds have an **aperiodic waveform**. As a working generalization, vowels are essentially periodic and consonants are aperiodic. You will encounter more refined descriptions of speech sounds in your phonetics courses.

Complex sounds may be analysed into their component parts to give a **sound spectrum** (Figure 22.1). This shows the frequencies present in the sound as a series of spikes. The relative height of the spikes indicates the relative contribution of each frequency to the overall sound. The fundamental frequency will produce the biggest spikes and increasingly higher harmonics (also called **formants** by phoneticians) will produce progressively lower spikes. The detected spectrum of complex sounds is essential for differentiating vowel sounds. Speech works on a **source-filter model**. A source generates a variety of frequencies which are modulated so that selective frequencies are attenuated (reduced or eliminated completely) by filters whilst others pass through. Low pass filters attenuate high frequencies and high pass filters do the reverse. A band pass filter allows frequencies falling in a limited range to pass through. Speech sounds generated in the larynx or vocal tract are filtered in the vocal tract so that some frequencies are amplified by resonance and others are cut off by filtering. As these frequencies are gained or lost, the net result is that the sound spectrum is changed and thus the quality or timbre of the sound is altered.

The essentials of the ear

The ear is divided into three parts, the outer, middle and inner ears (Figure 22.2). The first two parts collect sound waves and transmit them to the inner ear where sound is transduced into electrical signals carried by nerves to the brain. Because the ear is a very complex structure, an overview of the basic features is presented below. It is followed by a more detailed description of the features of each part of the ear.

The **pinna** or auricle, the ear you can see on each side of your head, collects the sound waves and channels them into the **external auditory meatus**, an air-filled tube going deep into the petrous temporal bone, the densest part of the skull. Stretched across the far end of this tube is the **tympanic membrane** (Figure 22.3). Its common name, the ear drum, is an accurate descriptive name. The tympanic membrane is moved by sound

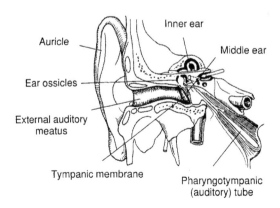

Figure 22.2 The ear.

waves; an increase in pressure pushes it inwards and as pressure drops it moves outwards again. The pinna, external auditory meatus and tympanic membrane constitute the outer ear.

The ear drum separates the outer ear from a slit-like cavity, the **middle ear**. The middle ear is also filled with air because it is connected via the **auditory tube** to the pharynx. It contains three tiny bones (**ossicles**) linked to each other by joints so that they move in a chain reaction. These bones are the **malleus**, **incus** and **stapes**, the Latin for hammer, anvil and stirrup respectively. The malleus and stapes certainly have some resemblance to a hammer and stirrup but the incus was probably called the anvil because it is struck by the hammer; it looks more like a misshaped tooth than an anvil. The malleus is attached to the tympanic membrane so that it moves as the membrane does. The malleus moves the incus and the incus moves the stapes and this chain reaction carries the sound waves across the middle ear to the inner ear where sound transduction takes place, which is separated from the middle ear by a thin membrane called the **oval window**. The stapes fits exactly into this window so that vibrations in the ossicular chain will set up vibrations in the fluid-filled inner ear. The ossicular chain is designed to transfer sound waves from air to fluid without loss of energy. The ossicles are also cleverly arranged so that the vibration of the tympanic membrane is amplified by their leverage at certain frequencies. In addition, the oval window is about 15 times smaller than the tympanic membrane so that sound is amplified by this factor as it is propagated along the ossicular chain.

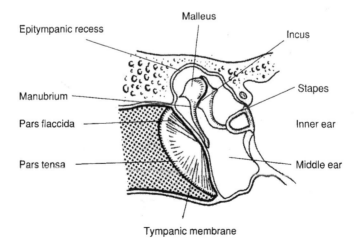

Figure 22.3 The tympanic membrane and middle ear showing the ear ossicles.

The **inner ear** must rank highly in any list of the seven wonders of the human body. Generally the epigram 'form is related to function' applies to all parts of the body: in other words, the structure of a particular cell, tissue or organ matches its function. Nowhere is this more apt than in the inner ear. There are several examples of beautiful pieces of design in the inner ear which occur nowhere else in the body; this is not unexpected as the ear fulfils the very specialized functions of hearing and balance. The inner ear is a complex structure that enables us to detect sounds over a wide range of pitch and intensity and conveys their subtleties to the brain.

The inner ear is located inside the petrous temporal bones, the densest parts of the skull. This location is important. The inside of the head is a very noisy environment with, for example, pulsatile blood flow in nearby arteries supplying the brain contributing to the noise. You can verify this easily by blocking off your ears with ear plugs or your fingers. As external sounds are cut out, you will become aware of the noises inside your own head. Try it! Sensory transduction inside the ear depends upon very small movements, and therefore the vibratory structures need to be isolated from sources of movement other than those produced by sound. The location of the inner and middle ear within dense bone helps to isolate them from the noisy internal environment of the head and from random movements.

The inner ear is enclosed in series of bony tubes called the **bony labyrinth** (Figure 22.4). This consists of a **vestibule** immediately inside of the oval window. Leading off from the vestibule are the **semicircular canals** which are involved in balance and the **cochlea**, a shell like structure which houses the sensory receptors for hearing. Within the bony labyrinth, a series of membranes, the **membranous labyrinth**, houses the special sensory receptors for balance and hearing. The space between the bone and membranous labyrinth is filled by a fluid called **perilymph**. The membranous labyrinth contains **endolymph**, a fluid of different ionic composition. **Hair cells,** the sensory receptors for hearing, have minute extensions called **stereocilia** on their apical surfaces which, at first glance, look like tiny hairs. The hair cells are supported by other cells which, as well as providing mechanical support, are functionally important in hearing. The complex of hair cells and support cells is known as the **spiral organ of Corti**.

The membranous labyrinth is set vibrating by the inward and outward movements of the oval window causing movement in the fluid of the inner ear. These vibrations are detected by the hair cells. The spiral organ follows the turns of the cochlea and hair cells at different distances from the vestibule respond to different frequencies. The human ear is capable of detecting frequencies between 20 and 20 000 Hz, although speech

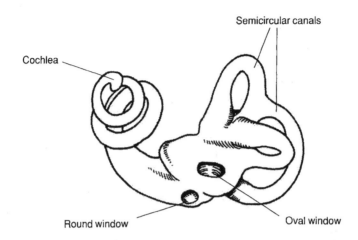

Figure 22.4 The membranous labyrinth and organ of Corti.

generally falls within the range of about 400–8000 Hz. Hair cells also have some astounding electrical properties which enables them to send information about the frequency and phase of incoming sound waves to the brain.

Although the ear consists anatomically of three parts, functionally it can be considered as only two parts: a **conducting mechanism** and a **sensorineural system**. The conducting mechanism, the outer and middle ear, is designed to ensure the delivery of sound energy at high efficiency to the sensorineural system, the inner ear. The sensorineural part of this system transduces sound energy into electrical energy in the form of action potentials within the sensory axons innervating the inner ear. These sensory axons travel to the brainstem within the **vestibulocochlear** (VIIIth cranial) **nerve** and synapse in the **cochlear nuclei** within the pons and medulla. Sensory information passes from the cochlear nuclei of the brainstem through the superior olivary nuclei and inferior colliculi to the medial geniculate bodies of the thalamus. From the medial geniculate body information is relayed to the primary and auditory association cortices. Decoding of the sound signal begins long before the auditory cortex: some distinction of tone takes place in the inner ear and the brainstem nuclei of the auditory pathways can discriminate loudness and direction of sound to some degree. The central auditory pathways are described in Chapter 23.

That concludes the overview. We now need to revisit some of the features described above to understand the details of how sound is conducted and transduced in the ear.

The external ear

The external ear comprises the pinna located on the side of the head, the external auditory meatus which is a blind-ending tube extending medially and the tympanic membrane that closes off the external auditory meatus from the middle ear. The external ear collects and channels sound vibrations on to the tympanic membrane which then vibrates and moves the ossicles within the middle ear. The external ear is also involved in sound localization and, through its resonant frequencies, enhances the energy of lower frequency sounds.

The **pinna**, or **auricle**, consists of a framework of elastic cartilage covered with skin containing sebaceous glands and hair follicles. The lateral surface of the pinna is slightly concave and bears a number of convexities, cavities and curvatures. The pinna develops from six separate components around the first pharyngeal cleft which accounts for the wide individual variation in the shape, size and disposition of cavities and convexities in the auricle. The pinna is attached to the side of the head by the continuity of its cartilaginous plate with the cartilage of the lateral part of the external auditory meatus and ligaments and muscles. The muscles are vestigial in man and do not serve the function, as in some mammals, of moving the pinna to face the direction of the sound source to aid sound localization.

The external auditory meatus is an oval S-shaped tube about 3 cm long and, on average, 6 mm wide. Its lateral one-third is cartilaginous and the medial two-thirds are enclosed in the temporal bone. In the adult, its overall inclination is downwards and backwards but it is nearly horizontal at its medial end. In young children, before craniofacial growth is complete, the external auditory meatus is directed upwards rather than downwards from medial to lateral with the degree of inclination gradually changing as growth proceeds. In addition, before the child can raise its head, the external auditory meatus is short. The meatus only deepens as the mastoid process develops as the supporting muscles of the neck, including the sternocleidomastoid, acquire more strength. The tympanic membrane is thus relatively superficial in neonates and babies and this must be borne in mind when conducting certain hearing tests which involve insertion of probes into the external auditory meatus (see below).

The lateral cartilaginous part of the tube is lined with skin continuous with that of the pinna. The subcutaneous tissue contains numerous **ceruminous glands** which secrete cerumen, or wax. The cerumen is waterproof and helps to prevent damage to the tissues of the meatus from water trapped inside. Excess build up of wax can impede the conduction of sound waves, leading to partial deafness, but it can be removed by having the external ear syringed with warm water. The medial end of the bony part lies obliquely with the anterior end being a few millimetres more medial than the posterior end. It is grooved where the tympanic membrane is attached. The bony part is lined with a stratified squamous epithelium that continues onto the tympanic membrane.

The oval, thin and semi-transparent **tympanic membrane**, separating the external ear from the middle ear, is concave facing the external auditory meatus (Figure 22.3). The apex of the concavity is the umbo. The membrane is only about 0.1 mm thick. It consists of a fibrous layer sandwiched between the outer stratified epithelium and the mucosal internal layer in the tympanic cavity. The tympanic membrane lies obliquely conforming to the bony end of the canal (see above). Its oblique orientation and concave shape both minimize reflection of sound waves. The **manubrium** of the malleus, the first bone in the ossicular chain, is embedded in the tympanic membrane with its tip at the umbo. Movements of the membrane are transmitted to the ossicles through the tight attachment between the tympanic membrane and the malleus. The tympanic membrane above the attachment of the manubrium is lax (the **pars flaccida**) whereas the remainder of the tympanic membrane is tense (the **pars tensa**).

The main function of the tympanic membrane is to transmit, as faithfully as possible, movements of air produced by sound waves to the ossicles of the middle ear. The membrane therefore needs to be sensitive to all frequencies and to transmit them equally. The tympanic membrane can transmit very small changes in pressure produced by low-intensity sounds. Such frequencies probably displace the membrane by molecular dimensions. It also acts as a barrier to protect the delicate structures in the middle ear.

The tympanic membrane is also part of an important mechanism that ensures the vibrations in the air within the tympanic cavity are very effectively damped. It is vital for hearing acuity that, as far as possible, the ossicles move only in response to air movements produced by sound. To this end, the walls of the tympanic cavity, including the tympanic membrane, are irregularly shaped to minimize reflection of pressure waves. This reduces the chance of competing extraneous sound sources or pressure changes within the middle ear interfering with the detection of pressure changes produced by sound energy. The integrity of the tympanic membrane is important for sound transmission. If it is torn or ruptured, it does not vibrate as faithfully as an intact eardrum, therefore some acuity is lost. If air pressure on either side of the tympanic membrane becomes unequal, such as when diving into deep water, it can be damaged or even burst resulting in temporary deafness in the affected ear. The auditory tube is involved in the mechanisms which equalize pressure. Mechanisms operating in the middle ear help protect the tympanic membrane and other parts of the ear against potential damage from excessively loud sounds (see below).

The middle ear (tympanic cavity)

The irregular and complexly shaped tympanic cavity is located deep within the petrous temporal bone (Figure 22.1). It is a slit-like cavity and at its narrowest point, which corresponds to the level of the deepest part of the concavity of the tympanic membrane, is only 2 mm across. There is an upward extension, the epitympanic recess, which allows for movement of the ear ossicles (Figure 22.3). The main contents of the tympanic cavity are three small bones united by synovial joints to form the **ossicular chain**. Two small muscles are attached to two of these bones and can modify the movements of the ossicular chain as a whole.

Essentially, the tympanic cavity is the remains of the depth of the first pharyngeal pouch (see Chapter 20). The rest of the pouch forms the auditory (Eustachian) tube which connects the tympanic cavity with the nasopharynx. As a result of this communication, the tympanic cavity is air-filled. The tympanic cavity is also in communication with the air cells in the mastoid process of the temporal bone. It is, in fact, a dilation of the tube by which the mastoid air cells communicate with the nasopharynx.

The tympanic cavity has a roof, floor, anterior, posterior, medial and lateral walls. The lateral wall is largely formed by the tympanic membrane. The thin roof is perforated by the entrance to the mastoid air cells. The floor of the tympanic cavity is another thin plate of bone separating the tympanic cavity from the internal jugular vein; it varies in thickness and may even be absent. The most obvious structure on the medial wall of the tympanic cavity is the **oval window** (fenestra vestibuli or ovalis) which is occupied by the footplate of one of the ossicles, the stapes. The oval window connects the tympanic cavity to the inner ear. The round window (fenestra cochlea or rotunda), closed by the secondary tympanic membrane, is inferior and posterior to the oval window. It also communicates with the cochlea. The facial nerve passes across the upper part of the medial wall as it travels from the internal auditory meatus to the stylomastoid foramen.

The ossicles

Three ossicles, the malleus, incus and stapes, bridge the tympanic cavity at its narrowest point from the tympanic membrane to the oval window.

The **malleus** is the largest of the ossicles. It consists of a head, a neck, one large and two small processes and vaguely resembles a hammer. The head of the malleus lies within the epitympanic recess and articulates with the incus. The neck joins the head to the largest process, the manubrium (handle), which extends inferiorly and is firmly attached to the tympanic membrane with its tip at the umbo.

The **incus**, the middle of the three ossicles, has a body and two processes. The roughly cuboid body articulates with the head of the malleus through a saddle-shaped joint. Its two processes are orientated almost at right angles to one another. The long process of the incus is about half the length of the manubrium of the malleus. It runs medial and parallel to the manubrium to end in a short curved spur whose rounded end articulates with the head of the stapes.

The **stapes** is the smallest and most medial of the ossicles. Its small head articulates with the incus. Two limbs diverge from the neck to join the oval footplate. This fits into the oval window and is attached to its margins by a ligament. The ligament is not of uniform thickness being thicker anteriorly and inferiorly. The thicker portions act like a hinge so that the stapes is rocked on the oval window rather than acting like a piston.

There are two synovial joints in the ossicular chain, the **incudomalleolar** joint between the malleus and the incus and the **incudostapedial joint** between the incus and the stapes. At normal ranges of sound intensity, the incus and malleus move as a single unit but at higher intensities some gliding movement occurs at the saddle-shaped incudomalleolar joint. Motion is quite free at the incudostapedial joint. The joint capsules contain an abnormally large quantity of elastic tissue. Ligaments support the ossicles within the tympanic cavity and strengthen the joints.

Movements of the tympanic membrane produced by sound pressure waves are transferred to the oval window by movements of the ossicles and thus displace fluid in the cochlea. The manubrium of the malleus is so firmly bound to the tympanic membrane that when the tympanic membrane moves, the manubrium faithfully follows it. As the tympanic membrane moves medially in response to the increased air pressure, the manubrium moves medially causing the head of the malleus to rotate. Normally the malleus and incus are locked together by their smaller processes, thus moving as a single unit; malleolar rotation produces a similar rotation of the incus. Larger movements produced by loud sounds unlock the two bones allowing the malleus to glide a little on the incus. This prevents the stapes being pulled off the oval window. Rotation of these two bones is about an anteroposterior axis and the head of the malleus and the body of the incus rotate laterally within the epitympanic recess (Figure 22.3). This causes the long process of the malleus to move medially in parallel with the manubrium of the malleus. As a result, the stapes is pushed medially into the oval window. The precise movements made by the footplate of the stapes vary. The main motion appears to be a hinge movement about a fulcrum located on the anteroinferior border of the oval window likened to the opening of a door. Whatever the precise mode of movement, the footplate pushes on the oval window causing fluid displacement in the membranous labyrinth. Because fluid cannot be compressed, this displacement ultimately causes the secondary tympanic membrane closing the round window to bulge laterally into the tympanic cavity.

The centre of gravity of the ossicular chain lies very close to the axis of rotation at the incudomalleolar joint. This is an important factor in ensuring that ossicular movements are rapidly damped; in other words, movements stop quickly when sounds stop. If undamped, the ossicles would exhibit a pendulum-like movement continuing beyond the end of a sound which would produce spurious pressure changes in the cochlea leading to sound distortion.

Functions of the middle ear

The tympanic cavity ensures the efficient transfer of energy from air to the aqueous fluids of the inner ear with as little loss as possible. When sound waves meet a denser medium they are reflected with a loss of sound. In theory, only about 1 per cent of the vibrational energy at the tympanic membrane should be transferred to the inner ear at the oval window. In reality, it is reduced by only about 50 per cent. This conservation of energy is achieved in three ways:

- The area of the tympanic membrane is about 15 times greater than the oval window. Pressure at the tympanic membrane is all concentrated into a much smaller area therefore amplifying the pressure at the oval window.
- The arrangement of the ossicles exerts a lever action which also amplifies the vibrations at the oval window, although this only makes a small contribution to the gain.
- The tympanic membrane is not a perfect drumskin; part of it is lax and part is stiff. Furthermore, the manubrium restricts vibration in the middle part of the tympanic membrane. The result is that the pars tensa of the tympanic membrane buckles rather than vibrating uniformly.

There are two small muscles within the tympanic cavity, the tensor tympani and the stapedius. Both these muscles modify ossicular movements in response to certain sounds. The **tensor tympani** muscle lies in a canal above and parallel to the auditory tube in the anterior wall. Its tendon emerges from the canal on the medial wall and turns laterally over a small bony process to attach to the manubrium of the malleus. The tensor tympani pulls the malleus medially and anteriorly. The muscle is supplied by a branch of the mandibular trigeminal nerve. The **stapedius** muscle is smaller than the tensor tympani. It lies in a canal in the posterior wall of the tympanic membrane. Its tendon attaches to the neck of the stapes. The stapedius draws the stapes posteriorly at right angles to the direction of rotation of the ossicular chain. The stapedius muscle is innervated by a branch of the facial nerve.

Both muscles have special features in common. Their fibres are arranged so that they can exert considerable force of contraction without excess shortening. Both muscles are contained in bony canals within the walls of the tympanic cavity; only the muscle tendons, which contain elastic fibres, enter the cavity itself. These two features help to isolate muscle vibration from ossicular vibration and allow for slower onset of contraction so that their activity does not generate spurious sound signals.

In general, both muscles contract simultaneously to pack the ossicles tightly together and to increase the stiffness, or impedance, of the whole ossicular chain. They contract reflexly in response to loud sounds, low frequency sounds, vocalization, speech, tactile stimulation of the head or general movement of the body. Their precise function is uncertain, but it seems likely that they offer some protection against loud sound and that they may regulate the transmission of low frequency sounds through the ossicular chain. Both muscles contract reflexly in response to sounds of greater than 80–90 dB, typically with latencies of between 50–150 msec. Clearly, this mechanism offers only limited protection to the ear against damage by loud sounds of sudden onset such as an explosion because reaction time is too slow. Therefore they probably function better in response to continuous loud noise. When you first enter a noisy pub or club, the noise may be deafening, but within a minute or two, it becomes more bearable. This is because contraction of these muscles may reduce transmission at low frequencies and attenuate transmission at high intensity. Movements of the ossicles will be greater at low frequencies, and if the sound pressures moving the ossicles are greater than the forces holding them together, then the ossicles will tend to separate when attempting to move in response to low frequency sounds of high intensity. This tendency is opposed by both muscles co-contracting to stiffen the ossicular chain. Stiffness is augmented by the elasticity of the tympanic membrane, the ligaments supporting the ossicles and the resistance to movement by the air in the tympanic cavity. Contraction of the tensor tympani pulls the tympanic membrane medially, thus increasing the force needed to move it, while contraction of both tensor tympani and stapedius will increase tension in the ligaments holding the ossicles. Increasing the stiffness of the ossicular chain reduces the transmission of low frequency sound. Another function of tensor tympani and stapedius may be to improve the response of the ossicular chain and to reduce the masking effect of low frequency sounds on high frequency sounds.

The **auditory tube** (pharyngotympanic or Eustachian tube) is an air-filled tube that runs downwards, forwards and medially from an opening low down on the anterior wall of the tympanic cavity to the lateral wall of the nasopharynx. Its structure and function have already been described in Chapter 21.

Conductive hearing loss

Hearing loss, whether mild or severe, is a condition that has profound consequences for the individual. Peripheral hearing loss is of two main types: conductive and sensorineural deafness.

Conductive hearing loss occurs due to damage to structures in the outer or middle ear. Common causes include:

- the immobilization or degeneration of one or more bones in the ossicular chain (**otosclerosis**) due to bone disease such as arthritis
- deformities or absence of the ossicles in first arch syndromes (see Chapter 20)
- middle ear infections – the accumulation of infected material in the middle ear means that the ossicles are trying to operate in a medium of the consistency of treacle
- excess build up of wax in the outer ear (see above).

Conductive hearing loss causes a generalized loss of hearing but the loss of low frequency acuity is often more noticeable. Speech is usually audible at high intensities. Although the conductive part of the ear is affected, the sensorineural mechanisms are still intact. If sound can find an alternative route to the inner ear, it can still be detected. This forms the basis of tests used to detect conductive hearing loss and to distinguish it from sensorineural hearing loss. In **Rinne's test**, a tuning fork is struck and held close to each ear in turn, If the client is deaf, nothing will be heard. The tuning fork is then placed on the mastoid process behind each ear; its vibrations will be conducted through the temporal bone to the inner ear. If conductive hearing loss is present, the tuning fork will now be heard in the affected ear(s) but if it is still unheard, sensorineural deafness must be investigated (see below). **Weber's test** is very similar to Rinne's test except the tuning fork is held against the frontal bone. Conductive deafness may also be detected in pure tone hearing tests used to investigate sensorineural hearing loss (see below) and other more sophisticated tests.

The treatment for conduction deafness depends upon the cause. Antibiotic treatment of middle ear infections or syringing to remove wax may be sufficient. A hearing aid can often help increase auditory ability in cases which cannot be dealt with by medical intervention. Occasionally surgery is employed, for example, to replace a damaged ossicle with a prosthesis.

The inner ear

The inner ear is located within the petrous part of the temporal bone and consists of a series of interconnected canals called the **bony labyrinth**. It is composed of three parts, the **vestibule**, the **semicircular canals**, and the **cochlea**. The bony labyrinth is filled with a fluid called **perilymph**. The bony labyrinth contains the **membranous labyrinth** which consists of a series of interconnected ducts and canals joined together via two centrally-placed sacs. The membranous labyrinth is filled with fluid of a different composition from perilymph called **endolymph**. The inner ear is involved in two sensory functions. The vestibular system monitors balance and head movement. The cochlea is concerned with hearing.

The bony labyrinth

The vestibule lies medial to the tympanic cavity at the centre of the bony labyrinth between the cochlea anteriorly and the semicircular canals posteriorly (Figure 22.4). The oval window is centrally placed on its lateral wall and covered by the footplate of the stapes. The round window is inferior to the oval window. The vestibule has openings into the semicircular canals and cochlea.

The **cochlea** is a helical coiled tube resembling a snail shell. The bony tube of the cochlear consists of $2\frac{3}{4}$ turns of a spiral around a central bony hollow pillar called the **modiolus**. A narrow, thin bony ledge, the **spiral osseous lamina**, projects from this central core but falls short of the outer wall of the cochlea by a variable margin. The width of the osseous spiral lamina is greatest at the base of the cochlea and decreases steadily towards the apex.

The membranous labyrinth

The membranous labyrinth is a continuous series of ducts within the bony labyrinth filled with endolymph and containing the sensory receptors for balance and for hearing. The membranous labyrinth is separated from the walls of the bony labyrinth by perilymph. The **cochlear duct** is contained with the bony cochlea and joins the membranous labyrinth components of the vestibular apparatus in the semicircular canals to form a closed system.

The cochlear duct

The cochlear membranous labyrinth is known as the cochlear duct. It is approximately triangular in shape and bridges between the modiolar and outer cochlear walls along the whole length of the cochlea. Two membranes enclose the cochlear duct above and below and its outer wall is formed by the bony wall of the cochlea between the attachments of the two membranes (Figure 22.5). The **organ of Corti**, a highly specialized sensory epithelium which transduces sound, is located within the cochlear duct.

The floor of the cochlear duct is formed by the **basilar membrane**, which is attached to the osseous spiral lamina on its modiolar side and extends to the outer wall of the cochlea. It is attached to the outer wall by the **osseous spiral ligament**. The **vestibular (Reissner's) membrane** forming the roof of the cochlear duct also extends from the osseous spiral lamina to the outer wall of the cochlea. It too is attached to the osseous spiral lamina but its attachment onto the outer wall is above that of the basilar membrane.

The cochlea duct and the osseous spiral lamina divide the bony cochlear tube into three chambers or scalae. The **scala vestibuli** lies above the cochlear duct between the vestibular membrane and the bony roof of the cochlea. The **scala tympani** lies beneath the basilar membrane and the floor of the bony wall of the cochlea. The cochlear duct between

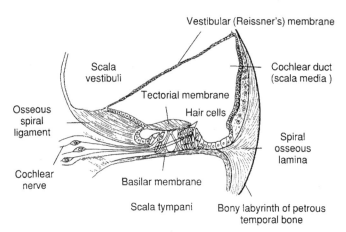

Figure 22.5 The cochlear duct.

them is known as the **scala media**. The scala vestibuli is continuous with the vestibule whereas the scala tympani ends blindly at the round window. They communicate at the apex of the cochlea via a small pore, the **helicotrema**, forming a continuous endolymph-filled chamber that spirals all the way up to the apex of the cochlea and back down again. Vibrations from the oval window pass through the vestibule and into the scala vestibuli (Figure 22.6).

The organ of Corti lies on the basilar membrane between the osseous spiral lamina and the spiral ligament. The basilar membrane is composed of collagenous fibres oriented in a predominantly radial direction. The medial part of the membrane is thin and extends beneath the organ of Corti. The thick lateral part extends from the organ of Corti to the spiral ligament. The basilar membrane is about 35 mm long and increases in width throughout its length from 150–200 μm at the base to 450–500 μm at its apex. The cochlea itself tapers in the opposite direction being broadest at its base. Changes in the width of the basilar membrane towards the apex of the cochlea are paralleled by a decrease in the width of the osseous spiral lamina and a reduction in the size of the spiral ligament.

The organ of Corti

The sensory receptors within the organ of Corti are the **hair cells**. There are two groups, the inner and outer hair cells, named from their position with respect to the modiolus. The apex of each cell carries 50–100 **stereocilia**. The stereocilia are stiff bristle-like structures formed from tightly

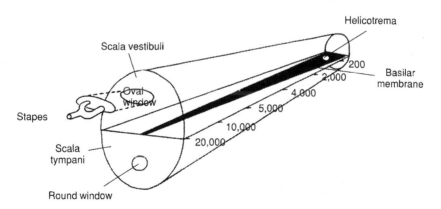

Figure 22.6 A schematic diagram of the inner ear showing the relationships of the scalae, the relative width of the basilar membrane and the location of frequency distribution along the basilar membrane.

packed parallel arrays of filaments. The hair cells are flanked by a variety of support cells, some of which structurally support the hair cells and others which aid their function. The organ of Corti is covered by the **tectorial membrane**, an acellular structure of keratin-like fibres embedded in a gelatinous matrix.

There are approximately 3500 inner hair cells that form a single row on the edge of the osseous spiral lamina close to the attachment of the basilar membrane. The **inner hair cells** are flask-shaped (Figure 22.7). They do not rest directly on the osseous spiral lamina: their bases are separated from it by up to eighteen sensory nerve terminals that contact the base of each hair cell. Efferent nerves are intermingled with the sensory nerves beneath the hair cells but these do not contact the hair cells directly:

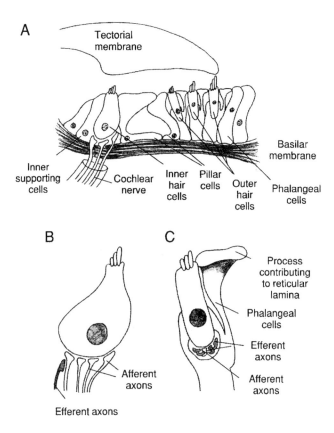

Figure 22.7 (A) The structure of the organ of Corti showing the relationship of the hair cells to the supporting cells and membranes. (B) Detail of an inner hair cell. (C) Detail of an outer hair cell and phalangeal cell.

instead they make presynaptic contacts on to the afferent nerves. The apex of each hair cell carries three or four arcs of stereocilia that gradually increase in height towards the spiral lamina. The stereocilia extend into the space beneath the tectorial membrane although it is not believed that the stereocilia actually contact the underside of the tectorial membrane. The apices of the inner hair cells are supported by a filamentous reticular membrane attached to the neighbouring inner supporting cells and the inner pillar cells (see below).

Outer hair cells (Figure 22.7C) are more numerous than the inner hair cells and twice as tall. There are some 12 000 outer hair cells arranged in three rows near the base of the cochlea but increasing up to five rows near the apex. They increase progressively in height from the base to the apex of the cochlear duct, the cells nearest that spiral lamina being tallest at any one point. The stereocilia of the outer hair cells increase in height from the base to the apex of the cochlear and are arranged in three or more W-shaped rows on each cell. The tips of the stereocilia of the tallest outer rows do make contact with the underside of the tectorial membrane. Afferent nerve terminals contact the bases of the outer hair cells but in smaller numbers than those found on the inner hair cells. More efferent terminals are present, however. The bases of the outer hair cells are cupped in a depression in the apices of outer supporting (phalangeal) cells. A finger-like process extends from each outer supporting cell at this point upwards to the apex of the outer air cell where it terminates in a flat plate which forms a tight junction with the hair cells. The plates of the supporting cells form a **reticular lamina** that is continuous with that supporting the apices of the inner hair cells.

There are two rows of pillar cells, the inner and outer pillar cells, between the inner and outer hair cells (Figure 22.7). The bases of the **inner pillar cells** rest partly on the osseous spiral lamina and partly on the basilar membrane while the bases of outer pillar cells rest solely on the basilar membrane. The apices of the pillar cells contribute to the reticular lamina. The reticular lamina forms a rigid support around the apices of the inner and outer hair cells. The hair cells are thus held rigidly between the basilar membrane and the reticular lamina; they are mechanically coupled to the basilar membrane so that they move in concert with the membrane. The stereocilia project above the reticular lamina and are therefore free to move.

The structure of the inner ear may appear to be ultracomplex on first reading and it is – but the arrangement of the membranous labyrinth, the hair cells and their supporting cells in the organ of Corti is crucial for the transduction of all facets of sound signals.

Hearing

The cochlea analyses and relays to the cochlear nuclei in the brainstem information about the frequency, intensity, onset, duration and cessation of sounds and, at low frequencies, information about phase. These functions are aided by active amplification occurring within the cochlea. Movements of fluids within the cochlea result in the movements of the vestibular and basilar membranes and hair cells, ultimately causing the hair cell stereocilia to bend. This generates action potentials in afferent axons in the auditory nerve. When sounds from the two ears are combined in the brainstem, information about the location of stationary and moving sound sources can also be extracted. Information is then relayed from the cochlear nuclei to the auditory cortex via the central auditory pathways. Analysis of stimuli continues at various relay stations in the central auditory pathways. The sensitivity of the cochlea to sound can be modified by descending (efferent) pathways originating in some of the relay stations; efferent axons terminate on or near the hair cells. This mechanism allows the nervous system to regulate what afferent information is relayed to it by the cochlea.

Movements of the basilar membrane

Vibrations transmitted from movement of the oval window to the cochlea set up pressure waves in the fluids within its different compartments. Because fluids are incompressible, the pressure waves are dissipated by compensatory outward movements of the round window. As vibrations move through the fluid, differential pressures occur between the scala vestibuli and tympani due to the time taken to reach different areas. Vibrations can be transmitted to the round window by one of two routes. They can either pass from the scala vestibuli into the scala tympani through the helicotrema or can pass directly across the cochlear duct through the vestibular and basilar membranes. Vibrations reaching the round window via the latter route will, of necessity, result in displacement of the basilar membrane and therefore movement of the organ of Corti that rests upon it. This will result in movement of the hair cells. The cell bodies of the hair cells are held rigidly in the organ of Corti by the reticular lamina. Thus, when the basilar membrane is displaced, the hair cells follow this movement faithfully rather than being deformed. In contrast, the stereocilia that project from the hair cell apices are not rigidly supported and are free to bend. The tips of the stereocilia lie close to, or actually touch, the underside of the tectorial membrane.

As the hair cell stereocilia bend in response to displacement of the basilar membrane, the hair cells are excited. The bending is caused by shear forces between the basilar membrane and the tectorial membrane. There are two reasons for this. The tectorial membrane and the basilar membrane form an outside and inside curvature. Since the radii of these two curvatures are different, when the basilar membrane moves the smaller radius will come under tension and the larger radius will be compressed causing a shear force. Additionally, the basilar membrane and the tectorial membrane have different points of attachment to the modiolar side of the cochlear duct so that when the basilar membrane is displaced, there will be a shear force between it and the tectorial membrane because of their different pivot points. In both cases, these forces bend hair cell stereocilia. It is relatively easy to understand how this comes about for the hair cells whose stereocilia are in direct contact with the tectorial membrane. It is less clear how shear forces bend the stereocilia not in direct contact with it, but the most likely possibility is that displacement is caused by generation of small movement of endolymph bathing the stereocilia as a consequence of viscous drag. The bending of stereocilia on the outer hair cells in contact with the tectorial membrane is in proportion to the height of the displacement of the basilar membrane. The bending of stereocilia of the inner hair cells is proportional to the speed at which the basilar membrane moves.

Protein filaments connect the tips of stereocilia in one row to the bases of stereocilia in the next row on the shorter side. As these protein filaments are moved by the bending of the stereocilia, they cause ion channels to open resulting in a depolarization of the hair cell (see below). When the stereocilia move back to their rest position, the channels are closed and the cells become hyperpolarized. This generates an electrical potential called a **generator potential** within the hair cell which stimulates the afferent fibres of the auditory nerve that innervate them. In reality, hair cells have spontaneous oscillations in membrane potential all the time; mechanical activation by stereocilial movement amplifies the spontaneous potential. Only mechanical deformations that generate large changes in the potential stimulate the nerves supplying the hair cells.

Frequency responses in the cochlea

The cochlea shows a graded change from its base to its apex in response to different sound frequencies (Figure 22.6). The base of the cochlea responds maximally to high frequency sounds while the apex of the cochlea responds maximally to low frequency sounds. The analysis of the frequency components of complex sounds takes place at many locations within the auditory pathway but actually begins within the cochlea. Part of the reason for this differential frequency response by the cochlea is the way in which the basilar membrane responds to sound. The vibration of the basilar membrane in response to a single frequency pure tone is maximal at a particular point along its length; the relationship between frequency and the point of maximum vibration parallels the frequency response of the cochlea as a whole. The basilar membrane responds to sounds in this way as a consequence of interaction between the mechanical properties of the membrane and those of the cochlear duct. However, the response of the cochlea as a whole to sounds of different frequencies is not completely explained by frequency variations in passive vibrations of the basilar membrane: another active process is thus involved (see below).

Because the basilar membrane is not uniform in structure throughout its length, its mechanical properties vary from region to region. The basilar membrane is narrower, thicker and more taut at the base of the cochlea whereas at the apex it is five times as wide but also thinner and more lax. When the oval window is stimulated at a particular frequency, the basilar membrane is progressively displaced from base to apex and the movement is in the form of a travelling wave. As the wave advances, it grows in amplitude and once it reaches a maximum, at a point on the membrane characteristic for that frequency, its amplitude quickly declines. The wave travels more slowly, changing the phase and producing a longer delay between movements of the oval window and the basilar membrane, and increases in wavelength. This mode of vibration means that, although all parts of the basilar membrane complete one cycle, they do so with different amplitudes, and at any one time different parts of the membrane are at different points in the cycle. As a wave comes in to the beach from the sea, it increases in height (amplitude) until it breaks and decays; this is similar to the behaviour of waves travelling up the basilar membrane. The maximum amplitude of the wave is greatest near the base of the cochlea for high frequency sounds and greater near the apex for low frequency sounds. The relationship between the frequency of a sound and the point on the basilar membrane at which the amplitude of vibration is at a maximum is not linear, but varies with the logarithm of the frequency. The human ear can detect frequencies between 20 Hz to 20000 Hz. About one-third of the length of the basilar membrane from base to apex covers each of the three ranges from 20–200 Hz, 200–2000 Hz and 2000–20000 Hz but in reverse order, so the basal third responds to the highest and the apex to the lowest frequencies. The basilar membrane is therefore optimally responsive to different frequencies causing mechanical displacement at different points along its length. The hair cells in the organ of Corti above these points respond maximally to the same frequencies.

The point at which the maximum amount of pressure passes across the cochlear duct to produce the greatest deflection of the basilar membrane depends upon the frequency of vibration. As frequency increases, so does the velocity of the particles within the medium conveying that vibration. However, because of inertia (resistance to movement), more energy is needed to move an object quickly than to move it slowly. The other factor preventing movement of the basilar membrane is its own stiffness, so the point of maximum vibration represents a balance between these two forces. At high frequencies the resistance to movement matches the greater stiffness near the base of the membrane producing maximum amplitude near the base. Beyond that point, the increasing laxity of the basilar membrane is readily overcome by movement and the peak of the wave will decline. This point is progressively nearer the cochlear apex as the frequency is reduced; very low frequency sounds will simply reach the round window through the helicotrema. Another way of explaining this is that there are two forces opposing movement of the basilar membrane, the stiffness of the membrane itself and the resistance to movement of the cochlear fluids. The point of maximum amplitude of vibration results from the interaction of these two forces.

The selectivity of this mechanism in situations where the basilar membrane is allowed to vibrate passively in isolation is actually rather poor, especially at low frequencies where there is a gradual and quite shallow reduction in amplitude from the point of maximum to the cochlear base. Selectivity is better at high frequencies where there is a much steeper decline of amplitude from the maximum. However, the sensitivity of the cochlea and of the auditory nerve fibres to different frequencies of sound is far greater than that of the basilar membrane. This implies that the cochlea must also amplify the sound energy to increase the ability to discriminate between two frequencies that only differ by a small amount (see below).

Hair cell response to sound

Mechanical bending of the hair cell stereocilia as the organ of Corti is moved by the travelling wave in the basilar membrane causes an electrical excitation of the hair cells. More is known about the excitation of inner hair cells than outer hair cells.

Inner hair cells have a resting membrane potential of −45 mV. The spontaneous voltage fluctuation, mentioned above, oscillates around the resting level. Different hair cells have different oscillation frequencies which match the frequencies at which they respond best to mechanical displacement. When the basilar membrane moves upwards towards the tectorial membrane and the stereocilia are bent, ion channels at the apices of the hair cells open. These ion channels are examples of a special kind of channel called **mechanically-gated ion channels** that open when the cell membrane changes in shape. The upward movement of the basilar membrane depolarizes the hair cell to produce an electrical response of up to −25 mV, the **generator potential**. As the basilar membrane moves in the opposite direction, these ion channels close and so the responses of the hair cells follow the oscillatory movements of the basilar membrane, albeit in a distorted way. Depolarization of the inner hair cells causes the release of the neurotransmitter, **glutamate**, causing excitation of the auditory nerves that innervate them.

The response of hair cells to different frequencies varies along the basilar membrane in a way that corresponds to the way in which the basilar membrane itself responds to a particular frequency of sound. Thus, an inner hair cell at any point along the basilar membrane will respond to a range of frequencies but will respond best to a sound of a particular frequency. The response of an individual inner hair cell to different frequencies can be plotted in what is called a **tuning curve** (Figure 22.8). The curve is produced by plotting the intensity of a pure tone at a given frequency that just produces a response in the hair cell. When this is performed over a range of frequencies, a curve is produced which is V-shaped with the apex of the V corresponding to the frequency at which the hair cell just responds to a pure tone of the lowest intensity. This is the **characteristic frequency** at which that particular hair cell gives its most sensitive response. The overall shape

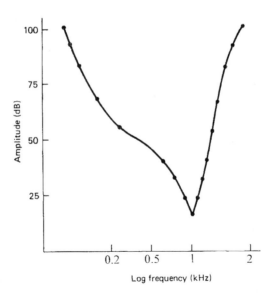

Figure 22.8 A tuning curve from an inner hair cell.

of the tuning curve is similar to that for the mechanical response of the basilar membrane at any point along its length to a range of sound frequencies. It shows a shallow slope on the low frequency side and a steeper slope on the high frequency side. Cells adjacent to one another on the basilar membrane can show differences in characteristic frequency as little as 0.2 per cent, a remarkably small difference in sensitivity. In comparison, adjacent notes on a piano differ in frequency by 6 per cent; approximately 400 inner hair cells would be needed to encompass an octave in change of pitch.

Inner hair cells also respond to changes in sound intensity. At the characteristic frequency, inner hair cells show a linear response at low intensity that becomes non-linear as intensity is increased. Outer hair cells have similar responses to inner cells both in terms of their sensitivity to different frequencies and their response to the sound intensity although they have higher resting membrane potentials of –70 mV.

Innervation of the hair cells

In the cochlear nerve in man there are 30–40 000 axons with a mixture of afferent and efferent fibres. The cell bodies of afferent axons are located in the **spiral ganglion** situated within the modiolus. They are bipolar; the peripheral processes innervate the hair cells by passing through fine holes in the spiral lamina and the central processes go to the brainstem. They leave the cochlea as a series of fine filaments which join together to form the cochlear part of the eighth cranial nerve. It joins the vestibular part of the eighth nerve in the internal auditory meatus where the nerve travels alongside the facial nerve to join the brainstem at the pontomedullary junction. The efferent axons originate from neurons in the periolivary nuclei of the superior olivary complex (see Chapter 23).

Approximately 90–95 per cent of afferent axons innervate the inner hair cells. These are **type I axons** arising from similarly named neurons in the spiral ganglion. Each inner hair cell receives up to 20 afferents and it is believed that a single type I afferent axon innervates just a single cell. Thus, the innervation pattern of inner hair cells is divergent with one hair cell communicating with the cochlear nuclei via a number of axons. Type I afferent fibres show a similar pattern of response to inner hair cells, in that they have a characteristic frequency at which they respond to sounds of the lowest intensity. The remaining 5–10 per cent of afferent axons are **type II axons** which innervate the outer hair cells. Each type II axon innervates as many as 10 outer hair cells, and each outer hair cell in turn receives afferents from several type II axons. Thus, the afferent innervation of the outer hair cells differs from that of the inner hair cells in being convergent as well as divergent.

The efferent innervation of the inner and outer hair cells also differs. The efferent axons to inner hair cells originate ipsilaterally from the superior olivary complex (see Chapter 23) and end presynaptically on type I afferent axons. Efferent axons end directly on the outer hair cells and originate contralaterally. Outer hair cells receive a much denser efferent innervation than inner hair cells with several efferent axons ending on the base of each cell.

The afferent innervation of the cochlea is thus dominated by axons from the inner hair cells, with each inner hair cell projecting directly to neurons within the cochlear nuclei of the brainstem. For this reason it is believed that the inner hair cells provide the main, and possibly the sole source, of afferent information upon which any subsequent analysis of sound within the brainstem nuclei and auditory cortex is based.

Responses of cochlear nerve axons

The response of an individual type I axon closely resembles that of the inner hair cell it innervates. The relationship between the sound intensity required to produce a detectable number of action potentials at a particular frequency can be plotted against that frequency to produce a tuning curve which is very similar in shape to that obtained from the corresponding inner hair cell. Type I axons also encode for the intensity of a sound by increasing their firing rate, the number of action potentials per second. As the sound becomes more intense, the firing rate eventually reaches a maximum. This poses a difficulty for the central nervous system: based upon the firing rate of an individual axon, it cannot distinguish whether a single axon is transmitting action potentials at a particular rate in response to a quiet sound at its characteristic frequency or a louder sound at another frequency. However, information about the frequency of sound is also transmitted to the brain by type I axons by another means. At low frequencies up to about 500 Hz, type I axons transmit action potentials at a rate linked to the frequency of a sound. About 1000 Hz corresponds to the maximum number of action potentials an axon can produce per second. Above this frequency, type I axons cannot produce an action potential per cycle. What actually happens is that an axon propagates an action potential once every 2–3 cycles. Furthermore, when the axon produces an action potential, it does so at exactly the same point in the cycle, thus conveying additional information about the phase of a sound. This **phase locking** is important also for the localization of low frequency sound (see below).

The brain thus receives information about the frequency of a sound in two ways, one that is dependent upon inner hair cell position on the basilar membrane and one that is independent of that position. Position-dependent frequency coding is needed at high frequencies, while the firing-rate-dependent frequency code is needed at low frequencies, because positional coding on the basilar membrane is less able to resolve low frequencies near the apex of the cochlea.

Information about the properties of a sound is conveyed to the brain by populations of axons rather than by single axons and it is the **population responses** that are analysed by neurons within the central auditory pathway. Information about the pitch (frequency) of a sound is produced by activity in groups of axons that is modified or modulated by the sound itself. Information about higher frequencies, including the quality or timbre, is relayed by axons innervating the inner hair cells near the base of the cochlea. Information about the intensity of sounds is probably relayed through the total amount of neural activity within the cochlear nerve reaching the brainstem.

Type I axons in the cochlear nerve also provide information about onset and duration of sounds at particular frequencies by their pattern of action potentials. When the sound starts, there is an intense burst of activity above the spontaneous discharge rate. This is followed by a lower rate of discharge although still higher than the spontaneous rate. At the end of the sound, the discharge rate falls briefly below the spontaneous rate before the axon resumes its spontaneous discharge rate.

Although the tuning curves of inner hair cells and type I cochlear axons parallel the mechanical response of the basilar membrane to sound of a particular frequency, there is one very obvious difference. The tuning curve for a single type I axon is much more selective in its frequency response, responding to a smaller band of frequencies than does the basilar membrane. The mechanical properties of the basilar membrane cannot, by themselves, account for the frequency discrimination that is seen in type I axons of the cochlear nerve. Increase in selectivity of response in cochlear nerve axons is observed only if the temporal bone is intact, and therefore it must involve some form of active and selective amplification of the response to sound within the cochlea itself.

The actual mechanism is still open to question but a role for the outer hair cells is strongly implicated. Although some afferent axons synapse with the outer hair cells, their main brainstem connections are through efferent pathways from superior olivary complex neurons. Outer hair cells systematically increase in size along the length of the basilar membrane from base to apex. Furthermore, when outer hair cells are stimulated, they respond by changing shape: the cell bodies become shorter when they are depolarized and longer when they are hyperpolarized, suggesting that the main function of the outer hair cells is quite different to that of the inner hair cells. It is believed that the outer hair cells act as auditory effectors, rather than sensory transducers, by changing shape to augment the movements of the basilar membrane and improving the frequency selectivity of the organ of Corti to a narrower band of frequencies. As the cells change shape, they pull down or push up the reticular lamina which affects movements of the inner hair cells in response to mechanical deformation of the basilar lamina. The movements of the outer hair cells must themselves be frequency selective for this mechanism to function efficiently. The efferent axons ending on the outer hair cells appear to be frequency tuned since they also respond maximally to a narrow band of frequencies. They end on outer hair cells at a point on the basilar membrane corresponding to that tuned frequency. This also indicates that efferent axons have a selective frequency response. Although outer hair cells are prime candidates for the active and selective amplification of basilar membrane movement in order to produce the high degree of frequency selectivity of the cochlear nerve, there may be other mechanisms yet to be clarified.

A summary of how the ear distinguishes frequency, loudness, timbre and onset

- Frequency is coded by place along the basilar membrane and inner hair cells at a particular location respond maximally to a particular frequency as shown by their tuning curve. However, the sharpest tuning is at low frequencies and broadens at higher frequencies. This may be counteracted to some extent through amplification by outer hair cell mechanisms but it is not certain how effective this mechanism really is. At low frequency, hair cells and their associated cochlear axons can fire at a rate proportional to frequency but above about 1000 Hz phase locking is used to convey this information, with hair cells generating action potentials only at a particular phase in the cycle.
- Timbre, a function of the overtones and harmonics (formants), is a refined analysis of all frequency information generated.
- Loudness is probably monitored by summating the activity at different frequencies over the whole cochlea.
- Onset is signalled by increased numbers of action potentials and cessation by a fall of activity below the spontaneous firing rate.

Otoacoustic emissions

Otoacoustic emissions are sounds produced by the cochlea itself. It is believed that they are the by-product of the active amplification in the cochlea described above. Otoacoustic emissions are of more than theoretical interest: they are also a useful tool for assessing hearing loss. There are two main types, spontaneous and evoked.

Evoked otoacoustic emissions are produced as the response to a brief auditory stimulus such as a click. After a delay, one or more sounds can be recorded from the ear with the highest frequency sounds having the shortest delays. **Spontaneous acoustic emissions** occur in the absence of any external stimulation. In a quiet location, a sensitive microphone, close to or within the external auditory meatus, will detect sounds coming from the ear. Sometimes in neonates or young children such sounds can be heard without electronic amplification. In clients suffering from **tinnitus**, a high pitched continuous noise in one or both ears, this noise can also be heard by someone else listening in a quiet place close to the sufferer's ear. The cause of these emissions is believed to be feedback from the amplification system in the ear. An apt analogy is the annoying feedback that affects amplifiers when the volume is set too high. Normally the ear is adjusted so that feedback is kept at a low, inaudible level but occasionally it produces sounds that can be heard.

Most hearing loss involves damage to outer hair cells, and when this damage occurs it affects evoked otoacoustic emissions. Defined stimuli in the form of wide frequency band clicks are played and a lightweight probe is placed in each external auditory meatus in turn. The evoked otoacoustic emissions are measured to assess hearing loss. The **transient evoked acoustic emission test** (TEOEA) can be used to detect hearing loss even in neonates and babies who are, of course, unable to report what they hear. It must be borne in mind that this test cannot be used successfully if middle ear function is impaired because the sound generated in the cochlea must be transmitted in the reverse direction through the middle ear.

The sooner hearing loss is detected, the sooner suitable remedial programmes can be started and the more effective they will be. Hearing loss in infants is particularly important because of the effect on language acquisition. Furthermore, any degree of hearing loss means they cannot monitor their own utterances by **auditory feedback** which is why the speech of people with congenital hearing loss is distorted.

Sensorineural hearing loss

Sensorineural hearing loss occurs within the cochlea or the cochlear nerve. Damage to the cochlear nerve is often the result of a tumour compressing the nerves within the internal auditory meatus or at their entry into the brainstem. In such cases, the facial nerve is almost always involved because of the close proximity of the facial and vestibulocochlear nerves throughout their course. However, damage within the cochlea itself is the most common cause. The hair cells are particularly vulnerable to damage; like neurons, they are incapable of cell division and cannot be replaced if they die. Most frequently it is the outer hair cells that are affected, resulting in a loss of sensitivity plus a reduction in the ability to resolve different frequencies of sound. Common causes of hair cell loss in adults include:

- trauma, including noise-induced hearing loss from noisy work environments or failure to wear ear protectors
- infection
- the administration of **ototoxic drugs**, such as the antibiotics neomycin or streptomycin or anti-cancer drugs, which kill outer hair cells
- **presbyacusis** – hearing loss due to ageing and degeneration of hair cells.

In many cases there may be no obvious cause.

Some of these factors may affect children but the most common causes of hearing loss in infants are

- congenital deafness due to abnormal development of the inner ear. Maternal **rubella** (German measles) in first two months of pregnancy is one such cause of ear defects. This accounts for about 85 per cent of permanent bilateral hearing loss in children which may be mild, severe or profound. The incidence is about 1.1 per 1000 live births; at the current birth rate, about 850 children a year are affected in the U.K.
- infections and trauma account for the other 15 per cent, meningitis being a major cause.

Sensorineural hearing loss can be tested for by otoacoustic emission tests for babies or young children. However, **pure tone audiometry threshold tests** are commonly used for compliant clients who are old enough to understand the tests. Most speech occurs within the frequency range of 400 to 4000 Hz and tests are usually carried out at frequencies between 250 to 8000 Hz in octave steps; for each octave there is a doubling of frequency, e.g. from 250 Hz to 500 Hz or 4000 to 8000 Hz. The client is provided with earphones connected to a sound generator that is linked to a computer. The generator produces pure tones of specific frequencies. The system can be adjusted so that intensity can be altered and the tone can be directed through either the left or right earpiece. A high frequency is played into one ear at 45 dB and the client indicates whether they can hear it. The intensity is increased or decreased as appropriate. It is then decreased in 10 dB steps until they report the sound is no longer audible; the intensity is increased by 10 dB to check that this is the hearing threshold. The test is repeated over the desired decreasing frequency range for both ears and a graph is plotted of threshold level of hearing (the lowest intensity detectable) against the frequency. Using this test, differences in threshold for both ears can be compared across a range of frequencies. This test can also be used to detect conductive hearing loss at the same time by placing a microphone over the mastoid process; a difference of greater than 15 dB between the airborne and conduction thresholds (the **air-bone gap**) is indicative of conductive hearing loss.

There are several other tests used in conjunction with pure tone audiometry threshold tests, including speech audiograms, and auditory brainstem response tests (see Chapter 23). **Speech audiograms** are obtained from children or adults by testing their ability to distinguish closely related words played at different frequencies and intensities and comparing them with a curve of normal hearing levels.

The range of frequency and intensity loss varies considerably depending on the cause of sensorineural hearing loss. Noise-induced hearing loss usually has raised thresholds at many frequencies but especially around 4000 to 6000 Hz, and the affected person has difficulty with speech discrimination even at high intensities and in sound localization. Clients with presbyacusis have difficulty understanding conversation even if people speak loudly (their thresholds are raised), especially in the presence of background noise, and have more difficulty hearing children's or women's voices (hearing loss is most obvious at higher frequencies); neither can they enjoy music anymore as there is poor discrimination of frequency, intensity and timing of sounds, all of which are essential to decode a complex sound like a symphony orchestra or even a five piece band.

Hearing aids are of limited value in treating sensorineural hearing loss because they can only amplify sounds and do not aid their resolution. Cochlear prostheses (**cochlear implants**) are sometimes used instead. An electronic device analyses sounds into their individual frequency components and delivers the results to one or more electrodes implanted in the scala tympani at an appropriate point on the basilar membrane to stimulate cochlear nerve axons. This exploits the frequency coding by position on the basilar membrane. The effectiveness of these implants varies: with training, some clients find that they can understand speech whereas others find implants do not help. This variability is probably due, in part, to the state of the cochlea when the implant is made. If there is extensive degeneration of the cochlea or the cochlear nerves, then no amount of stimulation will help.

Hearing speech

Detection of speech has several problems related to the nature of speech sounds. Voiced phonemes are produced by high frequency vibrations of the vocal folds. These, in turn, induce resonant vibrations in the supralaryngeal vocal tract but these are at such low frequencies (about 10 Hz) that they are below the threshold of hearing. However, these vibrations also produce formants which are above the hearing threshold. The cochlea can decode the complex waveforms thus produced and pass the information to the brain by altered firing patterns in afferent axons. We are all familiar with the terms AM and FM from our radio dials. AM means amplitude modulation and FM means frequency modulation. Essentially what happens is that a high frequency carrier wave is used to send the signal which is encoded within it. This is achieved in two ways. Either the amplitude of the wave is varied at frequencies in the audible range of 400–4000 Hz (amplitude modulation) or the frequency of the carrier wave is modulated by slowly decreasing the frequency (frequency modulation). There is evidence that the ear acts as both an AM and FM receiver to select audible information from complex carrier signals generated during speech.

CHAPTER 23

The central auditory pathways

Auditory information is relayed from the cochlea to the cerebral cortex by the cochlear nerve and a group of pathways within the brain called the central auditory pathways (Figure 23.1). These pathways have relays in three main locations in the brainstem. The three main pairs of nuclei within the auditory part of the brainstem are:

- the **cochlear nuclei**
- the **superior olivary complex**
- the **inferior colliculi**.

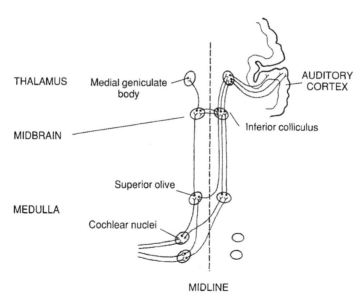

Figure 23.1 The central auditory pathways.

In the forebrain, the auditory pathways relay in the **medial geniculate bodies** of the thalamus, before reaching their destination, the **primary** and **auditory association cortex**.

Certain aspects of the analysis of simple and complex sound stimuli occur in the ear itself (see Chapter 22) and within the auditory pathways as well as the auditory cortex. Speech is constituted of some of the most complex sounds and this aspect of auditory function is still not fully understood.

Some important principles underlie auditory system organization. Any auditory stimulus possesses a number of features, all of which must be analysed if a sound is to be interpreted:

- A stimulus may have a single frequency or be composed of a number of frequencies, heard as its pitch.
- It has an intensity, which is heard as the degree of loudness.
- It starts at a particular time and only lasts for a certain duration.
- Stimuli originate from a particular point in space and must be localized, e.g. we need to know where the car engine noise is coming from if we are to cross the road safely.

Any of these features may be constant or may vary throughout the duration of the sound. Thus, a sound may change frequency or intensity or may come from a moving source. These discrete features of an auditory stimulus are analysed in parallel by different parts of the central auditory system. Although some analysis begins within the cochlea, some features require combined information from both ears, therefore analysis can only occur in the central auditory pathways. The principle of **parallel processing** of multiple features is exhibited by many sensory systems. Processing begins in the cochlear nuclei, the first relay nuclei of the auditory system, in which different cell types respond to different stimulus parameters.

The second important principle that underlies auditory system organization is one of **tonotopic localization**. Within every nucleus, information about a particular frequency, or tone, is localized at a specific region of that nucleus, continuing the frequency location established in the cochlea. Again, this organizational principle is found in many sensory systems, e.g. somatotopic organization in somatosensory systems (see Chapter 9).

There is extensive interaction between the information received by right and left ears throughout most of the auditory system and this extensive bilateral representation is continued throughout the central auditory pathway. Consequently, unilateral damage in the auditory pathways seldom results in deafness, although localization of sounds is often impaired.

The cochlear nuclei

The cochlear nuclei are the first relay stations in the auditory pathways. They are located dorsolaterally in the brainstem in the region of the pontomedullary junction. On each side, there are two separate nuclei joined together, the **dorsal cochlear nucleus** and the **ventral cochlear nucleus**. The latter is further subdivided into the **anteroventral cochlear nucleus** and **posteroventral cochlear nucleus**.

Afferent axons from the inner hair cells of the organ of Corti travelling in the cochlear division of the vestibulocochlear nerves enter the ventral cochlear nuclei. The axons bifurcate as they enter each nucleus with one branch ascending to enter the anteroventral cochlear nucleus and a second branch descending to enter, successively, the posteroventral and the dorsal cochlear nucleus. Thus, each incoming cochlear nerve axon synapses in all three parts of the cochlear nucleus and, in the process, with a number of neurons in all three parts of the cochlear nucleus. As described in Chapter 22, cochlear nerve afferent fibres are tuned to respond preferentially to a narrow frequency band. This frequency response determines the sites of terminations of the afferent axon within the three divisions of the cochlear nucleus. Axons responding preferentially to low frequencies bifurcate close to their point of entry in the cochlear nucleus and synapse with neurons in the ventrolateral parts of all three nuclei. Axons that respond preferentially to higher frequencies bifurcate at successively greater distances from their point of entry and terminate in successively more dorsomedial parts of all three nuclei. All three divisions of the cochlear nuclear complex are tonotopically organized with coding for any single frequency being represented at three loci within the cochlear nucleus. There are a number of cell types upon which the incoming afferents of the cochlear nerve can form a synapse. These cell types are classified by their shape, size and arrangement of dendrites and their physiological responses.

Within the ventral cochlear nucleus the main cell types found are bushy, stellate and octopus cells. **Bushy cells** exhibit physiological responses to the frequency, intensity and duration of sounds that are very similar to those of the cochlear nerve fibres that synapse upon them. There are two subtypes of bushy cells, one responding to lower frequencies, the other to higher frequencies. **Stellate cells** are found in the anteroventral and posteroventral cochlear nuclei. These cells respond to the onset or termination of a sound or to a change in its frequency or intensity. **Octopus cells** are located mainly in the posteroventral cochlear nucleus and respond to sound over a much wider range of frequencies than the responses shown by cochlear nerve fibres; they are less sharply tuned. The dorsal cochlear nucleus has only one main cell type, the fusiform cell, whose responses are unknown.

The output from the cochlear nuclei is directed to the inferior colliculi in the midbrain. There are both direct and indirect pathways: **direct pathways** travel to the colliculi without an intermediate synapse whereas **indirect pathways** synapse in the superior olivary complex en route. Axons from the dorsal cochlear nucleus decussate and ascend to the contralateral interior colliculus via a pathway called the **lateral lemniscus** (see below). Outputs from octopus cells join the contralateral lateral lemniscus. Stellate cell axons and some bushy cell axons also join the contralateral lateral lemniscus. These all contribute to the direct pathways from the cochlear nucleus to the inferior colliculus via the lateral lemnisci. Axons from bushy cells in the anteroventral cochlear nucleus terminate in the nuclei of the superior olive on both sides forming the indirect pathway. Axons from superior olivary neurons then join the lateral lemniscus to complete the indirect pathway to the inferior colliculus. The direct pathways encode onset and cessation of sounds and changes in their frequency and intensity together with, probably, sound localization in the vertical axis. The indirect pathway encodes sound localization in the horizontal axis.

The superior olivary nuclear complex

The superior olivary group of nuclei are also located at the pontomedullary junction but lie just below the ventral surface of the brainstem so are anterior to the cochlear nuclei. Each superior olive consists of three main nuclei plus a number of smaller associated nuclei. The main nuclei are the **medial superior olive**, the **lateral superior olive** and the **medial nucleus of the trapezoid body**. These main nuclei are surrounded by small **periolivary nuclei**. The main nuclei play an important role in sound localization while the neurons in the periolivary nuclei are the source of efferent axons forming the olivocochlear bundles (see below).

The **medial superior olive** receives input from the low frequency bushy cells of the anteroventral cochlear nuclei of both sides. It thus receives input from both ears and its function is to locate the source of a sound. It carries out this function by comparing the small difference in time taken by a sound to reach both ears. A sound originating from a source on one side of the head will reach the ear nearer the source sooner than that ear further away. Head size is such that the maximum delay will be approximately 700 μs. The delay declines to zero when the sound is delivered from directly in front or directly behind the listener. Axons conveying information from one ear are relayed to an array of neurons in the contralateral nucleus. These neurons also receive ipsilateral input from the other ear so their pathways must be shorter. The neurons respond when action potentials generated by the sounds reaching the ear furthest away from the source arrive at the same time as those from the nearer ear, due to the different time taken for conduction in the brainstem. This method of localizing sound is most effective for sounds of lower frequencies which are refracted around the head rather than reflected off it.

The **lateral superior olive** is also involved in sound localization but it locates the source of high frequency sounds. Timing differences between the two ears cannot be used to locate high frequency sounds because they are reflected off the head. This creates a sound shadow in which the ear furthest away from a high frequency source located to one side of the head receives a lower intensity of sound than the nearer ear. The lateral superior olive compares these intensity differences between the two ears with neurons connected together in such a way that they respond when the intensity of sound in one ear exceeds that in the other ear. Input reaches the lateral superior olive from the high frequency bushy cells of the ipsilateral anteroventral cochlear nucleus and indirectly from the contralateral nucleus via a synapse in the medial nucleus of the trapezoid body. Axons from neurons in the medial and lateral superior olivary nuclei join the lateral lemniscus to project to higher nuclei in the auditory pathways. The main site of termination of their axons is the inferior colliculus.

The **periolivary nuclei** contain neurons whose axons form efferent **olivocochlear bundles** returning to the ear. The axons of the medial olivocochlear bundle terminate on the outer hair cells predominantly in the contralateral cochlea. Efferent axons of the lateral olivocochlear bundle form another efferent pathway that terminates in the ipsilateral spiral ganglion. The function of these pathways is to regulate the response of the cochlea to sound, probably by fine tuning (see Chapter 22).

The majority of axons in the lateral lemniscus project to the ipsilateral inferior colliculus although some decussate to reach the contralateral inferior colliculus. En route to the inferior colliculi, collateral axons branch from the lateral lemniscus to the trigeminal and facial nerve motor nuclei where they form the afferent limb of a reflex arc. The efferent limb consists of the motor nerves supplying the tensor tympani and stapedius muscles. Although both muscles are involved, this reflex is usually called the **stapedial reflex** and its effects have been described in Chapter 22.

The inferior colliculi

The inferior colliculi are situated in the midbrain tectum. Each colliculus is composed of three main nuclei: the **main** (or central) **nucleus**, the **pericentral nucleus** and the **external nucleus**. Only the main nucleus appears to be solely auditory in function.

This nucleus receives inputs from both the ipsilateral and contralateral lateral lemniscus. The internal structure of the nucleus is complex with many layers. Its functions are still not fully understood but it is likely to be involved in sound localization. Outputs from the central nuclei terminate in the medial geniculate bodies of the thalamus. The functions of the pericentral and external nuclei remain unclear. They receive somato-sensory inputs in addition to those from the auditory system and project to the medial geniculate body.

The inferior colliculi also have important connections to the motor nuclei of the cranial nerves controlling the eye muscles, the ventral horn of the cervical spinal cord innervating the neck muscles and also to the ventral horns lower down that direct postural muscles. These connections enable moving sound sources to be tracked by coordination of eye, head and body movements.

The medial geniculate bodies

The medial geniculate bodies are specific auditory relay nuclei in the thalamus. Each medial geniculate body is divided into three parts: the ventral, dorsal and medial divisions.

Axonal input to the ventral division comes from the central nucleus of the ipsilateral inferior colliculus. Neurons in this division not only retain a high degree of frequency selectivity, but also remain sensitive both to timing and intensity differences between sound received at the two ears. Output from the ventral division reaches the primary auditory cortex via the internal capsule.

The other divisions of the medial geniculate body are probably not exclusively auditory in function. As with the external and pericentral nuclei of the inferior colliculi, both the dorsal and medial divisions of the medial geniculate bodies receive other sensory inputs in addition to auditory input. Neurons of the dorsal division project to the auditory association cortex. The medial division receives inputs from other sensory systems and projects to more widespread areas of the cortex, including non-auditory as well as auditory areas. It is believed that the dorsal division may play a role in auditory attention while the medial division could be part of a neuronal system regulating arousal.

The auditory cortex

The primary auditory cortex is located on each side in the **transverse temporal gyri** (Heschl's gyri) on the superior surface of the temporal lobe. It is surrounded by a number of auditory association areas that extend into the temporal lobe.

Primary auditory cortex

There are typically one to three transverse gyri (see Figure 13.1) and sometimes four but the number is frequently different on the left and right sides although there are no systematic left–right asymmetries between individuals. The most important input source to the auditory cortex is from the ventral divisions of the medial geniculate bodies. There have been extensive animal studies on the organization and functioning of the auditory cortices but it is hard to extrapolate these studies to man because human invasive investigations are impossible and areas specialized for language perception are unique to humans. What various studies have shown is that, as with the rest of the auditory pathways, there is a **tonotopic localization** in the auditory cortex. Neurons that respond preferentially to low frequencies are situated anterolaterally and neurons tuned to high frequencies lie posteromedially. The working assumption is that a similar tonotopic pattern exists in humans. At right angles to the bands of neurons responding to a particular frequency, there are bands containing neurons that respond to input from both ears, although the input from the contralateral ear usually exerts a stronger effect: these neurons respond maximally to stimulation from both ears and are known as **summation columns**. They alternate with bands known as **suppression columns** in which neurons are excited when receiving input from one ear but inhibited when receiving input from the other ear. Again, the assumption is made that this is also true of humans.

The auditory cortex is the origin of **efferent pathways** that descend through the brainstem in parallel with the ascending auditory pathways. Efferent axons probably descend from all levels of the auditory pathways joining in with those from the cortex. As described above, these descending pathways converge on the periolivary nuclei from which the olivocochlear bundles run to the ears to fine tune the hair cells in the organ of Corti in response to incoming sound.

Auditory association cortex

The auditory association cortex (see Figure 13.1) consists of several areas that surround the primary auditory cortex and receive inputs from it. The majority of these areas have tonotopic maps. At present, there is not a clear demarcation between auditory association areas that analyse sounds other than speech and those concerned with speech processing, although there are indications that some regions of both the primary and association auditory cortices in humans may be specialized for reception and perception of speech sounds. Experimental evidence is accumulating to identify all these areas and elucidate their functions although much remains to be done. Some aspects of this recent research have been mentioned in Chapter 13.

In summary, the auditory pathways are complex in comparison to some other sensory pathways. The important principles to grasp are that the multiple features that go to make up a sound area are analysed by different parts of the central auditory pathways working in parallel and that throughout the auditory system there is extensive left–right representation. The significance of the anatomical complexity of these pathways is still not clearly understood, neither is the physiological significance of how neuronal responses in particular cells at one level influence and interact with those at other levels.

Clinical anatomy of the central auditory pathways

Because the inputs from both ears cross and recross at virtually all levels of the pathways, information from both ears reaches all levels on both sides. Hearing loss is therefore not a consequence of unilateral damage to the central auditory pathways. However, lesions in the region of the superior olivary complex lead to poor sound localization despite the ability of other areas to cooperate in this function. Lesions which disrupt the collateral connections from the auditory pathways to the fifth and seventh nerve nuclei abolish or diminish the stapedial reflex, which also involves the tensor tympani (see Chapter 22). As a result, even quiet sounds can seem unbearably loud. In the auditory cortex itself, the major problems are a loss of frequency discrimination coupled with blurring of sound stop and start cues and loss of sound localization. Clients so affected find it difficult or impossible to appreciate music.

Auditory brainstem evoked responses (ABR) can be used as a test for hearing loss and can discriminate between conductive hearing loss, sensorineural hearing loss and damage in the auditory pathways above the cochlear nuclei. These highly reliable tests are carried out by presenting wide frequency range clicks into each ear in turn and the resulting electrical responses in the lower parts of the central auditory pathways are measured using surface electrodes. The equipment required is expensive and the tests require highly skilled audiologists so, at present, are not in widespread use. However, these are the tests preferred for assessment of hearing loss in babies in neonatal intensive care and special care baby units. For neonatal screening of hearing in well babies, evoked acoustic emission tests (see Chapter 22) are preferred.

Further Reading

We hope that the material presented in this book is comprehensive and comprehensible. You may wish to consult other sources for background reading to further your knowledge in specific areas or to consult some of the primary literature used during the writing of this book.

Chapters 2 – 7
These chapters are introductions to the various systems of the body. If you are new to biology or your biological knowledge is a little rusty, a good place to start is with one of the many excellent course books and revision notes for GCSE or A level Human Biology in the U.K. or a fundamental level textbook covering human biology in the U.S.A. *Fundamentals of Anatomy and Physiology* by F. H. Martini (5th edition 2001: Prentice Hall) gives excellent coverage of the fundamentals of the subjects, is profusely illustrated and also contains a comprehensive and useful glossary of terms.

Anatomy is very difficult to appreciate just from a textbook even though we have tried to make our illustrations of the major structures as accurate as possible. For those students who do not have access to a dissecting room or prepared human dissections during their course, the next best thing is an <u>atlas of human anatomy</u>. These are usually illustrated with photographs of human dissections but everything visible tends to be labelled so use with care. There are several atlases available but the two below are popular with students in other subjects that we teach.

Human Anatomy: colour atlas and text by G. A. Gosling, et al (3rd edition 1996; Mosby-Wolfe) covers the whole body but is still extremely useful.

A Color Atlas of Head and Neck Anatomy by R.M. H., McMinn, R.T. Hutchings, and B. M. Logan, (2nd edition 1994; Mosby-Wolfe) deals specifically with the head and neck.

Acland's Video Atlas of Human Anatomy. The head and neck (Tapes 4 and 5 2000; Lipincott, Williams and Wilkins) covers all aspects of head and neck anatomy. Beautiful dissections of unenbalmed human cadavers are shown with a commentary. Video techniques are used to deconstruct and reconstruct areas layer by layer so that you can really appreciate their three dimensional relationships. The use of unenbalmed material means that actions of muscles can be shown very clearly. Each tape is indexed by time making different sections easy to locate.

Chapters 8 to 12
There are several excellent neuroscience textbooks that vary in scope and complexity.

Neuroanatomy; an illustrated colour text by A.R. Crossman and D. Neary (2nd edition 2000; Churchill Livingstone) provides simple summaries of various aspects of the nervous system illustrated with full colour diagrams.

Clinical Neuroanatomy for Medical Students by R. S. Snell (5th Edition 2001; Lippincot Raven) is more complex; it contains useful clinical problems and true-false test questions but, as the title suggests, is aimed at medical students rather than speech and language therapy students.

Principles of Neural Science by E. R. Kandel, J. H. Schwartz and T.M. Jessell (4th edition 1999; McGraw Hill) is extremely comprehensive and up to date if you wish to get into the real detail of neuroscience.

Neuroanatomy: a text and atlas by J. H. Martin (2nd edition 1996; Appleton Lange)

Chapter 13
This field of human communication science is extremely fast moving to the point that some aspects of our account will be out of date in the few months that have passed between writing and publication.

Chapter 59 on 'Language and the aphasias' in *Principles of Neural Science* by Kandel et al (see above) is a good up to date summary of the subject.

For those interested in this area, there are some useful reviews.

J. R. Binder, et al (1997) Human brain language areas identified by functional magnetic resonance imaging *Journal of Neuroscience* **17** 353–362.
J. R. Binder, (2000) "The new neuroanatomy of speech perception" (Editorial) *Brain* **123** 2371–2372

S. E. Petersen, (1988) "Positron emission tomographic studies of the cortical anatomy of single word processing" *Nature* 331 585–589

C. J. Price, (2000) "The anatomy of language: contributions from functional neuroimaging" *Journal of Anatomy* 197 335–359

R. J. S. Wise, et al (2001) "Separate neural subsystems within 'Wernicke's area'" *Brain* 124 83–95

Chapters 14 and 15
The anatomy and physiology of the respiratory system is covered in any standard textbook but speech breathing is rarely covered in any depth, if at all. There are several books containing useful information on speech respiration.

Respiratory Function in Speech and Song by T. J. Hixon (1987; Taylor and Francis)

Control of Breathing in Man edited by B. J. Whipp (1987; Manchester University Press)

Breathing, Speech and Song by D. F. Proctor (1980, Springer Verlag)

Principles of Physiology by R.M. Berne and M.N. Levy, (4th edition 2000; Mosby) is a comprehensive physiology book that probably contains too much information on general physiology for speech and language therapists. However it contains useful material on respiration and speech respiration.

Chapter 16 and 17
The larynx is one of the most complex aspects of functional anatomy we can think of and there is much still uncertain and conjectural.

Some interesting insights into normal structure of the larynx and some common and not so common pathologies can be obtained in glorious colour from two colour atlases:

A Colour Atlas of Fibreoptic Endoscopy of the Upper Respiratory Tract by J.D. Shaw and J. M. Lancer (1987; Mosby Wolfe)

A Histological Color Atlas of the Human Larynx by M. Hirano and K. Sato (1993; Singular Publishing Group)

Organic Voice Disorders; assessment and treatment Edited by W. S. Brown, B. P. Vinson and M. A. Crary" (1996; Singular Publishing Group

Inc) is a clinical textbook containing useful chapters on common vocal fold pathologies.

Understanding voice problems by R. Colton and J. K. Casper (2nd edition 1996; Williams and Wilkins) is also a clinical textbook you may well encounter in other course modules but contains useful chapters on phonatory physiology, neuroanatomical control of voice mechanisms and laryngeal pathology.

The *Concise Encyclopaedia of Language Pathology* edited by F. Fabro (1999; Elsevier) has chapters on neuromuscular aspects of speech and functional and clinical anatomy of speech mechanisms to highlight just two from this useful publication.

The Phonetic Description of Voice Quality by J. Laver (1980; Cambridge University Press) is still regarded as a classic work of its kind.

Vocal Fold Physiology by I. R. Titze (1993; Whurr) is a more academic work covering research aspects of the subject. Although published a few years ago, some areas have received little coverage elsewhere since then.

Chapters 18 and 19
If you do not have access to the real thing, look in the atlases listed above to gain an impression of the structures mentioned and their relative scale. There are several textbooks of orthodontics available which deal with some of the subject matter of chapter 19.

Chapter 20
"The Embryonic Disk" by J.E. Cook and M.K. Osmond (2nd edition 2001) is a CD-ROM with descriptions, illustrations, video clips and animations of early embryology. It also contains a section written specifically for speech and language therapists covering embryology of the face, larynx and respiratory tract including cleft palate. The CD-ROM is available from www.ucl.ac.uk/innovations/embryonic

Langman's Medical Embryology by T. W. Sadler and J. Langman (8th edition 2000; Williams and Wilkins) covers basic embryology of the whole body.

Craniofacial Embryology by G. H. Sperber (3rd edition 1980; John Wright and Sons) has more detail on development of the head and neck.

R. E. Stark, "Prespeech segmental feature development" (In Fletcher, P and Garman, M (Eds) "Language Acquisition" (2nd Edition 1986; Cambridge

University Press) mainly covers the subject matter of the title but does contain important material on development of the vocal tract.

Chapter 21
Again, you are recommended to the atlases of anatomy for the general aspects of this subject. Dysphagia is a relatively new subject in the speech and language therapy curriculum.
Evaluation and Treatment of Swallowing Disorders by J. A. Logemann (2nd edition 1998: College Hill Press) is a good general textbook.

Principles of Physiology by R.M. Berne, and M.N. Levy, (see above) also contains useful material on the physiology of swallowing.

There are some useful review articles:

Diamant, N.E. (1995) "A glimpse at the central mechanism for swallowing?" Editorial in *Gastroenterology* 109 1700–1702
Hamdy, S. and Rothwell, J. C. (1998) "Gut feelings about recovery after stroke: the organisation and reorganisation of human swallowing motor cortex" *Trends in Neuroscience* 21 278–282
Kirshner, H. S. (1989) "Causes of neurogenic dysphagia" *Dysphagia* 3 184–188
Kirshner, H. S. (1997) "Disorders of the pharyngeal and esophageal stages of swallowing in Parkinson's disease" Editorial in *Dysphagia* 12 19–20
Sellars, C. et al (1999) Swallowing abnormalities after acute stroke: a case control study" *Dysphagia* 14 212–218

Chapters 22 and 23
Bases of Hearing Science by J. D. Durrant and Lovinic. J.H. (1995; Williams and Wilkins) is a good basic textbook.

An Introduction to the Physiology of Hearing By J. O. Pickles (2nd edition 1988; Academic Press) is more advanced.

Chapter 32 'Hearing' in *Principles of Neural Science* by E.R. Kandel et al (see above) gives a good current summary of hearing and central auditory pathways.

Clinical aspects of the different areas covered in this book are dealt with in more detail in textbooks on these subjects which will be on your reading lists for other course components or in the relevant academic and professional journals if you are already qualified.

Index

Where there are several entries for a subject, the main coverage of a topic is shown in **bold** typeface

Printed in Great Britain
by Amazon.co.uk, Ltd.,
Marston Gate.